Methods in Molecular Biology™

Series Editor
John M. Walker
School of Life Sciences
University of Hertfordshire
Hatfield, Hertfordshire, AL10 9AB, UK

For further volumes:
http://www.springer.com/series/7651

Transplantation Immunology

Methods and Protocols

Second Edition

Edited by

Andrea A. Zachary and Mary S. Leffell

Immunogenetics Laboratory, Department of Medicine
Johns Hopkins University School of Medicine, Baltimore, MD, USA

Humana Press

Editors
Andrea A. Zachary
Immunogenetics Laboratory
Department of Medicine
Johns Hopkins University School of Medicine
Baltimore, MD, USA

Mary S. Leffell
Immunogenetics Laboratory
Department of Medicine
Johns Hopkins University School of Medicine
Baltimore, MD, USA

ISSN 1064-3745 ISSN 1940-6029 (electronic)
ISBN 978-1-4939-6015-6 ISBN 978-1-62703-493-7 (eBook)
DOI 10.1007/978-1-62703-493-7
Springer New York Heidelberg Dordrecht London

Printed on acid-free paper

Humana Press is a brand of Springer
Springer is part of Springer Science+Business Media (www.springer.com)

Preface

Transplantation of organs, tissues, peripheral blood stem cells, and bone marrow affords many patients the opportunity for life-saving and life-altering treatment. The need for such transplants is steadily increasing, due both to growing numbers of patients who could benefit from the traditional indications for transplantation, such as end-stage organ failure, and to the more recent applications of transplantation for other clinical conditions. For patients with end-stage organ failure, the wait list in the USA alone is now over 100,000 candidates. This includes patients in need of kidney, pancreas, liver, heart, lung, and intestine allografts, as well as patients waiting for multiorgan transplants, such as combined kidney/pancreas and heart/lung transplants. Autologous or allogeneic hematopoietic stem cell transplantation (HSCT) is a potentially curative treatment for chemotherapy-incurable hematologic malignancies, conditions for which over 10,000 patients are diagnosed each year. Blood or marrow transplantation also offers a potential cure for certain immunodeficiency diseases, such as RAG2-deficient severe combined immunodeficiency; for hemoglobinopathies, such as sickle cell disease; and for some solid tumors, such as metastatic melanoma and metastatic renal cell carcinoma. Advances are being made with the application of allogeneic HSCT in autoimmune disorders, including systemic lupus erythematosus and multiple sclerosis, and HSCT, in conjunction with solid organ transplantation, may offer a means to achieve a state of transplant tolerance. One of the more dramatic and recent advances in clinical transplantation has been the development of composite tissue transplantation that is offering patients the opportunity for reconstructive facial and upper extremity allografts.

These advances in clinical transplantation have resulted from decades of research and have been facilitated in recent years by new techniques which are permitting even further understanding of immune mechanisms underlying immune recognition of allografts, as well as a more accurate and thorough evaluation of histocompatibility between donors and recipients. This volume in the series of *Methods in Molecular Biology* is focused on transplantation immunology and begins with seven chapters that provide overviews of some key areas of current research and clinical application. The first chapter reviews current understanding of the molecular basis of alloreactivity through structural analyses of the interactions of T lymphocyte receptors with different polymorphic molecules encoded within the major histocompatibility gene complex. Aspects of both humoral and cellular mechanisms in allograft injury are covered in two chapters: one dealing with the effects of antibodies on allograft target tissues and the other with different mechanisms of cell-mediated injury. A long-standing goal in transplantation has been to alleviate the side effects of immunosuppression by achievement of a state of tolerance to transplanted organs and tissues. The overview of tolerance discusses both the advances and limitations of current assays to assess a tolerant state. The chapter on composite tissue transplantation reviews the developments in microsurgery that have permitted face and hand transplants and also discusses some of the unique biologic features faced in these transplants. The last two chapters in Part I address some of the issues encountered in thoracic organ transplantation and in the transplantation of sensitized patients. These final overviews further provide guidelines for the application of laboratory assays that can facilitate successful transplantation.

Methods in histocompatibility testing historically were cell based, both for typing of HLA antigens and for detection of HLA-specific antibodies. These methods were fraught with limitations, including problems with cell viability and a lack of specificity and sensitivity. The molecular techniques in current use permit much more accurate definition of HLA antigens and alleles, as well as improved detection and characterization of clinically relevant antibodies. Part II covers four major areas that are being applied in histocompatibility evaluations and ongoing transplantation immunology research. These include genotyping methods for the HLA and KIR systems and for determination of chimerism between donors and recipients; assays for detection and identification of donor reactive antibodies; methods for measuring cellular immune function and alloreactivity; and lastly, protein array and RNA expression analysis methods being applied in transplantation research and immune monitoring.

The extreme genetic polymorphism of the HLA system confounds histocompatibility matching, since as of this writing, there are over 9000 recognized HLA alleles. Groups of related HLA alleles often share extensive sequences and may encode the same or very similar protein sequence, while other alleles encode immunologically distinct proteins. HLA typing can, therefore, be performed at what is referred to as a lower resolution or "antigen" level and at higher resolution or an "allele" level. For solid organ transplantation, HLA typing is generally performed at an antigen level; however, in some cases, allele level typing may be needed to define the presence or absence of a relevant mismatch, such as an allele in a patient's own antigen group. For HSCT, high-resolution definition of HLA alleles is considered essential. Allele-level HLA typing is a daunting task, however, since to resolve many HLA alleles adequately, the typing method must cover five to eight exons that encode the signal peptide, extracellular domains, a transmembrane region, and a cytoplasmic tail. In some cases, intronic regions must also be considered, resulting in extremely long DNA sequences that must be targeted for allelic resolution. Three methods currently in use are presented for HLA typing: a sequence specific primer method (SSP), sequencing based typing (SBT), and next generation HLA sequencing which holds the promise of high-throughput HLA typing that resolves many of the issues with typing assignment ambiguities encountered with other methods. All the chapters provide excellent discussions of the issues and technical problems in HLA typing. The reader is also referred to a previous volume of the *Methods in Molecular Biology* edited by Christiansen and Tait for an excellent chapter on microbead-based HLA typing by reverse sequence-specific oligonucleotide hybridization [1]. In HSCT, chimerism testing is needed to assess whether engraftment of the donor hematopoietic stem cells has occurred or if the patient's underlying disease has relapsed. Although HLA typing can be used to monitor donor chimerism, this section of the methods chapters includes a description of a sensitive and quantitative polymerase chain reaction using insertion and deletion (Indel) genetic markers to assess chimerism.

In addition to HLA alleles, another genetic system encoding the KIR or killer cell immunoglobulin-like receptors may impact outcomes in both HSCT and solid organ transplantation. The KIR gene family is also polymorphic and is thought to have coevolved with the HLA system, since certain HLA class I molecules serve as ligands for KIR. KIR are expressed on natural killer cells and some T lymphocytes and they have been implicated in contributing to the outcomes of allogeneic solid organ and HSCT. Thus, in addition to being a topic for transplantation research, KIR genotyping may become a routine histocompatibility consideration along with HLA alleles.

A major barrier to allogeneic transplantation is humoral sensitization to HLA alloantigens, i.e., HLA antigens encoded by alleles that differ between donors and recipients. Antibodies to HLA antigens and alleles have been clearly associated with increased risk of rejection and reduced long-term graft survival in solid organ transplantation and affect many candidates sensitized through transfusion, pregnancy, or prior transplantation. For example, approximately one-third of renal transplant candidates on the wait list in the USA are known to have HLA-specific antibodies that may preclude transplantation with donors having the corresponding HLA antigens. While consideration of HLA-specific antibodies is not an issue for HSCT between HLA identical individuals, there is increasing use of partially HLA-mismatched donors since the majority of patients lack a suitable, fully HLA-matched donor. The presence of donor HLA specific antibodies has been associated with increased risk of stem cell engraftment failure, presumably through antibody-mediated rejection. Therefore, evaluation of HLA-specific antibodies is indicated for HLA-mismatched HSCT. The development of solid phase immunoassays using solubilized HLA antigens as targets revolutionized antibody screening for transplantation; however, cell-based assays are still routinely employed for crossmatch tests of recipient serum against donor lymphocytes prior to transplantation. Two chapters in this volume are devoted to the complement-dependent cytotoxicity crossmatch and a flow cytometric crossmatch technique. The solid phase immunoassays are highly sensitive, but not without limitations. For a thorough review of these assays, the reader is referred again to the previous edition of this series to the chapter on detection of HLA antibodies by solid phase immunoassays [2]. Despite their limitations, the solid phase antibody assays afford the opportunity for modifications to determine functional antibodies. In this regard, we have included chapters on two modifications to determine the capability of HLA antibodies to activate complement, one that measures antibody binding of the complement component, C1q, and the other that detects deposition of the complement split product, C4d.

In addition to HLA-specific antibodies, antibodies to non-HLA antigens and some autoantigens may impact transplant outcomes. Antigens expressed on endothelial cells that have yet to be clearly defined appear to be targets for both antibody and cell-mediated injury to renal allografts, contributing to both acute and chronic rejection. Antibodies to the angiotensin II-type 1 receptor (AT1R), which may be both an autoantigen as well as an alloantigen, have been implicated in renal allograft rejection and several autoantigens, including vimentin, collagens, K-α1 tubulin, and myosin have been associated with decrease survival of heart, lung, and liver transplants. These potential areas in transplantation immunology are addressed in three chapters: one describing a method for detection of endothelial cell reactive antibodies in a flow cytometric assay; another providing a method for detection of antibodies to AT1R; and the third giving approaches to detection of antibodies to several autoantigens.

While there is currently much interest in both the impact of HLA- and non-HLA-specific antibodies in transplantation, ongoing research and clinical monitoring of transplant outcomes must still address aspects of the cell-mediated response. Three excellent chapters provide methods for assessing T lymphocyte functionality and their potential roles in promoting either rejection or immune regulation. The functional state of T lymphocyte can be evaluated by their release of cATP following mitogen stimulation, as well by the intracellular production of cytokines. The third chapter discusses the detection of tolerogenic dendritic cells and their potential to induce T lymphocyte-mediated suppression. The final two methods chapters describe innovative methods in proteomics and genomics that are being used to discover the protein targets of alloantibodies and to define molecular mechanisms that may define the elusive state of tolerance.

From a review of the topics and methods covered in this volume of the *Methods in Molecular Biology* series devoted to transplantation immunology, it should be apparent that this is a dynamic field, both in the practice of histocompatibility testing and in transplantation research. While this volume is certainly not inclusive of all areas of transplantation research nor of all the methods in use, it contains topics of much current interest and potential for future applications. We thank our contributors for their excellent manuscripts and the series editor, John M. Walker, and Humana Press for the opportunity to edit this volume.

1. Trajanoski D, Fidler SJ (2012) HLA typing using bead-based methods. Methods Mol Biol 882:47–65

2. Zachary AA, Vega RM, Lucas DP, Leffell MS (2012) HLA antibody detection and characterization by solid phase immunoassays: methods and pitfalls. Methods Mol Biol 882:289–308

Baltimore, MD, USA

Andrea A. Zachary
Mary S. Leffell

Contents

Contributors

ELHAM ASHOURI • *Endocrinology and Metabolism Research Center, Shiraz University of Medical Sciences, Shiraz, Iran*

JESSICA L. BADDERS • *Immunogenetics Laboratory, Department of Medicine, Johns Hopkins University School of Medicine, Baltimore, MD, USA*

GERALD BRANDACHER • *Department of Plastic and Reconstructive Surgery, Johns Hopkins University School of Medicine, Baltimore, MD, USA*

ROBERT A. BRAY • *Department of Pathology, Emory University Hospital, Atlanta, GA, USA*

COLIN BRINKMAN • *Departments of Surgery and Microbiology and Immunology, University of Maryland School of Medicine, Baltimore, MD, USA*

JONATHAN S. BROMBERG • *Departments of Surgery and Microbiology and Immunology, University of Maryland School of Medicine, Baltimore, MD, USA*

MIKE BUNCE • *Biofortuna Ltd, Bromborough, Wirral, UK*

BRYNA BURRELL • *Departments of Surgery and Microbiology and Immunology, University of Maryland School of Medicine, Baltimore, MD, USA*

REBECCA CHAPPEL • *Microarray and Next Generation Sequencing Core Facility, The Scripps Research Institute, La Jolla, CA, USA*

GE CHEN • *Histocompatibility, Immunogenetics & Disease Profiling Laboratory, Department of Pathology, Stanford University School of Medicine, Palo Alto, CA, USA*

DUSKA DRAGUN • *Clinic for Nephrology and Intensive Care Medicine, Charité—Campus Virchow-Klinikum, Berlin, Germany*

SIDONIA B.G. ECKLE • *Department of Microbiology & Immunology, University of Melbourne, Parkville, VIC, Australia*

DONNA FITZPATRICK • *Histocompatibility (HLA) Laboratory, Department of Pathology, Massachusetts General Hospital, Boston, MA, USA*

LAIMA GAIDULIS • *HLA laboratory, City of Hope, Duarte, CA, USA*

TERRI GELBART • *Laboratory for Functional Genomics, Department of Molecular and Experimental Medicine, The Scripps Research Institute, La Jolla, CA, USA*

KETEVAN GENDZEKHADZE • *HLA laboratory, City of Hope, Duarte, CA, USA*

RYOICHI GOTO • *Transplantation Research Immunology Group, Nuffield Department of Surgical Sciences, John Radcliffe Hospital, University of Oxford, Oxford, UK*

STEVEN R. HEAD • *Microarray and Next Generation Sequencing Core Facility, The Scripps Research Institute, La Jolla, CA, USA*

GILBERTO HERNANDEZ • *Microarray and Next Generation Sequencing Core Facility, The Scripps Research Institute, La Jolla, CA, USA*

CHERIE L. HOLCOMB • *Department of Human Genetics, Roche Molecular Systems, Pleasanton, CA, USA*

CAROLYN KATOVICH HURLEY • *CW Bill Young Marrow Donor Recruitment and Research Program, Department of Oncology, Georgetown University Medical Center, Washington, DC, USA*

ANNETTE M. JACKSON • *Immunogenetics Laboratory, Department of Medicine, Johns Hopkins University School of Medicine, Baltimore, MD, USA*

KANTHI KARIYAWASAM • *CW Bill Young Marrow Donor Recruitment and Research Program, Department of Pediatrics, Georgetown University Medical Center, Rockville, MD, USA*

JON A. KOBASHIGAWA • *Cedars-Sinai Heart Institute, Los Angeles, CA, USA*

CHIH-HUNG LAI • *HLA Laboratory, Cedars-Sinai Medical Center, Los Angeles, CA, USA*

ANA LAZARO • *CW Bill Young Marrow Donor Recruitment and Research Program, Department of Pediatrics, Georgetown University Medical Center, Rockville, MD, USA*

MARY S. LEFFELL • *Immunogenetics Laboratory, Department of Medicine, Johns Hopkins University School of Medicine, Baltimore, MD, USA*

DONNA P. LUCAS • *Immunogenetics Laboratory, Department of Medicine, Johns Hopkins University School of Medicine, Baltimore, MD, USA*

JOHN LUNZ • *University of Pittsburgh Medical Center, Pittsburgh, PA, USA*

JAMES MCCLUSKEY • *Department of Microbiology & Immunology, University of Melbourne, Parkville, VIC, Australia*

T. MOHANAKUMAR • *Department of Surgery, Washington University School of Medicine, St. Louis, MO, USA; Department of Pathology and Immunology, Washington University School of Medicine, St. Louis, MO, USA*

TONY MONDALA • *Microarray and Next Generation Sequencing Core Facility, The Scripps Research Institute, La Jolla, CA, USA*

ROBERT A. MONTGOMERY • *Department of Surgery, Johns Hopkins University School of Medicine, Baltimore, MD, USA*

JENNIFER NG • *CW Bill Young Marrow Donor Recruitment and Research Program, Department of Pediatrics, Georgetown University Medical Center, Rockville, MD, USA*

PHILLIP ORDOUKHANIAN • *Microarray and Next Generation Sequencing Core Facility, The Scripps Research Institute, La Jolla, CA, USA*

BEN PASSEY • *Biofortuna Ltd, Bromborough, Wirral, UK*

JIGNESH K. PATEL • *Cedars-Sinai Heart Institute, Los Angeles, CA, USA*

JEREMY RYAN PEÑA • *Histocompatibility (HLA) Laboratory, Department of Pathology, Massachusetts General Hospital, Boston, MA, USA*

RAJA RAJALINGAM • *Department of Pathology and Laboratory Medicine, UCLA Immunogenetics Center, David Geffen School of Medicine at UCLA, University of California at Los Angeles, Los Angeles, CA, USA*

ELAINE F. REED • *Department of Pathology and Laboratory Medicine, UCLA Immunogenetics Center, David Geffen School of Medicine, University of California, Los Angeles, CA, USA*

NANCY L. REINSMOEN • *HLA Laboratory, Cedars-Sinai Medical Center, Los Angeles, CA, USA*

MARLENE L. ROSE • *Transplant Immunology, Harefield Hospital, Imperial College, Harefield, UK*

JAMIE ROSSJOHN • *Department of Biochemistry and Molecular Biology, School of Biomedical Sciences, Monash University, Clayton, VIC, Australia; Institute of Infection and Immunity, School of Medicine, Cardiff University, Heath Park, Cardiff, UK*

Susan L. Saidman • *Histocompatibility (HLA) Laboratory, Department of Pathology, Massachusetts General Hospital, Boston, MA, USA*
Daniel R. Salomon • *Laboratory for Functional Genomics, Department of Molecular and Experimental Medicine, The Scripps Research Institute, La Jolla, CA, USA*
Nayan J. Sarma • *Department of Surgery, Washington University School of Medicine, St. Louis, MO, USA*
Minnie. M. Sarwal • *California Pacific Medical Center - Research Institute, San Francisco, CA, USA; BIOMARC Program for Personalized Medicine, Sutter Health Care, San Francisco, CA, USA*
Joseph Scalea • *Department of Surgery, University of Maryland School of Medicine, Baltimore, MD, USA*
David Senitzer • *HLA laboratory, City of Hope, Duarte, CA, USA*
Tara K. Sigdel • *California Pacific Medical Center - Research Institute, San Francisco, CA, USA; BIOMARC Program for Personalized Medicine, Sutter Health Care, San Francisco, CA, USA*
John D. Smith • *Transplant Immunology, Harefield Hospital, Imperial College, Harefield, UK*
Nicole Suciu-Foca • *Department of Pathology & Cell Biology, Columbia University, New York, NY, USA*
Venkataswarup Tiriveedhi • *Department of Surgery, Washington University School of Medicine, St. Louis, MO, USA*
Elizabeth A. Trachtenberg • *Children's Hospital & Research Center, Oakland, CA, USA*
Bin Tu • *CW Bill Young Marrow Donor Recruitment and Research Program, Department of Pediatrics, Georgetown University Medical Center, Rockville, MD, USA*
Dolly B. Tyan • *Histocompatibility, Immunogenetics & Disease Profiling Laboratory, Department of Pathology, Stanford University School of Medicine, Palo Alto, CA, USA*
Nicole M. Valenzuela • *Department of Pathology and Laboratory Medicine, UCLA Immunogenetics Center, David Geffen School of Medicine, University of California, Los Angeles, CA, USA*
George Vlad • *Department of Pathology & Cell Biology, Columbia University, New York, NY, USA*
Kathryn J. Wood • *Transplantation Research Immunology Group, Nuffield Department of Surgical Sciences, John Radcliffe Hospital, University of Oxford, Oxford, UK*
Yi Xiao • *CW Bill Young Marrow Donor Recruitment and Research Program, Department of Pediatrics, Georgetown University Medical Center, Rockville, MD, USA*
Ruyan Yang • *CW Bill Young Marrow Donor Recruitment and Research Program, Department of Pediatrics, Georgetown University Medical Center, Rockville, MD, USA*
Andrea A. Zachary • *Immunogenetics Laboratory, Department of Medicine, Johns Hopkins University School of Medicine, Baltimore, MD, USA*
Masaaki Zaitsu • *Transplantation Research Immunology Group, Nuffield Department of Surgical Sciences, John Radcliffe Hospital, University of Oxford, Oxford, UK*
Adriana Zeevi • *University of Pittsburgh Medical Center, Pittsburgh, PA, USA*

Part I

Overview Chapters

Chapter 1

Alloreactivity

Sidonia B.G. Eckle, Jamie Rossjohn, and James McCluskey

Abstract

The alloimmune response between individuals genetically disparate for antigens encoded within the major histocompatibility complex (MHC) remains a substantial barrier to transplantation of solid organs, tissues, and hematopoietic stem cells. Alloreactivity has been an immunological paradox because of its apparent contradiction to the requirement of MHC restriction for the induction of normal T lymphocyte mediated immune responses. Through crystallographic analyses and experimental systems utilizing murine CD8$^+$ cytolytic T cell clones, major advances have been achieved in understanding the molecular and structural basis of T cell receptor recognition of MHC–peptide complexes and the basis of T cell mediated alloreactivity. These studies have further provided an explanation for the relatively high frequencies of alloreactive T cells compared to the frequencies of T cells for microbial derived antigens.

Key words Alloreactivity, T cell receptor, Major histocompatibility complex, MHC restriction

1 Physiological Relevance and History of Alloreactivity

Clinical engraftment (transplantation) of histocompatibility mismatched hematopoietic stem cells, tissues, or organs between two genetically disparate individuals of the same species provokes allogeneic immune responses or allorecognition, which is the recognition of allo- (foreign) histocompatibility antigens by the host immune system. Allogeneic responses can be humoral (antibodies) or cellular (T cell mediated). Depending on the nature of the transplant, an alloresponse directed against the histocompatibility antigens of the transplant can be elicited that manifests itself clinically in graft rejection or graft-versus-host disease (GVHD) [1]. Alloreactivity was first demonstrated to be an immune system mediated reaction by Medawar in 1944 [2] and has ever since represented a longstanding paradox in immunology with regard to its biological meaning and its unexplained contradiction to the phenomenon of MHC restriction. The following sections provide an overview of T cell receptor (TCR) recognition of peptide laden

Andrea A. Zachary and Mary S. Leffell (eds.), *Transplantation Immunology: Methods and Protocols, Second Edition*, Methods in Molecular Biology, vol. 1034, DOI 10.1007/978-1-62703-493-7_1, © Springer Science+Business Media, LLC 2013

major histocompatibility complex (pMHC) molecules, the phenomenon of allorecognition, and the frequencies of alloreactive T cells, and discuss the structural basis of T cell mediated alloreactivity.

2 T Cell Receptor Recognition of Peptide-Major Histocompatibility Complex Molecules

In the adaptive cellular immune response, microbial derived (foreign) peptide antigen is displayed in complex with MHC molecules expressed on the cell surface of antigen presenting cells (APCs) to αβ T lymphocytes (T cells) [3, 4]. The central event of antigen recognition, that causes TCR signaling, is the highly specific interaction of αβ TCRs expressed on the surface of T cells with foreign peptide in the context of self-MHC molecules. T cells are selected during thymic development to react preferentially with the pMHC molecules of the host in which they developed, a concept termed MHC restriction [5]. Subsequent T cell activation involves clonal expansion (proliferation) and differentiation into effector T cells. Based on their effector function, usually two types of T cells can be distinguished that differ in co-receptor expression and differential MHC class reactivity. Cytotoxic T cells (CTLs) express the co-receptor CD8 and react with pMHC class I (pMHC-I), while helper T cells express the co-receptor CD4 and recognize pMHC class II (pMHC-II) [6–8]. MHC-bound peptides can also be derived from cellular protein and hence of self-origin [9] to which T cells are tolerant. Both, tolerance to self-peptides and self-MHC restriction are imprinted during thymic development of T cells where T cells are selected based on self-peptide bound to self-MHC molecules [10].

Given the need for a diverse immune response (within an individual and on a population scale) to ensure microbial recognition and adaptation to antigen escape variants within microbes, a large repertoire of peptides can be presented by the combination of MHC-I and MHC-II allotypes. This repertoire is conferred by (1) the polygenicity of the MHC-I and MHC-II genes encoded by three loci each, (2) the highly polymorphic nature of the MHC with approximately 5,458 allotypes within the human population, (3) the inheritance of sets of MHC alleles from both parents and their codominant expression allowing the simultaneous presence of gene products from up to six different MHC-I and MHC-II loci each, in each individual, and (4) the ability of one MHC allotype to bind a wide range of peptides of different amino acid sequences (a distinct set for each allotype), reviewed in [11]. MHC-I genes comprise in humans the subclasses HLA-A, HLA-B, and HLA-C and in mouse H2-D, H2-K, and H2-L; MHC-II genes comprise in humans the subclasses HLA-DP, HLA-DQ, and HLA-DR and in mouse H2-A (IA), H2-E (IE), and H2-P with H2-P being unproductive [12].

MHC-I and MHC-II molecules are heterodimers that exhibit different domain organizations, depicted in Fig. 1a in crystal structures of soluble pMHC-I and pMHC-II complexes: The MHC-I molecule consists of the MHC-I heavy chain comprising three N-terminal extracellular domains (α1, α2, α3), a transmembrane region, and a cytoplasmic tail, as well as the soluble non-polymorphic light-chain β_2-microglobulin (β_2m) subunit associated with the membrane proximal α3-domain of the MHC-I heavy chain to form a pedestal-like structure that supports the peptide binding groove created by the α1- and α2-domains. MHC-II molecules are composed of α- and β-chains comprising N-terminal extracellular membrane distal domains (α-chain: α1; β-chain: β1) and membrane proximal domains (α-chain: α2; β-chain: β2), a transmembrane region, and a C-terminal cytoplasmic tail. In MHC-II complexes, both the α- and β-chains make up the peptide-binding groove formed by the α1- and β1-domains, reviewed in [13].

The first crystal structures of pMHC-I molecules [14–16] and pMHC-II molecules [17] revealed that MHC-I and MHC-II peptide-binding grooves (Fig. 1c) consist of a main cavity with side-chains of polymorphic and conserved residues in the MHC α-helices and β-sheet creating unique pockets (denoted A to F in case of MHC-I) along the main cavity of the peptide-binding groove. By providing a variation in size, hydrophobicity, and electrostatic charge, the pockets of the peptide-binding groove determine which peptide side-chains are preferentially bound. The preferences are described by the specific peptide-binding motifs identified for each MHC allotype which determine a unique set of peptides with similar residues at particular positions (anchor residues) that interact with pocket residues [18], e.g., P2-Glu in case of HLA-B44.

While the MHC-I and MHC-II peptide-binding grooves are very similar, structural differences exist between these MHC classes. Most strikingly, MHC-I peptide-binding grooves are reduced in width at both ends and then closed up by bulky aromatic residues, restricting the length of peptides occupying the groove in an extended conformation to typically less than 10 amino acids (aa). MHC-II peptide-binding grooves on the contrary are open at both ends allowing for peptides longer than 10 aa to bind with the peptide ends protruding outwards. For both classes of MHC, peptides generally adopt an extended conformation along the length of the cleft with side-chains accommodated in the pockets. MHC-I-bound peptides can show a degree of flexibility and bulge away from the antigen-binding cleft, while MHC-II-bound peptides adopt a flatter polyproline-like conformation and are positioned deeper in the cleft, reviewed in [13, 19].

αβ TCRs consist of a heterodimer of α- and β-chains, which contain each a variable (V) and a constant (C) region (Fig. 1a).

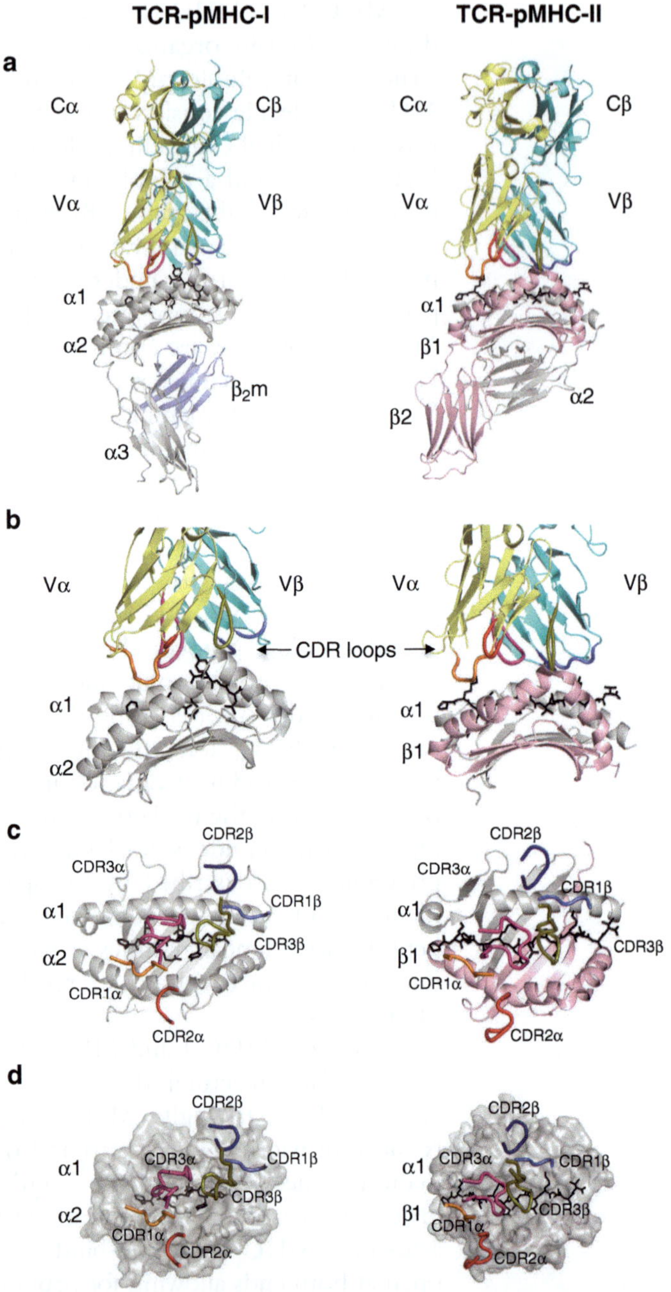

Fig. 1 Structural overview of the interaction between TCR and pMHC-I (LC13 TCR- FLR/HLA-B*08:01 [126], PDB ID: 1MI5) and pMHC-II (HA1.7 TCR-HA/DR4 [205], PDB ID: 1J8H). (**a**) Side view of the overall structures TCR-pMHC displayed as cartoon. The peptides are displayed as sticks. TCR and MHC domains are labeled. TCR α- and β-chains, β_2m, MHC-I MHC-II α- and β-chains share structural features that categorize them as members of the immunoglobulin superfamily (IgSF); MHC-I and MHC-II α- and β-chains are additionally members of the MHC superfamily (MhcSF), reviewed in [206]. Members of the IgSF (reviewed in [207]) share immunoglobulin domains, a structural feature which is characterized by a common immunoglobulin (Ig) fold in which two antiparallel β-sheets form a sandwich where

The TCR C-regions encode transmembrane regions and short cytoplasmic tails. The large range of clonal TCR specificities conferred by the TCR V regions is created during thymic development by somatic recombination of noncontiguous but linked gene segments: variable α (Vα/TRAV) and joining α (Jα/TRAJ) in case of the α-chain; and variable β (Vβ/TRBV), diversity (D) and joining β (Jβ/TRBJ) in case of the β-chain. Polygenicity allows for a total of 2,679 VJC combinations of the α-chain and 2,808 VDJC combinations of the β-chain and in total more than 7.5×10^6 TCR gene combinations in case of humans. Each TCR chain has three regions of hypervariability known as complementarity determining regions (CDR loops), which form a monovalent binding site and determine the specificity of the TCR. CDR1 and CDR2 are within the V gene and are entirely host-germ-line encoded, while CDR3 is located at the VJ junction in case of the Vα or the VDJ junction in

Fig. 1 (continued) the backbone switches repeatedly between the two β-sheets. The β-sheet sandwich is stabilized by hydrophobic interactions between the two β-sheets and a conserved disulfide bond. Based on size and function different categories of immunoglobulin domains exist, among them variable Ig domains (IgV), which contain nine β-strands and constant Ig domains (IgC), which contain seven β-strands. The TCR α- and β-chain V and C domains are IgV and IgC domains, respectively. β_2m, the MHC-I α3-domain, and the MHC-II α2- and β2-domains are IgC domains. MhcSF members (reviewed in [12]) are all of the G type, i.e., they have two MHC-like domains, each comprising four antiparallel β-strands (formed by the N-terminal segment) and one α-helix (formed by the C-term of the segment). Two membrane distal G-type (G for groove) domains together make up a three dimensional groove structure, which is formed by eight antiparallel β-strands (floor of the groove) and two α-helices (flanking sides of the groove). Within the G-type two domain categories exist: G-domains in case of MHC proteins and G-like domains for members other than MHC proteins. The MHC-I α1- and α2-domains and the MHC-II α1- and the β1-domains are G-domains. MHC-I has a conserved intradomain disulfide bond within the α2-domains. Similarly, the MHC-II β1-domain contains one conserved intradomain disulfide bond. In MHC-I molecules the 2 α-helices of the peptide-binding groove are nearly continuous, while the α-helix of the MHC-II α-chain is interrupted by a linear stretch of amino acids. (**b**) Close-up side view of the TCR CDR regions interacting with the pMHC molecules. (**c**, **d**) Top view on the pMHC in cartoon display (**c**), or surface display (**d**) with the footprint of isolated TCR CDR1, CDR2, and CDR3 loops displayed as loops over the surface and labeled. Within the surface display, the MHC α1- and α2/β1-helices are additionally indicated as cartoons. The same color scheme is used in all figures if not indicated otherwise: pMHC: peptide in *black*, MHC-I heavy chain in *grey*, β_2m in *grey-blue*, MHC-II α-chain in *grey*, MHC-II β-chain in *pink* (or *grey* in the other figures). TCR: TCR α-chain in *yellow*, TCR β-chain in *cyan*, CDR1, CDR2, and CDR3 loops in *orange*, *red*, and *magenta* in case of the TCR α-chain and in *slate blue*, *dark blue*, and *olive* in case of the TCR β-chain. If contact surfaces are displayed, they are colored in *yellow* and *cyan* for the TCR α- and β-chain, respectively; or in smudge for residues contacted by both, the α- and β-chains. All figures were generated using Pymol [208]

case of the Vβ and contains in addition to germ-line encoded also non-germ-line encoded residues (N) thus adding largely to TCR diversity [20] (Fig. 1b). The overall theoretical diversity of the TCR repertoire has been estimated to be up to 10^{15} [21]. While this diversity estimate applies to the population as a whole, the precursor pools differ between individuals [22]. Furthermore, the size of the repertoire decreases during thymic selection to approximately 2×10^7 in humans [23] and 2×10^6 in mice [24] because of failed positive selection for weak self-pMHC specificity (leading to apoptosis) and negative selection (deletion) of potent self-reactive specificities.

Co-crystal structures of TCR and pMHC complexes, as first determined by Garcia et al. [25, 26] and Garboczi et al. [27], have established that both MHC residues and solvent-exposed peptide residues of the peptide binding groove are contacted by the CDR loops of αβ TCRs during TCR engagement and a very approximate conserved binding geometry (also referred to as docking mode or footprint) is adopted by the TCR on the pMHC surface (Fig. 1c, d): Maximizing the contact surface with the bound peptide, TCRs often (but not exclusively) dock at the center of the peptide-binding groove with the TCR α-chain positioned over the peptide N-terminus and the MHC-I α2-helix or the MHC-II β1-helix, while the TCR β-chain is positioned over the peptide C-terminus and the MHC-I or MHC-II α1-helix. Accordingly docking angles range between 22° and 87°, reviewed in [28, 29].

Often the germ-line encoded CDR1 and CDR2 loops have been observed to contact MHC residues and CDR3 loops the peptide; at the same time examples where CDR1 and CDR2 loops mediate important peptide contacts (e.g., [30, 31]) and CDR3 loops MHC contacts (e.g., [32, 33]) exist, evaluated in [30].

3 The Phenomenon of Allorecognition

T cells are genetically restricted to recognize foreign antigen only presented by self-MHC molecules, referred to as MHC restriction [5]. Violating MHC restriction, the same T cell repertoire [34] can also recognize intact allogeneic MHC molecules, i.e., non-self/foreign MHC molecules of varying allotype than that encountered during thymic selection, referred to as direct allorecognition [35]. T cells can furthermore recognize peptides derived from allogeneic MHC molecules complexed with self-MHC molecules, termed indirect allorecognition [36], as well as minor histocompatibility antigens complexed with self-MHC molecules [37]. Despite their importance in graft rejection [38, 39], indirect allorecognition and the recognition of minor histocompatibility antigens are forms of conventional T cell recognition [36] and as such not further discussed here.

An alloresponse is a synergistic effort of the adaptive and innate immune system and involves CTLs, granulocyte activation, NK-cell activation, alloantibody production by B cells, and complement activation [1]. Alloantibody production is a consequence of indirect allorecognition and is dependent on donor-reactive T cell help, as it requires presentation of alloantigen recognized by the B cell receptor and presentation of processed alloantigen to T cells, which in turn activate B cell effector function [1]. Allograft destruction is mediated through a combination of CD4⁺ or CD8⁺ T cells that exert cytotoxicity upon recognition of allogeneic MHC molecules, alloantibodies that can opsonize grafted cells and thereby activate complement or antibody dependent cytotoxicity, and macrophage-mediated delayed type hypersensitivity stimulated by activated CD4⁺ and CD8⁺ T cells [40]. Several data supports the concept of direct stimulation of CD4⁺ or CD8⁺ T cells by "passenger" antigen presenting cells of the allograft [36, 41, 42]. In addition CD4⁺ or CD8⁺ T cells can be primed by intact MHC molecules that have been transferred from the allograft to recipient APCs, referred to as "semi-direct" pathway [43]. In vitro T cell alloresponses can be simulated in mixed lymphocyte reactions (MLRs) as first described by Hirschhorn et al. [44]. In fact MLRs are sometimes performed as one of the transplant matching strategies indicating compatibility of mismatched donor–recipient pairs; however, the reproducibility of these assays means they are rarely used as predictive tests in routine HLA laboratories.

While generally the extreme polymorphism of the MHC allotypes is responsible for allorecognition, the association of specific MHC mismatches with allograft survival varies, with some mismatches having a beneficial effect on graft survival, some being permissive, some associated with significant adverse affects and some highly associated with transplant rejection, referred to as taboo mismatches as for example evaluated for kidney transplants [45, 46], and hematopoietic stem cell transplants [47–49]. Such dominance hierarchies include interlocus hierarchies with greater responses toward HLA-B molecules than HLA-A, e.g., [50–53], and intralocus hierarchies, e.g., a larger response directed to HLA-B*44:03 compared to HLA-B*44:02 [50]. Hierarchy patterns for a particular mismatch are dependent on the nature and number of other mismatches present, suggested to reflect partly alloantigenic competition in responder cell responses [50]. Furthermore mismatches can be asymmetric. For example in HLA-B*44:02/03 mismatched individuals, allo-HLA-B*44:03 T cells give rise to a response of larger magnitude than allo-HLA-B*44:02 T cells [50]. Association with allograft survival is not necessarily related to the degree of MHC polymorphism between MHC mismatches. For example in the case of mismatched allotypes that differ in 20–30 aa, micropolymorphism of 1 aa such as between HLA-B*44:02 and HLA-B*44:03, exerts alloreactive responses of similar magnitude causing GVHD and transplant rejection [54, 55]. In fact, highly divergent MHC mismatches can be superior in transplant survival upon hematopoietic stem cell transplantation [56]. Instead, the mapping of alloreactive T cell epitopes (TCE) present on certain allotypes that either form direct T cell epitopes or indirectly impact on certain immunogenic allopeptides bound, as performed for HLA-DP allotypes, allowed to define groups of clinically relevant nonpermissive MHC matches [47, 48].

4 Frequencies of Naïve and Memory Alloreactive T Cells

Surprisingly the precursor frequency of alloreactive T cells within the naïve mature T cell repertoire is up to 10 %, 100- to 1,000-fold higher than the precursor frequency specific for any single pathogen derived epitope in context of autologous MHC [57–59]. In addition to naïve, also memory T cells, that have previously encountered antigen such as of viral and bacterial origin or from a previous transplant, mediate alloreactivity [60]. Memory T cells are generally more potent in eliciting an immune response based on qualitative features such as less activation requirements with regard to co-stimulation and antigen dose, broader homing properties, and the expression of molecules with effector function combined with clonal frequencies that are higher than naïve precursor frequencies [61]. As such, alloreactive memory T cells are suspected to be the major contributor in clinical transplant rejection [61]. Indeed a high frequency of approx. 45 % of viral specific memory T cells that exert direct alloreactivity in MLRs against at least one allogeneic HLA has been determined [62]. Amir et al. postulated that virtually all antigen-specific T cells are allo-MHC-I- or MHC-II-reactive as their study did not account for infrequent MHC molecules and tissue specific allopeptides [62]. Although there is one report showing that the presence of viral specific memory T cells does not exacerbate GVHD in vivo [63].

Impaired negative selection, as it takes place in mice expressing a single pMHC molecule, gives rise to T cells that have a significantly higher alloreactive potential as compared to those derived from mice with conventional thymic selection [64–66]. Also, alloreactivity frequencies across MHC classes are increased [64–66] which are largely absent under conventional thymic selection conditions when a self-MHC- and peptide-specific repertoire is created [57, 62, 64, 67, 68] and might in part reflect the role of co-receptors CD4/CD8, discussed in the context of MHC restriction. Nonetheless, a few examples of $CD8^+$ T cells that react with allogeneic MHC-II molecules in MLRs have been derived from human [62, 69–73] and murine PBMCs [74] under normal selection conditions. While generally, TCR α- and β-chains are subject to allelic exclusion so that a unique $\alpha\beta$ TCR type is expressed by a given T cell clone (also referred to as clonal distribution) dual TCR T cells exist which was not excluded as the underlying mechanism for dual MHC-I/II recognition of most of the systems, except [62, 69, 73]. In fact up to 30 % of mature human T cells [75] and up to 21 % of mature murine T cells [76] express a second TCR α-chain; 1–8 % of the second TCR α-chain in humans and mice also pair with the present TCR β-chain and give rise to dual TCR T cells [75, 77, 78]. Dual TCR T cells were shown to make up 50 % of the alloreactive repertoire and comprise up to 60 % of peripheral activated T cells during GVHD in a mouse model [79]. In addition to the presence of two receptors with different specificities, this was attributed to the less stringent thymic selection requirements of secondary TCRs [80, 81] which give rise to higher frequencies of alloreactivity [64, 68].

5 The Molecular Basis of Alloreactivity

The existence of alloreactive T cells in large numbers in the naïve T cell repertoire has been and still is one of the most intriguing questions in immunology and many models have been proposed to account for this. The molecular basis of T cell allorecognition has been informed by crystal structures of the soluble versions of alloreactive TCRs liganded with the soluble versions of self- and allogeneic pMHC complexes. Due to the difficulties involved in identifying allopeptides bound to the allogeneic MHC molecules, the number of structural studies addressing T cell allorecognition is limited. To date they include five systems of TCRs alloreacting with polymorphic MHC allotypes, reviewed in [82], and one system of a TCR alloreacting with a different class of MHC [83]. In the following, models of alloreactivity developed early on are being discussed in the context of functional and crystallographic data present to date. In addition the structural insights gained from three systems, namely, the 2C, LC13, and YAe62, are illustrated in detail in the section thereafter (Subheading 6).

5.1 The Relative Contribution of Peptide and MHC Molecule to Alloreactivity and the Phenomenon of Polyspecificity Underlying T Cell Alloreactivity

The contribution of peptide and MHC in direct allorecognition has been discussed historically in two non-mutually exclusive models. The "peptide-centric" model states that the TCR interacts in a mimicry approach with a set of residues shared by self- and allogeneic-MHC, so that alloreactivity depends crucially on the allopeptide, recognized as foreign ("altered self"), and "antigen frequency" drives allorecognition [84]. The "MHC-centric" model on the other hand states that alloreactive T cells focus on polymorphic residues of the allogeneic MHC molecule, while the peptide is largely irrelevant. In such a "peptide degenerate" interaction T cells with low affinity for allo-MHC are activated based on the high "antigen density" (of allo-MHC molecules) on engrafted cells. The repertoire and thus the frequencies of such T cells exceed the numbers of T cells that respond to conventional antigen where both peptide and MHC are recognized [85]. Obst et al. developed experimentally in vitro that the higher the homology/similarity between the donor and recipient allotypes the higher the proportion of "peptide-centric" versus "MHC-centric" alloreactive T cells that are more frequent in case of low similarity/homology between the donor and recipient allotypes [86].

There is some experimental support of T cell alloreactivity being independent of a particular peptide or any peptide at all [87–92]. Structural insight into peptide degenerate recognition has been provided by the autoimmune 3A6 TCR [93], as well as the highly peptide and MHC cross-reactive YAe62 TCR, derived from severely limited negative selection conditions, when liganded with both, pMHC-II [94] and allogeneic pMHC-I [83], as described below in detail (YAe62 system).

Most studies, however, demonstrate that inhibited presentation of endogenous peptide decreases alloreactive responses in vivo [95] and in vitro where alloreactive T cell clones specifically recognize peptide such as derived from certain fractions of cell material [96–100] or cell-type/tissue specific peptides [62, 69, 101, 102] and in fact in some instances the required allopeptides essential for allorecognition have been identified, e.g., [103–106]. Identification of allopeptides allows for the generation of allopeptide/MHC-tetramers which have been formally shown to bind to alloreactive T cells as they would to conventional antigen specific T cells [107], and as such can be used in the analysis, enrichment and isolation of alloreactive T cells, with recent advances reviewed in [108].

There is also direct support for the "peptide-centric" model in case of similar allo-MHC molecules as shown by Obst et al. [86] and further demonstrated in the crystal structures of the 2C TCR engaged with its syngeneic ligand dEV8/H-2-K^b and its allogeneic ligand dEV8/H-2-K^{bm3} in a molecular mimicry approach where the peptide albeit the same as in the syngeneic ligand (and hence not truly alloreactive) adopts a slightly different conformation induced by a polymorphic MHC residue and is thus recognized as foreign [109], explained in detail below (2C system). The same principal was suggested based on functional data involving alloreactivity directed against mutant versions of H2-K^b [110] and IA^b [111]. Alternatively, the allo-MHC molecule might bind self-peptides differing from the ones presented by self-MHC molecules and thus recognized as foreign as suggested by the allorecognition pattern of broadly mutated HLA-A*02:01 [112].

However, substantial functional and structural evidence has emerged, that allorecognition is mostly specific for both, peptide and MHC, as first established by Heath and colleagues who found that H-2K^b-specific alloreactive CTL clones were capable of lysing human Jurkat T cells transfected with H-2K^b only in the presence of a murine cell extract derived allopeptide [99]. Also, Allen and colleagues tested recently a large pool of IE^k-alloreactive T cell hybridomas, generated by immunizing mice with β-galactosidase, against a large pool of naturally processed peptides in context of IE^k. They observed clonally dependent highly specific responses to more than one peptide involving unique interactions with peptide and MHC molecule, as tested through mutagenesis of peptide and MHC residues [113]. These observations have been reconciled in a phenomenon termed polyspecificity, i.e., the inherent ability of a single TCR to be able to recognize multiple distinct but structurally related ligands while maintaining exquisite specificity for each, [114–116], reviewed in [117]. Other than being the underlying cause of most alloreactivity (or alloreactivity the by-product of polyspecificity), polyspecificity is relevant to many aspects of T cell biology, such as T cell selection, survival, and foreign-antigen recognition, which entail signal integration from the interaction of the TCR with numerous different peptide-self-MHC ligands [118]. Also, based on mathematical models, polyspecificity has been suggested to ensure that a sufficient number of T cells are recruited during an immune response [119, 120]. One mechanism of polyspecificity is molecular mimicry that has been a priori an attractive concept underlying alloreactivity [121]. In fact molecular mimicry has been observed in case of the LC13 TCR that interacts with the allopeptide and allo-MHC molecule in nearly an identical manner to that observed with the distinct cognate ligand [104], described in detail below (LC13 system).

However, polyspecificity can often involve structural changes in the TCR even when engaging ideal structural mimics such as in case of the yeast derived Tel1p peptide and the viral (human T cell leukemia virus-1 derived) Tax peptide in complex with HLA-A*02:01 [27, 122] or slightly imperfect structural mimics such as in case of the self-peptide derived from the neuronal protein HuD and Tax peptide in complex with HLA-A*02:01 [123] engaged by the A6 TCR, also arguing against the hypothesis by Obst et al. [86]. Such structural changes in the TCR, also referred to as TCR flexibility/plasticity, have been informed by the comparisons of crystal structures of unliganded with pMHC liganded TCRs and between pMHC liganded TCRs for which different mechanisms can be distinguished: (1) The CDR loops can undergo conformational changes in the backbone, as often observed for the CDR3 loops [25, 27, 83, 122–127], reviewed in [128]. (2) Varying inter-domain orientations between Vα and Vβ domains have been observed for different ligands, as recognized by Reiser et al. [129] and often observed [130]. (3) Recently, Yin et al. detected alternate TCR core conformations as the underlying mechanism of the alloreactive YAe62 TCR to engage with pMHC-I and pMHC-II molecules. Here, compared to a "closed conformer" in an "open conformer" the variable domain of either TCR chain can disengage from the J segment thus switching the position of the variable domain of one chain relative to the other chain [83], described in detail below (YAe62 system). Closed conformers are observed in most unliganded and liganded TCR structures. Open conformers are limited to a few TCR families, including mouse TRAV4 TCRs (bound to pMHC-I molecules), human TRAV4 TCRs (bound to pMHC-I molecules or unliganded) and in murine TRBV2 TCRs (bound to pMHC-I molecules) [83]. A TCR can thus potentially switch between three different core conformers or if both V-domains adopted switchable conformers at the same time four conformers would be possible (which has not been observed so far) [83].

While TCR plasticity can account for polyspecificity, TCRs can furthermore induce subtle changes in the peptide and the MHC complex albeit to a varying degree, depending on the inherent flexibility/plasticity of a given pMHC complex, e.g., [122, 127, 131, 132]. Observed changes in the peptide include side movements [93], altered backbone-, and side-chain conformations [27, 31, 104, 125, 131]. Less subtle can be the flattening of bulged peptides [133]. Changes in the MHC include displacements of the MHC helices [93, 134], changes in the helix structure [122, 135], and altered side-chain conformations of residues present in the helices [31, 134].

Illustrating another mechanism underlying polyspecificity, the alloreactive murine 2C TCR globally repositions on the allogeneic ligand QL9/H2-L^d compared to its syngeneic ligand, thereby preserving its structure [136], explained in detail below (2C system).

Due to a limited amount of TCR-pMHC structures it is unclear to which extent the emerging mechanisms of polyspecificity are unique to alloreactive or cognate interactions versus common between both types. Importantly, however, individual receptors can utilize combinations of the mechanisms named above as for example the molecular mimicry exhibited by the LC13 TCR involves a TCR induced conformational side-chain change of the allopeptide [104], and possibly other mechanisms that are not known yet [137]. Polyspecificity itself is not unlimited. Huseby et al. established that negative selection during thymic selection (although not occurring on allo-MHC molecules) limits the mature T cell repertoire in degenerate reactivity for MHC and peptide [64, 68], and αβ TCR chain pairing [138] and fine-tuning by CDR3 loops [139] have been identified as driving elements in limiting MHC cross-reactivity/creating MHC specificity. Based on the notion that most T cells are not alloreactive for a given MHC, e.g., [62], Allen and colleagues furthermore showed, that alloreactivity is limited by the endogenous peptide repertoire rather than the inability to interact with allogeneic MHC molecules albeit being specific for and critically dependent on interactions with the MHC molecule [140]. This was demonstrated by the addition of peptide mimotopes which allowed for specific allorecognition of certain MHC molecules that was otherwise not observed [140].

The question whether alloreactive T cells have an inherently higher degree of polyspecificity [141] has also been addressed in part when comparing the sequences of alloreactive versus non-alloreactive TCRs. While generally a broad use of germ-line encoded TCR segments is observed in polyclonal alloreactive responses [140, 142, 143] that also differs between individuals [62], skewing in non-germ-line encoded CDR3 regions of alloreactive versus non-alloreactive TCRs with a minimal overlap of sequences (<10 %) has been observed [140]. Conclusions from this are unclear, however, given that CDR3 length and sequence composition were indifferent so that no difference in flexibility, hydrophobicity, or charge in the loops was suspected [140]. Conclusions are furthermore exacerbated by the versatile role CDR3 loops play in contacting peptide and/or MHC [30] and their possible role in fine-tuning germ-line encoded MHC interactions [139].

5.2 Alloreactivity as a By-product of the Intrinsic Bias of TCRs to Interact with MHC Molecules

In explaining the origin of αβ TCR restriction for MHC, Jerne's theory that TCR germ-line encoded elements have been evolutionary selected to interact with MHC molecules regardless of MHC allotype or class [144], also referred to as the "hardwiring" of TCRs for MHC, provides another attempt in explaining the high frequency of alloreactive T cells. Based on the fact that self-MHC restriction is imprinted in the thymus, as experimentally first explored by Fink and Bevan [145] as well as Zinkernagel et al. [146], a contradicting view states that MHC restricted T cells are selected during thymic selection from a preselection repertoire with completely random specificities. MHC restriction could then be imprinted through interaction with MHC raising the question how T cells are guided to interact with MHC molecules in the presence of all the other proteins expressed by cells in the thymus such as the co-receptors CD4 and CD8; alternatively mature T cells could have been selected on other proteins than MHC whereby T cells with high affinity/avidity for those proteins died in negative selection calling for the existence of T cells which have low affinity for proteins other than MHC [147].

A strong a priori argument in favor of Jerne's theory came from the observation of the conserved TCR docking topology (as described above) and reviewed in [148–150]. However, other plausible explanations for the conserved docking topology could be external constraints, such as the co-receptors CD4 and CD8 [151], or CD3 interactions imposing steric requirements to allow for productive signaling of the TCR complex [152]. The first experimental support came indirectly from in vitro fused cells expressing randomly generated hybrid TCRs that showed frequent MHC reactivity not being a product of thymic selection [153]. Further evidence came from Zerrahn et al. [154] and Merkenschlager et al. [155], who determined in the preselection repertoire higher frequencies of T cells reacting with MHC than expected in case of random receptor specificity. Recently, also structural correlates of MHC restrictive elements have been identified:

Originally identified as the minimal structural requirements underlying MHC restriction in the crystal structure of the SB27 TCR in complex with the superbulged 13-mer peptide (LPEP) bound to HLA-B*35:08 [156], MHC-I contact residues 65 and 69 on the α1-helix and 155 on the α2-helix (the "triad") are structurally conserved among all TCR–pMHC-I interactions as established by comparative analysis of known structures [28, 30, 156]. Also, a similar set of residues has been identified for MHC-II molecules (residue 57 and 61 on the α1-helix and 70 on the β1-helix) [28]. Notably, differences occur in the CDR loop residues contacting the triad residues, and CDR3 residues have a dominant role in contacting the energetic hotspots [28, 30, 157]. Also, the interaction with the triad residues is characterized by different bonding properties [28] and thus their function in contributing energy to the interaction TCR-pMHC varies in different complexes and is not necessarily required for productive engagement [30, 157] and not all triad residues are necessarily contacted [158]. However, Burrows et al. also suggested that the restriction triad residues might play a more consistent role in thymic positive selection while they could persist to varying degrees in the interactions of the mature T cell repertoire accounting for the inherent TCR flexibility in pMHC-I recognition [30].

Furthermore, TCR residues repeatedly contributing in the interaction with IA have been identified in members of the mouse Vβ8.2 family (CDR2 Y46, Y48 and E54) and related families in mice and humans [94, 149, 150, 159]. The same residues were also used by the IA^b-specific YAe62 TCR (Vβ8.2) derived from a system of limiting negative selection [64] in contacting MHC-I H2-K^b [83]. Moreover, these residues are important in efficient thymic selection [160].

Garcia and colleagues furthermore identified precise MHC residues contacted and conserved throughout IA MHC allotypes (Lys39, Gln57 and Gln61), referred to as "pair-wise interaction motif" or "interaction codon" [136, 161–163]. Generalizing this observation they suggest that many different germ-line-derived TCR–MHC interaction codons exist for different sets of V regions interacting with specific MHC allotypes. Furthermore, influenced by CDR3 loops and MHC-bound peptide, several distinct codons exist for a given V segment to interact with a given MHC ("editing of the germ-line encoded interaction codons"), further enlarging the number of pairwise interaction-codons [150, 159, 164].

In contrast, Marrack, Kappler, and colleagues propose certain sites on the MHC that are often contacted, namely, areas around residue 69 on the α1-helix and 158 on the α2-helix in case of MHC-I molecules and areas around residue 64 on the α1-helix and residue 73 on the β1-helix in case of MHC-II molecules. These areas are located on the tops of the helices of all MHC molecules and are populated by small amino acids (alanine, glycine) exposing the backbone of the MHC helices and limited in size by adjacent side-chains thus allowing for some flexibility (along the helices) when accommodating CDR3 loops and MHC-bound peptide while at the same time preserving conserved and specific interactions. They furthermore acknowledge that TCRs, which have undergone conventional negative selection, most likely manifest when engaging pMHC only a few selected or even none of the hardwiring interactions, while others are modulated or prevented by the CDR3 loops, by the peptide [64, 94, 139, 149], and through differential V-chain pairing inducing altered binding-modes [138, 165], thus decreasing the dominating effect of the otherwise predominant contribution of those residues to the interaction.

In line with the models presented by both groups is the arrangement of the MHC contact sites or residues which occur opposite each other and hence impose a roughly conserved docking topology of the TCR onto the pMHC surface [94, 149, 150, 159]; whereby variability within the conserved mode would be due to peptide and CDR3 differences accommodated by the flexibility of the docking site [149] or the use of one of different interaction codons influenced by the CDR3 loops and peptide [150].

Another mechanism that was considered to govern inherent MHC restriction is a common thermodynamic signature. However, there is no uniform thermodynamic signature for TCR–pMHC-I interactions with some interaction characterized by favorable enthalpy (arising from interface contacts) combined with unfavorable entropy (anticipated from the ordering of CDR loops upon ligation) [166–168], while others are characterized by favorable enthalpy combined with favorable entropy [32, 169].

Experimental evidence for co-receptors imposing TCR specificity for MHC during thymic selection and MHC restriction in the periphery came from studies from Singer and colleagues [170–172]. Their study focused on Lck, which initiates TCR signaling in both immature and mature T cells and occurs in two forms in the cytoplasm, "free," or bound to the ITAMS of the co-receptors CD4 and CD8, whose extracellular domains bind to MHC-II and MHC-I molecules, respectively. Their studies, involving thymocytes at the double positive stage and peripheral T cells of quadruple-knockout mice (mice deficient in MHC-I, MHC-II, CD4, and CD8), suggested that the co-receptors CD4 and CD8 sequester Lck away, thus leaving insufficient amounts of "free" Lck required for co-receptor independent TCR signaling (that would also be MHC independent) and only allowing for signaling of TCRs (and the development of their corresponding T cells) that engage MHC molecules and thereby co-engage co-receptor bound Lck [170]. In contrast, T cells that had differentiated in the absence of MHC molecules and co-receptors exhibited a diverse repertoire and reacted with antigen independently of MHC in a TCR specific way, indicating a unique recognition repertoire [170, 171]. Notably, Singer and colleagues recently identified two TCRs from quadruple-knockout mice that recognize two different glycosylation-dependent conformational epitopes on CD155 with an affinity of ~200 nM affinity (10–100 times higher than conventional TCR recognize antigen in the context of MHC molecules) and do not recognize MHC molecules [171]. CD155 recognition was mediated by CDR3 residues but also required the identical CDR2β germ-line encoded residues that had previously been suggested to guide MHC bias, directly challenging inherent MHC restriction of TCRs [171]. Singer and colleagues do not dispute the existence of germ-line bias toward MHC recognition but rather consider that "the bias is not strong enough to have eliminated MHC-independent αβ TCRs" from the preselection repertoire and that it is the co-receptors that provide bias toward MHC recognition in the thymus [170, 171]. There are furthermore rare reports of αβ TCRs cloned from conventionally selected T cell populations which bind and are activated by ligands independently of MHC. Common to those ligands is the presence of multiple epitopes in close space either on one molecule with abundant regularly repeated antigenic epitopes [173] or through multimerization of the ligand [174, 175], or additional CD2–CD58 adhesive interactions [176], indicating the necessity of enhancement of the overall avidity of a low affinity interaction. That no high-affinity TCR reactivities for non-MHC ligands have been observed in case of conventionally selected T cells would be in line with the model from Singer and colleagues as they would have been prescreened for MHC specificity in the thymus [170, 171]. The hypothesis by Singer and colleagues also holds with regard to a report by Kim et al., who demonstrated that T cells could not be selected on the MHC-II like protein HLA-DM expressed in mice deficient in classical MHC (but expressing co-receptors) [177]; as well as the inverse scenario given by a study where β/β-homodimers of MHC-II molecules (comprising the CD4 binding site) were the single classical MHC molecules expressed in mice and allowed for appreciable levels of positive selection bearing T cells reactive with β/β-homodimer and classical pMHC-II molecules [178].

In contrast advocates of the "inherent bias for MHC model" would argue that HLA-DM like any other non-MHC ligand is not part of the evolutionary forces that have shaped the TCR–MHC interaction and thus not sufficient as a selecting ligand. Similarly, they would argue that MHC-II β/β-homodimers are structurally quite distinct from heterodimers which are yet recognized by selected T cells thus suggesting that TCR specificity is not dependent on normal positive selection but inherently present. Taken together, the evidence for an inherent bias of TCRs towards recognition of pMHC complexes is still only circumstantial when examined structurally and poorly generalized making this issue controversial among immunologists.

6 Structural Insights into Direct TCR Allorecognition

6.1 The 2C System

6.1.1 Overview of the System

The 2C system represents the murine $CD8^+$ CTL clone 2C for which several syngeneic and allogeneic ligands have been identified, a clonotype specific antibody has been cloned (1B2) and 2C TCR transgenic mice including $RAG1^{-/-}$ mice were generated, reviewed in [179]. This system was used in pioneering studies and contributed largely to our understanding in the characterization of naïve and memory T cells, thymic selection, alloreactivity including the cross-reactive potential of T cells with regard to allo- and syngeneic pMHC ligands, the relationships between binding parameters and T cell function including the impact of CD8, and insights into TCR structure being one of the first TCRs to be cloned (*TRAV3*, *TRBV8.2*) and crystallized yielding the first crystal structures of unliganded TCR (PDB ID: 1TCR) and TCR in complex with pMHC (PDB ID: 2CKB) [25, 26], reviewed in [179].

The 2C T cell clone was originally isolated from a BALB.B ($H\text{-}2^b$) mouse in an allogeneic response toward $H\text{-}2^d$ cells upon injection in the mouse [180]. The allogeneic response was identified to be specific for $H2\text{-}L^d$ in MLRs [180]. Subsequently two overlapping $H\text{-}2L^d$ restricted natural self-peptides derived from the enzyme α-ketoglutarate dehydrogenase (α-KGDH) were identified in HPLC fractions of trifluoroacetic acid (TFA) treated mouse spleens that when bound to $H2\text{-}L^d$ stimulated 2C T cells. Those peptides were p2Ca (LSPFPFDL) [103] and the N-terminal extended p2Cb (VAITRIEQLSPFPFDL) [181]. 20s proteasome degradation of p2Cb yielded furthermore a series of N-terminal truncated peptides of 9–13 residues in length which bound to $H2\text{-}L^d$ and as such were capable of stimulating 2C T cells [182]. One of the peptides, QL9 (QLSPFPFDL), had a higher affinity for $H\text{-}2L^d$ and was a stronger agonist for the 2C TCR compared to p2Cb [183].

Furthermore, in 2C transgenic mice, $H\text{-}2K^b$ was identified as a syngeneic ligand that allows for positive selection [184, 185] in complex with the naturally occurring peptide dEV8 (EQYKFYSV) derived from the enzyme NADH-ubiquinone oxidoreductase [186, 187], while 2C T cells are deleted during thymic selection in mice expressing H-2L^{d} [184]. Also H2-K^{bm3}, one of several naturally in vivo occurring allelic variants of the gene encoding H2-K^{b}, which differs from H2-K^{b} in two amino acids located in the α1-domain (Asp77Ser, Lys89Ala, reviewed in [188]), causes thymic deletion in 2C TCR transgenic mice mediated by the Asp77Ser mutation [184]. The dEV8 peptide also binds to H2-K^{bm3} from which it was in fact originally eluted and forms compared to when in complex with H2-K^{b} a stronger (but yet weak) agonist ligand for 2C that causes an alloreactive response [187, 189, 190]. Furthermore, as a potent activator of 2C T cells in context of H2-K^{b} the peptide SIYR (SIYRYYGL) was identified (from a synthetic octamer peptide library with fixed anchor residues) [191]; activation with this peptide was shown to be CD8 dependent, while activation with QL9/H-2L^{d} was similarly strong regardless of CD8 [192, 193]. Further naturally occurring or synthetic mutant and modified peptides that bind to H2-K^{b} or H2-L^{d} and stimulate 2C T cells were identified, reviewed in [179]. Additionally, the 2C TCR can be positively selected on nonclassical MHC-I molecules [194] and classical MHC-II molecules [195].

6.1.2 Structural Insights

The crystal structure of the 2C TCR in complex with its self-selecting ligand dEV8/H2-K^{b} [25, 26], PDB ID: 2CKB, and in complex with the two alloreactive ligands dEV8/H-2K^{bm3} [109], PDB ID: 1MWA, and QL9/H-2L^{d} [136], PDB ID: 2OI9, have been determined and compared [109, 136] as summarized below.

The selecting ligand dEV8/H2-K^{b} and the allogeneic ligand QL9/H2-L^{d} present similar but yet distinct surfaces to the 2C TCR: The peptides dEV8 (EQYKFYSV) and QL9 (QLDPFPFDL) are different in length, sequence and structure with the QL9 peptide bulging out of the groove (Fig. 2a, left and middle panels). Although being homologous, H2-K^{b} and H2-L^{d} comprise 34 polymorphic residues of which 7 are TCR accessible and 12 are located on the floor of the peptide-binding groove (Fig. 2b, left and middle panels). Rather than focusing on similarities the majority of contacts by the 2C TCR focus on differences of the two ligands and use dissimilar structural, chemical, and thermodynamic mechanisms, referred to as a divergent strategy. Much like a

Fig. 2 (continued) H-2L^{d}, H-2K^{b} and H-2K^{bm3}. Isolated 2C TCR CDR loops are displayed as loops over the surface. In case of dEV8/H-2K^{bm3} the 2C TCR footprint as on dEV8/H-2K^{b} is superimposed (*light green*). (**d**) Side-views of the 2C TCR in complex with QL9/H-2L^{d} and dEV8/H-2K^{bm3}. Depicted are the TCR variable domains (*ribbon* display) and the peptide-binding grooves (*cartoon* display) with the peptides. The structure of the 2C TCR as engaged with dEV8/H-2K^{b} is superposed (*light green, ribbon* display) in both cases, and the dEV8 peptide in case of dEV8/H-2K^{bm3} displayed (*light green*)

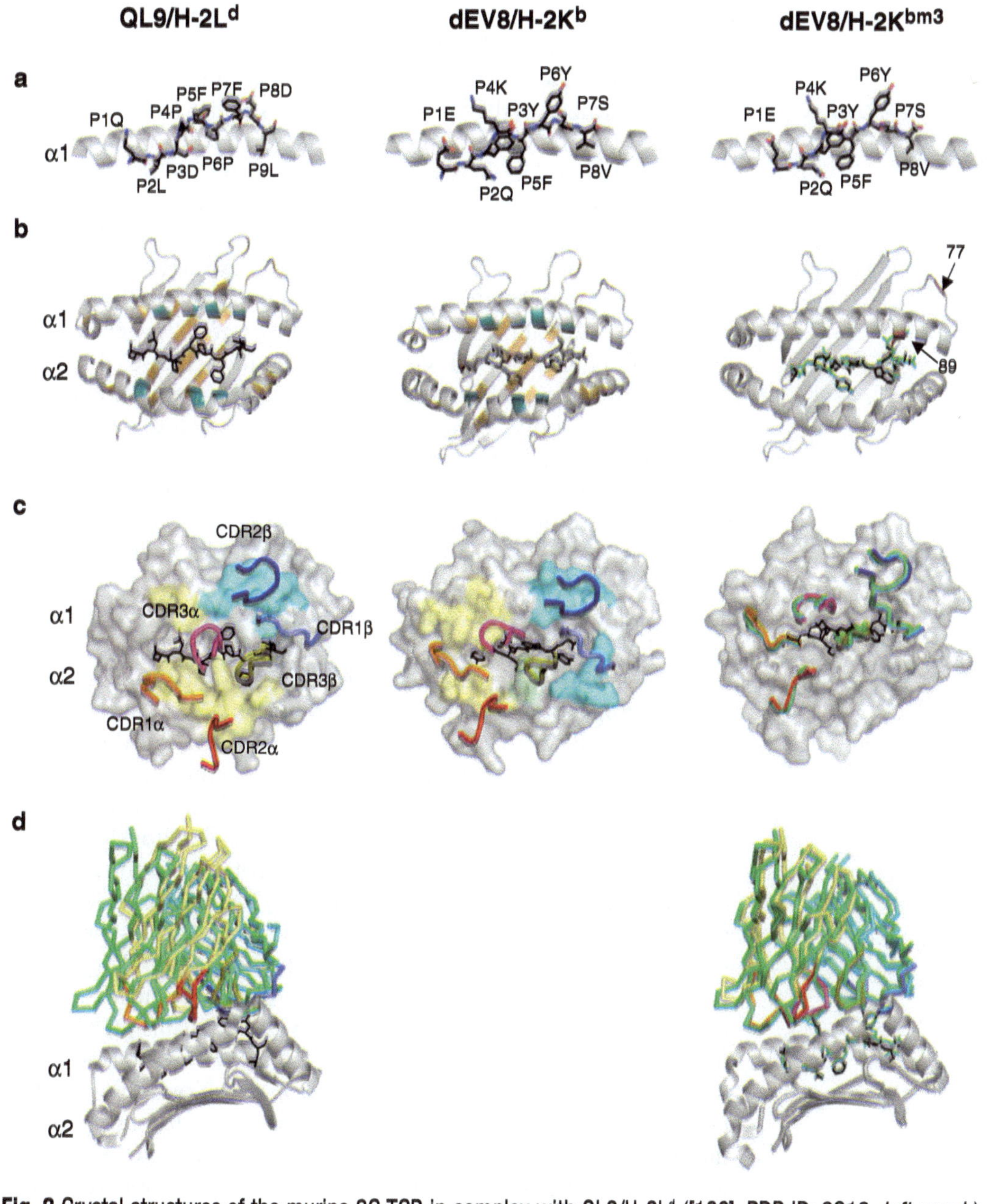

Fig. 2 Crystal structures of the murine 2C TCR in complex with QL9/H-2L^{d} ([136], PDB ID: 2019, *left panels*), dEV8/H-2K^{b} ([25], PDB ID: 2CKB, *middle panels*), and dEV8/H-2K^{bm3} ([109], PDB ID: 1MWA, *right panels*) (**a**) Side-view of the peptides QL9 (QLDPFPFDL) and dEV8 (EQYKFYSV) as bound in the peptide-binding grooves and when engaged with the 2C TCR. The peptide residues are labeled. (**b**) Top-view of the peptides and the peptide binding-grooves when engaged with the 2C TCR. Polymorphic residues (34) of homologous H-2K^{b} and H-2L^{d} that are TCR accessible (7, *turquoise*) or present in the floor of the peptide-binding groove (14, *sand color*) are highlighted in each complex. The two polymorphic residues that differ between H-2K^{bm3} and H-2K^{b} are highlighted in *brown* on dEV8/H-2K^{bm3}, and Ser77 as present in H-2K^{bm3} is indicated in *stick* display in *brown*, and Asp77 as present in H-2K^{b} in *light green*. dEV8 in the peptide-binding groove of H-2K^{b} in complex with the 2C TCR is shown (*light green*, *stick* display). (**c**) Footprints (top-view) of the 2C TCR on the surfaces of

conventional TCR, the 2C TCR mediates energetically important interactions with the MHC but also to a lower extent with the peptide of the allogeneic ligand (and the selecting ligand), considered as a synthesis of the "peptide-centric" and the "MHC-centric" hypothesis with a bias toward the MHC. The 2C TCR engages with a similar number of residues of the selecting and the allogeneic MHC complexes including a small number of shared residues and residues unique to either of the MHC complexes. Similarly, the residues used by the 2C TCR to contact the two MHC complexes are partly the same and partly unique and in total a similar number of residues (~23) approximately evenly distributed between the 2C TCR α- and β-chains (~11 Vα and ~12 Vβ) in each case contribute to the interactions. However, the actual pairwise interactions between CDR loop residues and MHC-helix residues (shared and unique ones) largely diverge as they are structurally and chemically distinct. When considering the peptide contacts, 2C TCR α- and β-chains contribute approximately equally in case of the dEV8 peptide (6 each), while β-chain contacts dominate the interaction with the QL9 peptide (4 Vα versus 9 Vβ). All CDR loops are involved in contacting the QL9 peptide, while the dEV8 peptide is not contacted by CDR2α, CDR2β, and CDR3α. The overall divergent mechanisms applied by the 2C TCR to contact the selecting versus allogeneic ligands results in different (or disparate/shifted) docking modes with regard to the positioning of the TCR on the pMHC (the TCR footprint) (compare Fig. 2c, left and middle panels): the docking orientation relative to the long axis of the pMHC groove on QL9/H2-L^d is ~20° more perpendicular (~44° docking angle) as compared to on dEV8/H2-K^b due to a rotation of the 2C TCR as a whole; also a lateral translation on QL9/H2-L^d towards the C-terminus occurs. The footprint on QL9/H2-L^d is predominantly limited to one helix of the MHC for each TCR chain; in contrast the footprint on dEV8/H2-K^b spans both helices. There is also a rotation of the 2C TCR α- and β-chains chains with respect to each other, while the individual CDR loop conformations are quite similar and move in a rigid body like fashion. Hence, TCR plasticity does not contribute to this allorecognition. In spite of the differences, the overall docking orientation on the allogeneic ligand (and the selecting ligand) is within the normal range observed to date. The binding orientation on the allogeneic ligand appears to be more optimal, being superior in shape complementarity (0.70 versus 0.41), with more atomic contacts (305 versus 104), albeit a smaller interface surface area buried (~1,770 $Å^2$ versus 2,095 $Å^2$) and yielded in a favored entropy compared to the syngeneic ligand.

The selecting dEV8/H2-K^b and the allogeneic dEV8/H2-K^{bm3} ligands vary minimally with the same peptide being presented (Fig. 2a, right and middle panels) and only two residues difference in the MHC molecules (residues 89 and 77, indicated in Fig. 2b, right panel) of which residue 89 does not contribute to the TCR-pMHC interface being located outside the binding groove. In contrast residue 77, an Aspartic acid in H-$2K^b$, is the only residue that ultimately confers alloreactivity when mutated to Serine, as present in H2-K^{bm3}. Being located on the α1-helix and pointing in the peptide-binding groove, residue 77 is not a direct TCR contact (Fig. 2b, right panel) and hence the mechanism of changed 2C reactivity is indirect as revealed in the crystal structure: To preserve the hydrogen bond of the hydroxyl group of Asp77 to the peptide backbone nitrogen at position 8, the shorter side-chain of Ser77 induces local rearrangements of the peptide which translate into a shift of the peptide backbone at three C-terminal residues toward the α1-helix of H-$2K^{bm3}$ and this way toward residue 77. The biggest movement of the peptide was measured for the carboxyl group at position 8 which is pulled towards the α1-helix and this way presents itself differently to the TCR (Fig. 2b, right panel). Movements in the vicinity of residue 77 allow for an additional TCR β-chain mediated hydrogen bond to the peptide as well as an increase in the number of van der Waals (vdw) contacts between the TCR and pMHC, accompanied by increased shape complementarity (0.61) involving largely the TCR β-chain with a nearly fourfold increase in contacts. The TCR β-chain mediated hydrogen bond and vdw contacts convert the α-chain dominated interaction observed for the syngeneic structure into a β-chain dominated one. Globally the subtle changes translate for the alloreactive compared to the syngeneic interaction into minimal deviations of individual structures (Fig. 2c, d, right panel), a slight increase in buried surface area (~2,100 $Å^2$) and an increased shape complementarity around residue 77 conveying functionally stronger agonism with decreased off-rates albeit similar affinities. Overall the 2C TCR engages the dEV8/H2-K^{bm3} and dEV8/H2-K^b ligands in superposable mimicry-based fashion with the majority of contacts being conserved and using the same diagonal orientation (Fig. 2c, d, right panel). In summary this system depicts how a single residue MHC polymorphism can cause subtle differences in the presentation of the same peptide which cause a slightly altered pMHC surface sensed by the 2C TCR as unique but engaged in an overall conserved docking mode underlying molecular mimicry.

6.2 The LC13 System

6.2.1 Overview of the System

The $CD8^+$ CTL LC13 T cell clone (*TRAV26-2*01,TRAJ52*01*; *TRBV7-8*03*, *TRBD1/D2*, *TRBJ2-7*01*) represents a publicly used T cell clone [196] in HLA-B*08:01$^+$ individuals in the memory T cell response to the immunodominant epitope FLR (FLRGRAYGL) derived from latent Epstein-Barr virus nuclear antigen 3A (EBNA3A) presented by HLA-B*08:01 [197, 198]. The LC13 T cell clone is deleted during thymic selection when HLA-B*44:02 or HLA-B*44:03 are coinherited in *trans* [196, 199] and alloreacts with HLA-B*44:02 [200] and HLA-B*44:05

[104] but not with HLA-B*44:03 as demonstrated in MLRs [199]. The three HLA-B*44 allotypes differ only at two positions which are located in the F pocket (residue 116) and the α2-helix/DE pocket (residue 156), respectively, and thus are unable to directly impact on TCR recognition (HLA-B*4405: 116-Tyr, 156-Asp; HLA-B*44:02: 116-Asp, 156-Asp; HLA-B*4403: 116-Asp, 156-Leu) (Fig. 3a, left panel). In the presence of HLA-B44 the immunodominant LC13 TCR usage is deleted; instead T cells with a diverse TCR repertoire mediate FLR/HLA-B*08:01 reactivity [196]. Fine-specificity analysis with FLR peptide analogs revealed that while the HLA-B*44:02 alloreactive LC13 TCR reacts with C-terminal peptide residues, many HLA-B44 tolerant TCRs focus on the peptide N-terminus, such as the CF34 T cell clone (*TRAV14*01,TRAJ49*; *TRBV11-2*03*, *TRBD2*01*, *TRBJ2-3*) or the center, such as the RL42 T cell clone [157]; other clones are sensitive to substitutions at the N- and the C-termini and some have a similar specificity profile as compared to the LC13 TCR [196, 201]. The peptide N-terminus, contacted by most HLA-B44 tolerant T cell clones, coincides with polymorphic regions between HLA-B*08:01 and HLA-B44, suggesting an evasion of an area that mimics a structure presented on HLA-B44 [196, 201] which was further informed by crystal structures (as discussed below).

Candidate allopeptides (mimotopes) of the LC13 mediated alloreactivity were identified using a baculovirus pMHC display library which was screened for interaction with recombinant, bivalent LC13 TCR [104]. The HLA-B*44:05 restricted mimotope

Fig. 3 (continued) Polymorphic residues (2) between HLA-B*44:02/03/05 are indicated (*brown*, *stick* display) on unliganded EEYLQ/HLA-B*44:05 (*left panel*). Polymorphic residues (5) between HLA-B*08:01 and HLA-B*44 are indicated (*brown*, *stick* display) on unliganded FLR/HLA-B*08:01 (*right panel*). (**b**) Side-view of the peptides EEYLQ (EEYLQAFTY) (*left panel*) and FLR (FLRGRAYGL) (*middle panel*) as bound in the peptide-binding grooves of unliganded HLA-B*44:05 and HLA-B*08:01, respectively. Peptide residues are labeled. The *right panel* displays EEYLQ (*light green*) and FLR (*black*) in the peptide-binding groove of HLA-B*08:01 upon superposition of unliganded EEYLQ/HLA-B*44:05 onto FLR/HLA-B*08:01. (**c**) Side-view of the peptides EEYLQ (*left panel*) and FLR (*middle panel*) (*pink*, *stick* display) as bound in the peptide-binding grooves of unliganded HLA-B*44:05 and HLA-B*08:01, respectively, superposed with the unliganded state (peptides in *black*) as shown in (**b**). The *right panel* displays EEYLQ (*light green*) and FLR (*black*) in the peptide-binding groove of HLA-B*08:01 upon superposition of LC13 liganded EEYLQ/HLA-B*44:05 onto FLR/HLA-B*08:01. (**d**) Footprints (top-view) of the LC13 TCR on the surfaces of EEYLQ/HLA-B*44:05 (*left panel*) and FLR/HLA-B*08:01 (*middle panel*). Isolated LC13 TCR CDR loops are displayed. The *right panel* displays the LC13 TCR footprint as on EEYLQ/HLA-B*44:05 (*light green*) superposed onto the LC13 TCR footprint on FLR/HLA-B*08:01 (as shown in the *middle panel*). (**e**) Side-view of the LC13 TCR as in complex with EEYLQ/HLA-B*44:05 (*light green*) superposed onto the LC13 TCR in complex with FLR/HLA-B*08:01. Depicted are the TCR variable domains (*ribbon* display) and the peptide-binding grooves with the peptides. (**f**) Side-view (*left panel*) and footprint (*right panel*) of the CF34 TCR in complex with FLR/HLA-B*08:01. Side-view: Depicted are the TCR variable domains (*ribbon* display) and the peptide-binding grooves with the peptides. Isolated CF34 TCR CDR loops are displayed

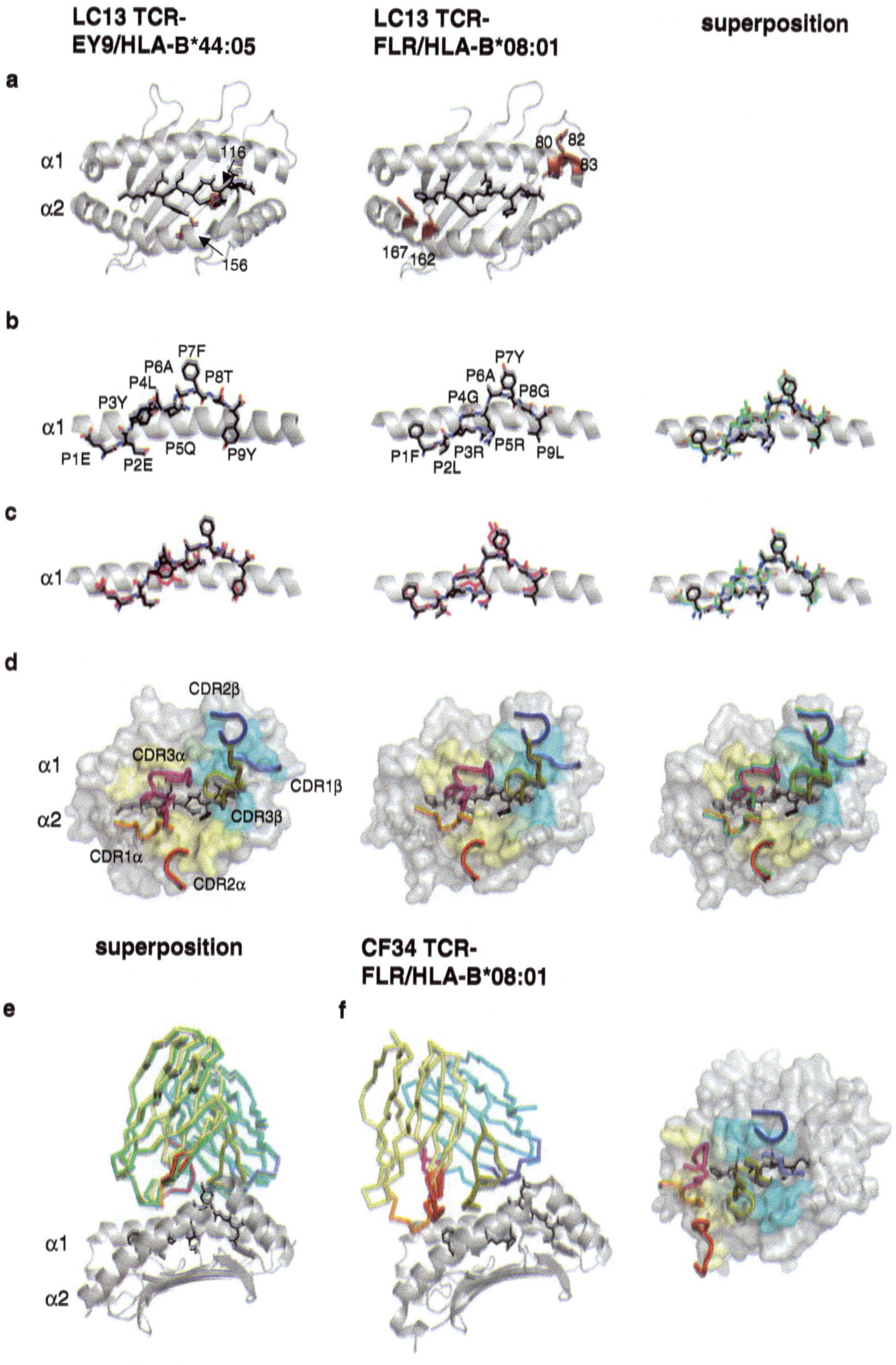

Fig. 3 Crystal structures of the human LC13 TCR in complex with EEYLQ/HLA-B*44:05 ([104], PDB ID: 3KPS) and FLR/HLA-B*08:01 ([126], PDB ID: 1MI5); crystal structures of the unliganded EEYLQ/HLA-B*44:05 ([104], PDB ID: 3KPP) and unliganded FLR/HLA-B*08:01 ([209], PDB ID: 1M05); crystal structure of FLR/HLA-B*08:01 in complex with the CF34 TCR ([201], PDB ID: 3FFC). (**a**) Top-view of the peptides and the peptide binding-grooves.

(EEYLKAWTF) shares 66 % homology with two human proteome analogs, of which only the peptide EEYLQAFTY (EY9), derived from an ATP binding cassette protein ABCD3, was capable of activating LC13 TCR+ T cells to a similar extent as the mimotope and super transfection and RNA interference knock-down experiments of the ABCD3 gene confirmed the allopeptide to be the natural alloantigen recognized by the LC13 TCR [104]. LC13 TCR affinities as determined by SPR were highest for FLR/HLA-B*08:01 (K_D ~ 10–15 μM for the LC13 TCR and ~8.9 μM for the CF34 TCR) [126, 157, 201], followed by EY9/HLA-B*44:05 (K_D ~ 49 μM) and EY9/HLA-B*44:02 (K_D ~ 189 μM), while the affinity exceeded 200 μM in case of EY9/HLA-B*44:03 [104], consistent with the lack of LC13 T cell alloreactivity on HLA-B*44:03.

6.2.2 Structural Insights

The crystal structures of the LC13 TCR in complex with FLR/HLA-B*08:01 [126], PDB ID: 1MI5, and in complex with the allogeneic ligand EY9/HLA-B*44:05 [104], PDB ID: 3KPS, have been determined and compared [104]. Furthermore, the crystal structure of the CF34 TCR in complex with FLR/HLA-B*08:01, has been determined and compared to the LC13 TCR-FLR/HLA-B*08:01 crystal structure [201], PDB ID: 3FFC. Both comparisons are summarized in the following.

The two pMHC complexes engaged by the LC13 TCR differ largely: There are 24 polymorphic residues between HLA-B44 and HLA-B*08:01, 5 of which map to the peptide-binding groove where they form clusters at the N-terminus (HLA-B*08:01 → HLA-B*44: Thr → Leu163 and Trp → Ser167) and C-terminus (HLA-B*08:01 → HLA-B*44: Asn → Thr80, Arg → Leu82, Gly → Arg83) of the α-helices, respectively (Fig. 3a, right panel). In addition the allotope and the viral epitope differ in sequence.

Despite those differences, the LC13 TCR alloreactivity is underpinned by HLA and peptide dependent molecular mimicry. Overall, the LC13 TCR superposes remarkably closely when liganded with FLR/HLA-B*08:01 and EQ9/HLA-B*44:05, including positioning and conformations of the CDR loops, docking angle (~60°) and C-terminal focus, and hence creates nearly identical footprints (Fig. 3d). These similarities are also reflected in comparable values for buried surface areas (2,290 Å² versus 2,320 Å²) and shape complementarities (0.59 versus 0.60) of the TCR- FLR/HLA-B*08:01 and EY9/HLA-B*44:05 interfaces, respectively. The overall mimicry approach by the LC13 TCR is retained on the molecular level, where it commits to similar numbers and types of interactions with EY9/HLA-B*44:05 and FLR/HLA-B*08:01, respectively (1 conserved salt bridge each, 146 and 135 vdw interactions, and 15 and 14 hydrogen bonds). The interactions are mediated in an unskewed manner by both, Vα- and Vβ-domains with all CDR loops contributing to the recognition of peptide and

MHC to a varying extent in a similar way in both ligands. In fact individual contacts between CDR loop residues and MHC are mostly conserved apart from rare contacts of non-conserved residues and contacts of conserved residues present only in either of the structures. When interacting with the respective peptides, the same three C-terminal positions bulged out form the cleft (P6–P8) and are critical for FLR/HLA-B*08:01 reactivity and EQ9/HLA-B*44:05 reactivity. FLR and EY9 adopt in the liganded states similar conformations within the respective peptide-binding grooves. However, when comparing the structures of unliganded (PDB ID: 3KPP) and liganded allotope/HLA-B*44:05 a conformational change of P3Y was observed (Fig. 3c). This TCR induced conformational change is unfavorably accommodated by HLA-B*44:03 in complex with the same allopeptide where a movement of the P3Y toward residue 156Leu places the hydroxyl group of Tyr3 into a hydrophobic pocket compared to the charged Asp of HLA-B*44:05 (Fig. 3a). Thus how a single residue HLA polymorphism affects the plasticity of the bound peptide and ultimately efficient engagement, further highlights the intrinsic specificity of the LC13 TCR in the molecular mimicry mediated allorecognition when discriminating between closely related HLA-B*44 allotypes.

Unlike the LC13 clonotype, the CF34 T cell clone is not deleted from the repertoire by adopting an altered docking mode which avoids an HLA-B*08:01 area that mimics a structure present on HLA-B*44. Instead the CF34 TCR interacts extensively with the N-terminal polymorphic cluster of residues of HLA-B*08:01 which are not contacted by the LC13 TCR and adopts thereby an extremely N-terminal focussed footprint (Fig. 3f). At the same time the conserved roughly diagonal docking mode (58° along the long axis of the peptide-binding groove) is preserved and positions 65, 69, and 155 of HLA-B*08:01 are contacted. Also a similar surface compared to the LC13 TCR is buried (~2,180 Å^2), the shape complementarity is similar (0.65) and a similar amount of interactions are made (127 vdw interactions, 12 hydrogen bonds, and no salt bridges). The Vβ domain shows a slight dominance in the interaction (contribution of 58.3 %) but nevertheless all six CDR loops contribute in contacts to the pMHC albeit to varying degrees. In line with the markedly different footprint of the CF34 TCR as compared to the LC13 TCR, also the contacts made with the MHC and the peptide are largely different with regard to the positioning and the relative contributions from the CDR loop residues.

6.3 The YAe62 System

6.3.1 Overview of the System

Severely limited negative selection as observed in mice genetically manipulated to express a single pMHC complex, such as the MHC-II molecule H2-IA^b covalently linked to the peptide SP (H2-IA^b-SP mouse), gives rise to T cells that cross-react extensively with regard to peptide, MHC allotype and MHC class [64, 65].

One such T cell clone, YAe62 (*TRAV4.12*, *TRAJ11*; *TRBV8.2*, *TRBD1*, *TRBJ2.4*) was isolated from IA^b-SP mice upon immunization with dendritic cells presenting IA^b covalently linked to a foreign peptide (p3K, FEAQKAKANKAVD) [64]. When expressed trans-genetically in $H2^b$ mice deficient in MHC-II, $CD8^+$ YAe62 T cells were positively selected on $H2^b$ MHC-I molecules [64] and mediated cytotoxic and proliferative responses toward MHC-II deficient cells bearing H2-K^b MHC-I molecules [64, 83]. An H2-K^b restricted mimotope, WIYVYRPM (pWM), recognized by YAe62 T cells was identified [83]. The affinity of the YAe62 TCR for pWM/H2-K^b (K_D ~ 15 μM) was slightly lower than for p3K/IA^b (K_D ~ 9.3 μM), as determined by SPR [83].

6.3.2 Structural Insights

The crystal structures of the YAe62 TCR in complex with p3K/IA^b [94], PDB ID: 3C60, and in complex with pWM/H-2K^b [83], PDB ID: 3RGV, have been determined and compared [83], as summarized in the following.

H2-K^b and IA^b are of different MHC class and as such largely differ in sequence as well as structure (as described above) (Fig. 4a). Also the two peptides, pWM and p3K differ in sequence and length (Fig. 4b). Nonetheless, the YAe62 Vα and Vβ germ-line encoded CDR1 and CDR2 loops adopt similar backbone conformations and mostly conserved side-chain conformations when engaging the two classes of MHC molecules. Moreover the same four conserved germ-line-encoded residues discussed in the context of MHC restriction (Y46, Y48, and E54 of CDR2β as well as Y29 of CDR1α; E54 in case of MHC-I interaction to a lesser extent) make critical contacts with both, the MHC-I and MHC-II complexes. Additionally, these residues contact the respective MHC helices at similar positions on the α1-domains (CDR2β) and β1/α1-domains (CDR1α), respectively, thus imposing an overall similar docking orientation of the YAe62 TCR onto H-2K^b and IA^b, with only a slight relative shift (Fig. 4c). Furthermore, the YAe62 TCR contacts both ligands dominantly in vdw interactions. In line with the observation that the YAe62 TCR is highly peptide degenerate, the number of peptide atoms contacted are small (16 contacts, each) and the ratio of MHC atoms to peptide atoms contacted is similarly large for both pMHC-II and pMHC-I ligands (3.6 and 3.2, respectively).

Otherwise the TCR uses different strategies in engaging the pMHC-I versus the pMHC-II complex, with TCR plasticity as the underlying mechanism: The number of atom to atom contacts in case of the allogeneic ligand is markedly decreased (171 versus 273) especially with regard to the Vβ contacts (128 versus 226 contacts) albeit a larger number of TCR residues involved in contacts (18 versus 14) and a larger buried surface area (1,500 $Å^2$ versus 1,200 $Å^2$) as compared to the syngeneic ligand (Fig. 4c). Furthermore CDR3 loop residues involved in contacts differ

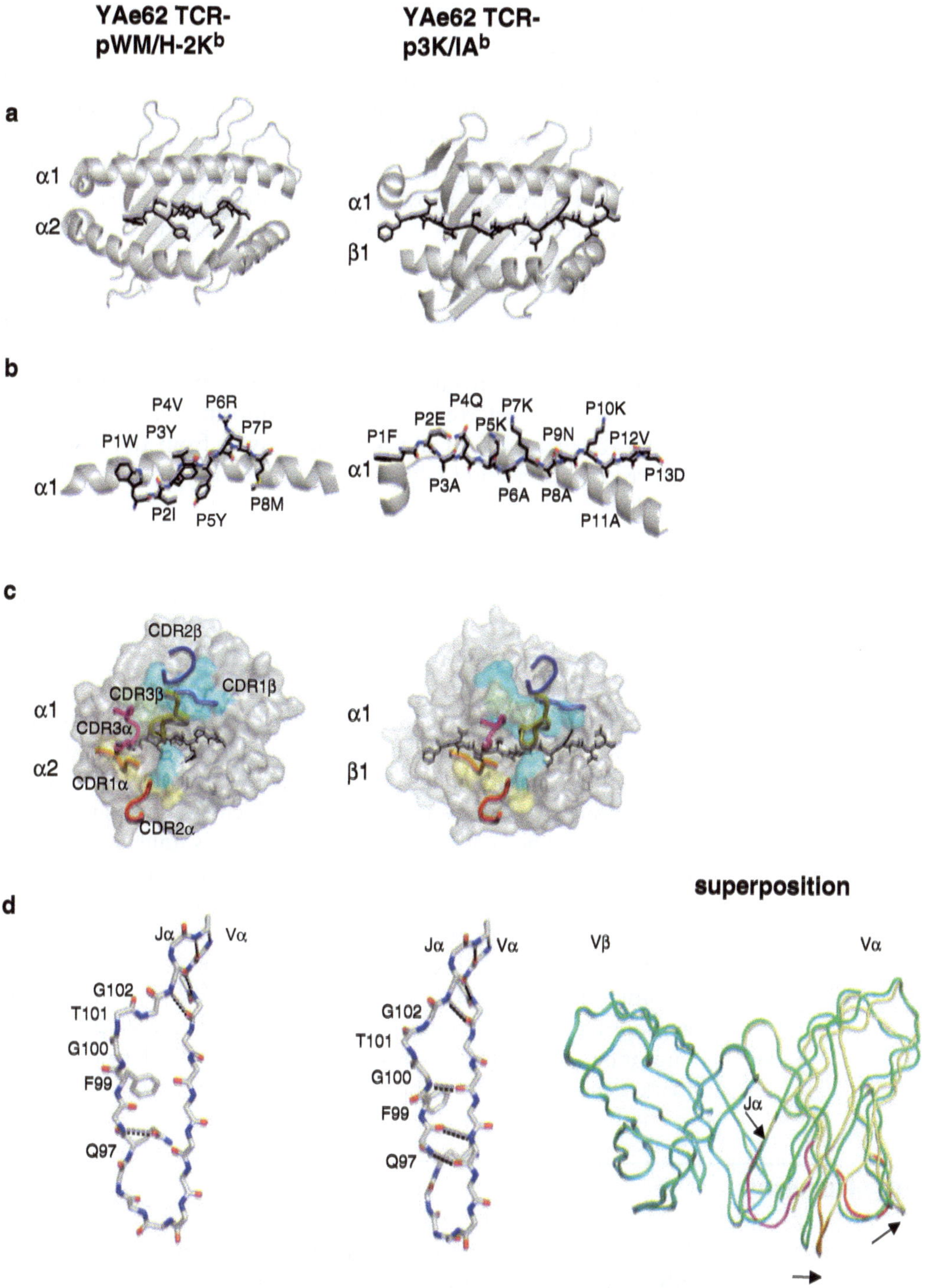

Fig. 4 Crystal structures of the murine YAe62 TCR in complex with pWM/H-2K^b ([83], PDB ID: 3RGV) and p3K/IA^b ([94], PDB ID: 3C60). (**a**) Top-view of the peptides pWM (WIYVYRPM) and p3K (FEAQKAKANKAVD) and the peptide binding-grooves in the TCR liganded state. (**b**) Side-view of the peptides pWM and p3K as bound in the peptide-binding grooves of liganded H-2K^b and IA^b, respectively. Peptide residues are labeled. (**c**) Footprints (top-view) of the YAe62 TCR on the surfaces of pWM/H-2K^b (*left panel*) and 3K/IA^b (*right panel*). Isolated YAe62 TCR CDR loops are displayed over the surface. (**d**) β-Strand interactions between Jα and Vα of the YAe62 TCR (*grey*, *stick* display of the backbone) when bound to pWM/H-2K^b (*left panel*) or p3K/IA^b (*middle panel*). The side chains of the FGXG motif and of Q97 are displayed. Backbone hydrogen bonds as well as the hydrogen bond involving the Q97 side-chain are indicated (*black*, *dotted lines*). Superposition of the YAe62 TCR when bound to pWM/H-2K^b and p3K/IA^b (*light green*) based on the Vβ-chains

largely for the two ligands, accomplished with considerable changes in CDR3 loop conformations (Fig. 4c). Most strikingly, the YAe62 TCR switches between alternate TCR core conformations, thereby altering the positions of the CDR1 and CDR2 loops of Vα relative to those of Vβ (Fig. 4d, right panel). A closed TCR core conformation was adopted when bound to pMHC-II (Fig. 4d, middle panel). However, when bound to pMHC-I, the Jα β-strand (strand 9 in the β-barrel) separated hydrogen bonds to the adjacent Vα β-strand 8 in the lower portion of the strand and rotated away from it, such that globally Vα CDR1 and CDR2 were swiveled away from Vα CDR3 (the loop between β-strands 8 and 9) and Vβ, referred to as open conformation (Fig. 4d, left panel). The rotation of the β-strand 9 away from the β-strand 8 occurred at the second Gly of the canonical J region FGXG motif (residues 99–102).

7 Implications of the Molecular Basis of Alloreactivity in Clinical Transplantation

Almost 60 years after the first groundbreaking experiments demonstrating acquired tolerance to alloantigens in mice by Medawar [202], the induction of clinical tolerance remains difficult. Given the inherent nature of T cell receptor mediated, peptide-, and MHC-specific allorecognition coupled with a very large number of polymorphic MHC molecules and MHC-bound peptides, specific blocking of the interaction is unlikely to form a therapeutic option in preventing allograft rejection. Instead, protocols favoring tolerance will most likely need to rely on immunosuppressive/tolerogenic mechanisms targeting inflammation and co-stimulation, and inducing peripheral tolerance mechanisms including regulatory T cells, reviewed in [203, 204]. To allow for appropriate interference, furthermore the development of "immune monitoring" protocols, that are validated assays or biomarkers predictive of tolerance, is essential [203, 204].

Acknowledgments

We acknowledge the following people for helpful discussions and advice: Stephanie Gras, Onisha Patel, Jérôme Le Nours, Alexander Theodossis, and Lars Kjer-Nielsen. We thank the staff at the MX1 and MX2 beamlines of the Australian Synchrotron for assistance with data collection on many of the structures described herein. This research was supported by grants from the National Health and Medical Research Council of Australia (NHMRC) and the Australian Research Council (ARC). J. Rossjohn was supported by an NHMRC Australia Fellowship. S. B. G. Eckle was supported by a Melbourne International Research Scholarship (MIRS) and a Melbourne International Fee Remission Scholarship (MIFRS).

References

1. Afzali B, Lechler RI, Hernandez-Fuentes MP (2007) Allorecognition and the alloresponse: clinical implications. Tissue Antigens 69:545–556
2. Medawar PB (1944) The behaviour and fate of skin autografts and skin homografts in rabbits: a report to the War Wounds Committee of the Medical Research Council. J Anat 78:176–199
3. Grey HM, Buus S, Colon S, Miles C, Sette A (1989) Structural requirements and biological significance of interactions between peptides and the major histocompatibility complex. Philos Trans R Soc Lond B Biol Sci 323:545–552
4. Townsend AR, McMichael AJ (1985) Specificity of cytotoxic T lymphocytes stimulated with influenza virus. Studies in mice and humans. Prog Allergy 36:10–43
5. Zinkernagel RM, Doherty PC (1997) The discovery of MHC restriction. Immunol Today 18:14–17
6. Goldrath AW, Bevan MJ (1999) Selecting and maintaining a diverse T-cell repertoire. Nature 402:255–262
7. Starr TK, Jameson SC, Hogquist KA (2003) Positive and negative selection of T cells. Annu Rev Immunol 21:139–176
8. von Boehmer H, Aifantis I, Gounari F, Azogui O, Haughn L, Apostolou I, Jaeckel E, Grassi F, Klein L (2003) Thymic selection revisited: how essential is it? Immunol Rev 191:62–78
9. Kisielow P, Blüthmann H, Staerz UD, Steinmetz M, von Boehmer H (1988) Tolerance in T-cell-receptor transgenic mice involves deletion of nonmature CD4+ 8+ thymocytes. Nature 333:742–746
10. Hogquist KA, Baldwin TA, Jameson SC (2005) Central tolerance: learning self-control in the thymus. Nat Rev Immunol 5:772–782
11. Trowsdale J, Parham P (2004) Mini-review: defense strategies and immunity-related genes. Eur J Immunol 34:7–17
12. Lefranc M-P, Duprat E, Kaas Q, Tranne M, Thiriot A, Lefranc G (2005) IMGT unique numbering for MHC groove G-domain and MHC superfamily (MhcSF) G-like-domain. Dev Comp Immunol 29:917–938
13. Madden DR (1995) The three-dimensional structure of peptide-MHC complexes. Annu Rev Immunol 13:587–622
14. Bjorkman PJ, Saper MA, Samraoui B, Bennett WS, Strominger JL, Wiley DC (1987) Structure of the human class I histocompatibility antigen, HLA-A2. Nature 329:506–512
15. Garrett TP, Saper MA, Bjorkman PJ, Strominger JL, Wiley DC (1989) Specificity pockets for the side chains of peptide antigens in HLA-Aw68. Nature 342:692–696
16. Saper MA, Bjorkman PJ, Wiley DC (1991) Refined structure of the human histocompatibility antigen HLA-A2 at 2.6 A resolution. J Mol Biol 219:277–319
17. Brown JH, Jardetzky TS, Gorga JC, Stern LJ, Urban RG, Strominger JL, Wiley DC (1993) Three-dimensional structure of the human class II histocompatibility antigen HLA-DR1. Nature 364:33–39
18. Falk K, Rötzschke O, Stevanović S, Jung G, Rammensee HG (1991) Allele-specific motifs revealed by sequencing of self-peptides eluted from MHC molecules. Nature 351:290–296
19. Yaneva R, Schneeweiss C, Zacharias M, Springer S (2010) Peptide binding to MHC class I and II proteins: new avenues from new methods. Mol Immunol 47:649–657
20. Cabaniols JP, Fazilleau N, Casrouge A, Kourilsky P, Kanellopoulos JM (2001) Most alpha/beta T cell receptor diversity is due to terminal deoxynucleotidyl transferase. J Exp Med 194:1385–1390
21. Davis MM, Bjorkman PJ (1988) T-cell antigen receptor genes and T-cell recognition. Nature 334:395–402
22. Bousso P, Casrouge A, Altman JD, Haury M, Kanellopoulos J, Abastado JP, Kourilsky P (1998) Individual variations in the murine T cell response to a specific peptide reflect variability in naive repertoires. Immunity 9:169–178
23. Arstila TP, Casrouge A, Baron V, Even J, Kanellopoulos J, Kourilsky P (1999) A direct estimate of the human alphabeta T cell receptor diversity. Science 286:958–961
24. Casrouge A, Beaudoing E, Dalle S, Pannetier C, Kanellopoulos J, Kourilsky P (2000) Size estimate of the alpha beta TCR repertoire of naive mouse splenocytes. J Immunol 164:5782–5787
25. Garcia KC, Degano M, Pease LR, Huang M, Peterson PA, Teyton L, Wilson IA (1998) Structural basis of plasticity in T cell receptor recognition of a self peptide-MHC antigen. Science 279:1166–1172
26. Garcia KC, Degano M, Stanfield RL, Brunmark A, Jackson MR, Peterson PA, Teyton L, Wilson IA (1996) An alphabeta T cell receptor structure at 2.5 A and its orientation in the TCR-MHC complex. Science 274:209–219
27. Garboczi DN, Ghosh P, Utz U, Fan QR, Biddison WE, Wiley DC (1996) Structure of the complex between human T-cell receptor, viral peptide and HLA-A2. Nature 384:134–141

28. Rudolph MG, Stanfield RL, Wilson IA (2006) How TCRs bind MHCs, peptides, and coreceptors. Annu Rev Immunol 24:419–466
29. Godfrey DI, Rossjohn J, McCluskey J (2008) The fidelity, occasional promiscuity, and versatility of T cell receptor recognition. Immunity 28:304–314
30. Burrows SR, Chen Z, Archbold JK, Tynan FE, Beddoe T, Kjer-Nielsen L, Miles JJ, Khanna R, Moss DJ, Liu YC, Gras S, Kostenko L, Brennan RM, Clements CS, Brooks AG, Purcell AW, McCluskey J, Rossjohn J (2010) Hard wiring of T cell receptor specificity for the major histocompatibility complex is underpinned by TCR adaptability. Proc Natl Acad Sci USA 107:10608–10613
31. Gras S, Chen Z, Miles JJ, Liu YC, Bell MJ, Sullivan LC, Kjer-Nielsen L, Brennan RM, Burrows JM, Neller MA, Khanna R, Purcell AW, Brooks AG, McCluskey J, Rossjohn J, Burrows SR (2010) Allelic polymorphism in the T cell receptor and its impact on immune responses. J Exp Med 207:1555–1567
32. Ely LK, Beddoe T, Clements CS, Matthews JM, Purcell AW, Kjer-Nielsen L, McCluskey J, Rossjohn J (2006) Disparate thermodynamics governing T cell receptor-MHC-I interactions implicate extrinsic factors in guiding MHC restriction. Proc Natl Acad Sci USA 103:6641–6646
33. Borg NA, Ely LK, Beddoe T, Macdonald WA, Reid HH, Clements CS, Purcell AW, Kjer-Nielsen L, Miles JJ, Burrows SR, McCluskey J, Rossjohn J (2005) The CDR3 regions of an immunodominant T cell receptor dictate the "energetic landscape" of peptide-MHC recognition. Nat Immunol 6:171–180
34. Hünig T, Bevan MJ (1981) Specificity of T-cell cones illustrates altered self hypothesis. Nature 294:460–462
35. Sherman LA, Chattopadhyay S (1993) The molecular basis of allorecognition. Annu Rev Immunol 11:385–402
36. Lechler RI, Batchelor JR (1982) Restoration of immunogenicity to passenger cell-depleted kidney allografts by the addition of donor strain dendritic cells. J Exp Med 155:31–41
37. Simpson E, Scott D, James E, Lombardi G, Cwynarski K, Dazzi F, Millrain M, Dyson PJ (2002) Minor H antigens: genes and peptides. Transpl Immunol 10:115–123
38. Dalchau R, Fangmann J, Fabre JW (1992) Allorecognition of isolated, denatured chains of class I and class II major histocompatibility complex molecules. Evidence for an important role for indirect allorecognition in transplantation. Eur J Immunol 22:669–677
39. Vella JP, Spadafora-Ferreira M, Murphy B, Alexander SI, Harmon W, Carpenter CB, Sayegh MH (1997) Indirect allorecognition of major histocompatibility complex allopeptides in human renal transplant recipients with chronic graft dysfunction. Transplantation 64:795–800
40. Le Moine A, Goldman M, Abramowicz D (2002) Multiple pathways to allograft rejection. Transplantation 73:1373–1381
41. Lafferty KJ, Bootes A, Dart G, Talmage DW (1976) Effect of organ culture on the survival of thyroid allografts in mice. Transplantation 22:138–149
42. Lechler RI, Batchelor JR (1982) Immunogenicity of retransplanted rat kidney allografts. Effect of inducing chimerism in the first recipient and quantitative studies on immunosuppression of the second recipient. J Exp Med 156(1835):41
43. Jiang S, Herrera O, Lechler RI (2004) New spectrum of allorecognition pathways: implications for graft rejection and transplantation tolerance. Curr Opin Immunol 16:550–557
44. Hirschhorn K, Bach F, Kolodny RL, Firschein IL, Hashem N (1963) Immune response and mitosis of human peripheral blood lymphocytes in vitro. Science 142:1185–1187
45. Doxiadis II, Smits JM, Schreuder GM, Persijn GG, van Houwelingen HC, van Rood JJ, Claas FH (1996) Association between specific HLA combinations and probability of kidney allograft loss: the taboo concept. Lancet 348:850–853
46. Maruya E, Takemoto S, Terasaki PI (1993) HLA matching: identification of permissible HLA mismatches. Clin Transpl. 511–520
47. Crocchiolo R, Zino E, Vago L, Oneto R, Bruno B, Pollichieni S, Sacchi N, Sormani MP, Marcon J, Lamparelli T, Fanin R, Garbarino L, Miotti V, Bandini G, Bosi A, Ciceri F, Bacigalupo A, Fleischhauer K (2009) Nonpermissive HLA-DPB1 disparity is a significant independent risk factor for mortality after unrelated hematopoietic stem cell transplantation. Blood 114:1437–1444
48. Zino E, Frumento G, Marktel S, Sormani MP, Ficara F, Di Terlizzi S, Parodi AM, Sergeant R, Martinetti M, Bontadini A, Bonifazi F, Lisini D, Mazzi B, Rossini S, Servida P, Ciceri F, Bonini C, Lanino E, Bandini G, Locatelli F, Apperley J, Bacigalupo A, Ferrara GB, Bordignon C, Fleischhauer K (2004) A T-cell epitope encoded by a subset of HLA-DPB1 alleles determines nonpermissive mismatches for hematologic stem cell transplantation. Blood 103:1417–1424
49. Kawase T, Morishima Y, Matsuo K, Kashiwase K, Inoko H, Saji H, Kato S, Juji T, Kodera Y, Sasazuki T (2007) High-risk HLA allele mismatch combinations responsible for severe

acute graft-versus-host disease and implication for its molecular mechanism. Blood 110:2235–2241
50. Mifsud NA, Purcell AW, Chen W, Holdsworth R, Tait BD, McCluskey J (2008) Immunodominance hierarchies and gender bias in direct T(CD8)-cell alloreactivity. Am J Transplant 8:121–132
51. Roelen DL, van Bree SP, van Beelen E, Schanz U, van Rood JJ, Claas FH (1994) Cytotoxic T lymphocytes against HLA-B antigens are less naive than cytotoxic T lymphocytes against HLA-A antigens. Transplantation 57:446–450
52. Zhang L, van Bree S, van Rood JJ, Claas FH (1990) The effect of individual HLA-A and -B mismatches on the generation of cytotoxic T lymphocyte precursors. Transplantation 50:1008–1010
53. Thorogood J, Persijn GG, Schreuder GM, D'Amaro J, Zantvoort FA, van Houwelingen JC, van Rood JJ (1990) The effect of HLA matching on kidney graft survival in separate posttransplantation intervals. Transplantation 50:146–150
54. Keever CA, Leong N, Cunningham I, Copelan EA, Avalos BR, Klein J, Kapoor N, Adams PW, Orosz CG, Tutschka PJ (1994) HLA-B44-directed cytotoxic T cells associated with acute graft-versus-host disease following unrelated bone marrow transplantation. Bone Marrow Transplant 14:137–145
55. Fleischhauer K, Kernan NA, O'Reilly RJ, Dupont B, Yang SY (1990) Bone marrow-allograft rejection by T lymphocytes recognizing a single amino acid difference in HLA-B44. N Engl J Med 323:1818–1822
56. Heemskerk MBA, Cornelissen JJ, Roelen DL, van Rood JJ, Claas FHJ, Doxiadis IIN, Oudshoorn M (2007) Highly diverged MHC class I mismatches are acceptable for haematopoietic stem cell transplantation. Bone Marrow Transplant 40:193–200
57. Lindahl KF, Wilson DB (1977) Histocompatibility antigen-activated cytotoxic T lymphocytes. II. Estimates of the frequency and specificity of precursors. J Exp Med 145:508–522
58. Suchin EJ, Langmuir PB, Palmer E, Sayegh MH, Wells AD, Turka LA (2001) Quantifying the frequency of alloreactive T cells in vivo: new answers to an old question. J Immunol 166:973–981
59. Macedo C, Orkis EA, Popescu I, Elinoff BD, Zeevi A, Shapiro R, Lakkis FG, Metes D (2009) Contribution of naïve and memory T-cell populations to the human alloimmune response. Am J Transplant 9:2057–2066
60. Selin LK, Brehm MA (2007) Frontiers in nephrology heterologous immunity, T cell cross-reactivity, and alloreactivity. J Am Soc Nephrol 18:2268–2277
61. Bingaman AW, Farber DL (2004) Memory T cells in transplantation: generation, function, and potential role in rejection. Am J Transplant 4:846–852
62. Amir AL, D'Orsogna LJ, Roelen DL, van Loenen MM, Hagedoorn RS, de Boer R, van der Hoorn MA, Kester MGD, Doxiadis IIN, Falkenburg JHF, Claas FHJ, Heemskerk MHM (2010) Allo-HLA reactivity of virus-specific memory T cells is common. Blood 115:3146–3157
63. Melenhorst JJ, Leen AM, Bollard CM, Quigley MF, Price DA, Rooney CM, Brenner MK, Barrett AJ, Heslop HE (2010) Allogeneic virus-specific T cells with HLA alloreactivity do not produce GVHD in human subjects. Blood 116:4700–4702
64. Huseby ES, White J, Crawford F, Vass T, Becker D, Pinilla C, Marrack P, Kappler JW (2005) How the T cell repertoire becomes peptide and MHC specific. Cell 122:247–260
65. Ignatowicz L, Kappler J, Marrack P (1996) The repertoire of T cells shaped by a single MHC/peptide ligand. Cell 84:521–529
66. Logunova NN, Viret C, Pobezinsky LA, Miller SA, Kazansky DB, Sundberg JP, Chervonsky AV (2005) Restricted MHC-peptide repertoire predisposes to autoimmunity. J Exp Med 202:73–84
67. Wise M, Zelenika D, Bemelman F, Latinne D, Bazin H, Cobbold S, Waldmann H (1999) CD4 T cells can reject major histocompatibility complex class I-incompatible skin grafts. Eur J Immunol 29:156–167
68. Huseby ES, Crawford F, White J, Kappler J, Marrack P (2003) Negative selection imparts peptide specificity to the mature T cell repertoire. Proc Natl Acad Sci USA 100:11565–11570
69. Rist M, Smith C, Bell MJ, Burrows SR, Khanna R (2009) Cross-recognition of HLA DR4 alloantigen by virus-specific CD8+ T cells: a new paradigm for self-/nonself-recognition. Blood 114:2244–2253
70. Aparicio P, Jaraquemada D, López de Castro JA (1987) Alloreactive cytolytic T cell clones with dual recognition of HLA-B27 and HLA-DR2 antigens. Selective involvement of CD8 in their class I–directed cytotoxicity. J Exp Med 165:428–443
71. Aparicio P, López de Castro JA (1989) CD8 is involved in both class I- and class II-induced proliferation of a cytolytic T-cell clone with dual specificity for HLA-B27 and HLA-DR2 antigens. Hum Immunol 24:295–299

72. López, D., Barber, D.F., Villadangos, J.A., López de Castro, J.A. (1993) Cross-reactive T cell clones from unrelated individuals reveal similarities in peptide presentation between HLA-B27 and HLA-DR2. Journal of immunology (Baltimore, Md. : 1950). 150, 2675-86.
73. Heemskerk MH, de Paus RA, Lurvink EG, Koning F, Mulder A, Willemze R, van Rood JJ, Falkenburg JH (2001) Dual HLA class I and class II restricted recognition of alloreactive T lymphocytes mediated by a single T cell receptor complex. Proc Natl Acad Sci USA 98:6806–6811
74. Schilham MW, Lang R, Benner R, Zinkernagel RM, Hengartner H (1986) Characterization of an Lyt-2+ alloreactive cytotoxic T cell clone specific for H-2Db that cross-reacts with I-Ek. J Immunol 137:2748–2754
75. Padovan E, Casorati G, Dellabona P, Meyer S, Brockhaus M, Lanzavecchia A (1993) Expression of two T cell receptor alpha chains: dual receptor T cells. Science 262:422–424
76. Heath WR, Carbone FR, Bertolino P, Kelly J, Cose S, Miller JF (1995) Expression of two T cell receptor alpha chains on the surface of normal murine T cells. Eur J Immunol 25:1617–1623
77. Alam SM, Gascoigne NR (1998) Posttranslational regulation of TCR Valpha allelic exclusion during T cell differentiation. J Immunol 160:3883–3890
78. Corthay A, Nandakumar KS, Holmdahl R (2001) Evaluation of the percentage of peripheral T cells with two different T cell receptor alpha-chains and of their potential role in autoimmunity. J Autoimmun 16:423–429
79. Morris GP, Allen PM (2009) Cutting edge: highly alloreactive dual TCR T cells play a dominant role in graft-versus-host disease. J Immunol 182:6639–6643
80. He X, Janeway CA, Levine M, Robinson E, Preston-Hurlburt P, Viret C, Bottomly K (2002) Dual receptor T cells extend the immune repertoire for foreign antigens. Nat Immunol 3:127–134
81. Zal T, Weiss S, Mellor A, Stockinger B (1996) Expression of a second receptor rescues self-specific T cells from thymic deletion and allows activation of autoreactive effector function. Proc Natl Acad Sci USA 93:9102–9107
82. Gras S, Kjer-Nielsen L, Chen Z, Rossjohn J, McCluskey J (2011) The structural bases of direct T-cell allorecognition: implications for T-cell-mediated transplant rejection. Immunol Cell Biol 89:388–395
83. Yin L, Huseby E, Scott-Browne J, Rubtsova K, Pinilla C, Crawford F, Marrack P, Dai S, Kappler JW (2011) A single T cell receptor bound to major histocompatibility complex class I and class II glycoproteins reveals switchable TCR conformers. Immunity 35:23–33
84. Matzinger P, Bevan MJ (1977) Hypothesis: why do so many lymphocytes respond to major histocompatibility antigens? Cell Immunol 29:1–5
85. Bevan MJ (1984) High determinant density may explain the phenomenon of alloreactivity. Immunol Today 5:128–130
86. Obst R, Netuschil N, Klopfer K, Stevanović S, Rammensee HG (2000) The role of peptides in T cell alloreactivity is determined by self-major histocompatibility complex molecules. J Exp Med 191:805–812
87. Müllbacher A, Hill AB, Blanden RV, Cowden WB, King NJ, Hla RT (1991) Alloreactive cytotoxic T cells recognize MHC class I antigen without peptide specificity. J Immunol 147:1765–1772
88. Villadangos JA, Galocha B, López de Castro JA (1994) Unusual topology of an HLA-B27 allospecific T cell epitope lacking peptide specificity. J Immunol 152:2317–2323
89. Smith PA, Brunmark A, Jackson MR, Potter TA (1997) Peptide-independent recognition by alloreactive cytotoxic T lymphocytes (CTL). J Exp Med 185:1023–1033
90. Elliott TJ, Eisen HN (1990) Cytotoxic T lymphocytes recognize a reconstituted class I histocompatibility antigen (HLA-A2) as an allogeneic target molecule. Proc Natl Acad Sci USA 87:5213–5217
91. Burrows SR, Silins SL, Khanna R, Burrows JM, Rischmueller M, McCluskey J, Moss DJ (1997) Cross-reactive memory T cells for Epstein-Barr virus augment the alloresponse to common human leukocyte antigens: degenerate recognition of major histocompatibility complex-bound peptide by T cells and its role in alloreactivity. Eur J Immunol 27:1726–1736
92. Janković V, Remus K, Molano A, Nikolich-Zugich J (2002) T cell recognition of an engineered MHC class I molecule: implications for peptide-independent alloreactivity. J Immunol 169:1887–1892
93. Li Y, Huang Y, Lue J, Quandt JA, Martin R, Mariuzza RA (2005) Structure of a human autoimmune TCR bound to a myelin basic protein self-peptide and a multiple sclerosis-associated MHC class II molecule. EMBO J 24:2968–2979
94. Dai S, Huseby ES, Rubtsova K, Scott-Browne J, Crawford F, Macdonald WA, Marrack P, Kappler JW (2008) Crossreactive T Cells spotlight the germline rules for alphabeta T cell-receptor interactions with MHC molecules. Immunity 28:324–334

95. Felix NJ, Brickey WJ, Griffiths R, Zhang J, Van Kaer L, Coffman T, Ting JP (2000) H2-DMalpha(-/-) mice show the importance of major histocompatibility complex-bound peptide in cardiac allograft rejection. J Exp Med 192:31–40
96. Heath WR, Kane KP, Mescher MF, Sherman LA (1991) Alloreactive T cells discriminate among a diverse set of endogenous peptides. Proc Natl Acad Sci USA 88:5101–5105
97. Guimezanes A, Schumacher TN, Ploegh HL, Schmitt-Verhulst AM (1992) A viral peptide can mimic an endogenous peptide for allorecognition of a major histocompatibility complex class I product. Eur J Immunol 22:1651–1654
98. Rötzschke O, Falk K, Faath S, Rammensee HG (1991) On the nature of peptides involved in T cell alloreactivity. J Exp Med 174:1059–1071
99. Heath WR, Hurd ME, Carbone FR, Sherman LA (1989) Peptide-dependent recognition of H-2Kb by alloreactive cytotoxic T lymphocytes. Nature 341:749–752
100. Wang W, Man S, Gulden PH, Hunt DF, Engelhard VH (1998) Class I-restricted alloreactive cytotoxic T lymphocytes recognize a complex array of specific MHC-associated peptides. J Immunol 160:1091–1097
101. Heath WR, Sherman LA (1991) Cell-type-specific recognition of allogeneic cells by alloreactive cytotoxic T cells: a consequence of peptide-dependent allorecognition. Eur J Immunol 21:153–159
102. Marrack P, Kappler J (1988) T cells can distinguish between allogeneic major histocompatibility complex products on different cell types. Nature 332:840–843
103. Udaka K, Tsomides TJ, Eisen HN (1992) A naturally occurring peptide recognized by alloreactive CD8+ cytotoxic T lymphocytes in association with a class I MHC protein. Cell 69:989–998
104. Macdonald WA, Chen Z, Gras S, Archbold JK, Tynan FE, Clements CS, Bharadwaj M, Kjer-Nielsen L, Saunders PM, Wilce MCJ, Crawford F, Stadinsky B, Jackson D, Brooks AG, Purcell AW, Kappler JW, Burrows SR, Rossjohn J, McCluskey J (2009) T cell allorecognition via molecular mimicry. Immunity 31:897–908
105. Amir AL, van der Steen DM, Hagedoorn RS, Kester MGD, van Bergen CAM, Drijfhout JW, de Ru AH, Falkenburg JHF, van Veelen PA, Heemskerk MHM (2011) Allo-HLA-reactive T cells inducing graft-versus-host disease are single peptide specific. Blood 118:6733–6742
106. Weber DA, Terrell NK, Zhang Y, Strindberg G, Martin J, Rudensky A, Braunstein NS (1995) Requirement for peptide in alloreactive CD4+ T cell recognition of class II MHC molecules. J Immunol 154:5153–5164
107. Moris A, Teichgräber V, Gauthier L, Bühring HJ, Rammensee HG (2001) Cutting edge: characterization of allorestricted and peptide-selective alloreactive T cells using HLA-tetramer selection. J Immunol 166:4818–4821
108. Davis MM, Altman JD, Newell EW (2011) Interrogating the repertoire: broadening the scope of peptide-MHC multimer analysis. Nat Rev Immunol 11:551–558
109. Luz JG, Huang M, Garcia KC, Rudolph MG, Apostolopoulos V, Teyton L, Wilson IA (2002) Structural comparison of allogeneic and syngeneic T cell receptor-peptide-major histocompatibility complex complexes: a buried alloreactive mutation subtly alters peptide presentation substantially increasing V(beta) Interactions. J Exp Med 195:1175–1186
110. Chattopadhyay S, Theobald M, Biggs J, Sherman LA (1994) Conformational differences in major histocompatibility complex-peptide complexes can result in alloreactivity. J Exp Med 179:213–219
111. Pierres M, Marchetto S, Naquet P, Landais D, Peccoud J, Benoist C, Mathis D (1989) I-A alpha polymorphic residues that determine alloreactive T cell recognition. J Exp Med 169:1655–1668
112. Santos-Aguado J, Crimmins MA, Mentzer SJ, Burakoff SJ, Strominger JL (1989) Alloreactivity studied with mutants of HLA-A2. Proc Natl Acad Sci USA 86:8936–8940
113. Felix NJ, Donermeyer DL, Horvath S, Walters JJ, Gross ML, Suri A, Allen PM (2007) Alloreactive T cells respond specifically to multiple distinct peptide-MHC complexes. Nat Immunol 8:388–397
114. Evavold BD, Sloan-Lancaster J, Wilson KJ, Rothbard JB, Allen PM (1995) Specific T cell recognition of minimally homologous peptides: evidence for multiple endogenous ligands. Immunity 2:655–663
115. Bhardwaj V, Kumar V, Geysen HM, Sercarz EE (1993) Degenerate recognition of a dissimilar antigenic peptide by myelin basic protein-reactive T cells. Implications for thymic education and autoimmunity. J Immunol 151:5000–5010
116. Wucherpfennig KW, Strominger JL (1995) Molecular mimicry in T cell-mediated autoimmunity: viral peptides activate human T cell clones specific for myelin basic protein. Cell 80:695–705
117. Wucherpfennig KW, Allen PM, Celada F, Cohen IR, De Boer R, Garcia KC, Goldstein B, Greenspan R, Hafler D, Hodgkin P, Huseby ES, Krakauer DC, Nemazee D, Perelson AS, Pinilla C, Strong RK, Sercarz EE (2007)

Polyspecificity of T cell and B cell receptor recognition. Semin Immunol 19:216–224
118. Morris GP, Allen PM (2012) How the TCR balances sensitivity and specificity for the recognition of self and pathogens. Nat Immunol 13:121–128
119. De Boer RJ, Perelson AS (1993) How diverse should the immune system be? Proc Biol Sci 252:171–175
120. Mason DA (1998) A very high level of cross-reactivity is an essential feature of the T-cell receptor. Immunol Today 19:395–404
121. Oldstone MB (1998) Molecular mimicry and immune-mediated diseases. FASEB J 12:1255–1265
122. Borbulevych OY, Piepenbrink KH, Gloor BE, Scott DR, Sommese RF, Cole DK, Sewell AK, Baker BM (2009) T cell receptor cross-reactivity directed by antigen-dependent tuning of peptide-MHC molecular flexibility. Immunity 31:885–896
123. Borbulevych OY, Piepenbrink KH, Baker BM (2011) Conformational melding permits a conserved binding geometry in TCR recognition of foreign and self molecular mimics. J Immunol 186:2950–2958
124. Reiser J-B, Darnault C, Grégoire C, Mosser T, Mazza G, Kearney A, van der Merwe PA, Fontecilla-Camps JC, Housset D, Malissen B (2003) CDR3 loop flexibility contributes to the degeneracy of TCR recognition. Nat Immunol 4:241–247
125. Mazza C, Auphan-Anezin N, Gregoire C, Guimezanes A, Kellenberger C, Roussel A, Kearney A, van der Merwe PA, Schmitt-Verhulst A-M, Malissen B (2007) How much can a T-cell antigen receptor adapt to structurally distinct antigenic peptides? EMBO J 26:1972–1983
126. Kjer-Nielsen L, Clements CS, Purcell AW, Brooks AG, Whisstock JC, Burrows SR, Mccluskey J, Rossjohn J (2003) A structural basis for the selection of dominant alphabeta T cell receptors in antiviral immunity. Immunity 18:53–64
127. Gagnon SJ, Borbulevych OY, Davis-Harrison RL, Turner RV, Damirjian M, Wojnarowicz A, Biddison WE, Baker BM (2006) T cell receptor recognition via cooperative conformational plasticity. J Mol Biol 363:228–243
128. Armstrong KM, Piepenbrink KH, Baker BM (2008) Conformational changes and flexibility in T-cell receptor recognition of peptide-MHC complexes. Biochem J 415:183–196
129. Reiser JB, Grégoire C, Darnault C, Mosser T, Guimezanes A, Schmitt-Verhulst AM, Fontecilla-Camps JC, Mazza G, Malissen B, Housset D (2002) A T cell receptor CDR3beta loop undergoes conformational changes of unprecedented magnitude upon binding to a peptide/MHC class I complex. Immunity 16:345–354
130. McBeth C, Seamons A, Pizarro JC, Fleishman SJ, Baker D, Kortemme T, Goverman JM, Strong RK (2008) A new twist in TCR diversity revealed by a forbidden alphabeta TCR. J Mol Biol 375:1306–1319
131. Archbold JK, Macdonald WA, Gras S, Ely LK, Miles JJ, Bell MJ, Brennan RM, Beddoe T, Wilce MCJ, Clements CS, Purcell AW, McCluskey J, Burrows SR, Rossjohn J (2009) Natural micropolymorphism in human leukocyte antigens provides a basis for genetic control of antigen recognition. J Exp Med 206:209–219
132. Fabian H, Huser H, Narzi D, Misselwitz R, Loll B, Ziegler A, Böckmann RA, Uchanska-Ziegler B, Naumann D (2008) HLA-B27 subtypes differentially associated with disease exhibit conformational differences in solution. J Mol Biol 376:798–810
133. Tynan FE, Reid HH, Kjer-Nielsen L, Miles JJ, Wilce MCJ, Kostenko L, Borg NA, Williamson NA, Beddoe T, Purcell AW, Burrows SR, McCluskey J, Rossjohn J (2007) A T cell receptor flattens a bulged antigenic peptide presented by a major histocompatibility complex class I molecule. Nat Immunol 8:268–276
134. Ishizuka J, Stewart-Jones GBE, van der Merwe A, Bell JI, McMichael AJ, Jones EY (2008) The structural dynamics and energetics of an immunodominant T cell receptor are programmed by its Vbeta domain. Immunity 28:171–182
135. Smith KJ, Reid SW, Stuart DI, McMichael AJ, Jones EY, Bell JI (1996) An altered position of the alpha 2 helix of MHC class I is revealed by the crystal structure of HLA-B*3501. Immunity 4:203–213
136. Colf LA, Bankovich AJ, Hanick NA, Bowerman NA, Jones LL, Kranz DM, Garcia KC (2007) How a single T cell receptor recognizes both self and foreign MHC. Cell 129:135–146
137. Yin Y, Mariuzza RA (2009) The Multiple Mechanisms of T Cell Receptor Cross-reactivity. Immunity 31:849–851
138. Stadinski BD, Trenh P, Smith RL, Bautista B, Huseby PG, Li G, Stern LJ, Huseby ES (2011) A role for differential variable gene pairing in creating T cell receptors specific for unique major histocompatibility ligands. Immunity 35:694–704
139. Rubtsova K, Scott-Browne JP, Crawford F, Dai S, Marrack P, Kappler JW (2009) Many different Vbeta CDR3s can reveal the inherent MHC reactivity of germline-encoded TCR V

regions. Proc Natl Acad Sci USA 106:7951–7956
140. Morris GP, Ni PP, Allen PM (2011) Alloreactivity is limited by the endogenous peptide repertoire. Proc Natl Acad Sci USA 108:3695–3700
141. Felix NJ, Allen PM (2007) Specificity of T-cell alloreactivity. Nat Rev Immunol 7:942–953
142. Garman RD, Ko JL, Vulpe CD, Raulet DH (1986) T-cell receptor variable region gene usage in T-cell populations. Proc Natl Acad Sci USA 83:3987–3991
143. Tjoa B, Kranz DM (1992) Diversity of T cell receptor-alpha chain transcripts from hyper-immune alloreactive T cells. J Immunol 149:253–259
144. Jerne N (1971) The somatic generation of immune recognition. Eur J Immunol 1:1–9
145. Fink P, Bevan M (1978) H-2 antigens of the thymus determine lymphocyte specificity. J Exp Med 148:766–775
146. Zinkernagel R, Callahan G, Althage A, Cooper S, Klein P, Klein J (1978) On the thymus in the differentiation of "H-2 self-recognition" by T cells: evidence for dual recognition? J Exp Med 147:882–896
147. Marrack P, Rubtsova K, Scott-Browne J, Kappler JW (2008) T cell receptor specificity for major histocompatibility complex proteins. Curr Opin Immunol 20:203–207
148. Bankovich A, Garcia K (2003) Not just any T cell receptor will do. Immunity 18:7–11
149. Marrack P, Scott-Browne JP, Dai S, Gapin L, Kappler JW (2008) Evolutionarily conserved amino acids that control TCR-MHC interaction. Annu Rev Immunol 26:171–203
150. Garcia KC, Adams JJ, Feng D, Ely LK (2009) The molecular basis of TCR germline bias for MHC is surprisingly simple. Nat Immunol 10:143–147
151. Mazza C, Malissen B (2007) What guides MHC-restricted TCR recognition? Semin Immunol 19:225–235
152. Adams JJ, Narayanan S, Liu B, Birnbaum ME, Kruse AC, Bowerman NA, Chen W, Levin AM, Connolly JM, Zhu C, Kranz DM, Garcia KC (2011) T cell receptor signaling is limited by docking geometry to peptide-major histocompatibility complex. Immunity 35:681–693
153. Blackman M, Yagüe J, Kubo R, Gay D, Coleclough C, Palmer E, Kappler J, Marrack P (1986) The T cell repertoire may be biased in favor of MHC recognition. Cell 47:349–357
154. Zerrahn J, Held W, Raulet DH (1997) The MHC reactivity of the T cell repertoire prior to positive and negative selection. Cell 88:627–636
155. Merkenschlager M, Graf D, Lovatt M, Bommhardt U, Zamoyska R, Fisher AG (1997) How many thymocytes audition for selection? J Exp Med 186:1149–1158
156. Tynan FE, Burrows SR, Buckle AM, Clements CS, Borg NA, Miles JJ, Beddoe T, Whisstock JC, Wilce MC, Silins SL, Burrows JM, Kjer-Nielsen L, Kostenko L, Purcell AW, McCluskey J, Rossjohn J (2005) T cell receptor recognition of a "super-bulged" major histocompatibility complex class I-bound peptide. Nat Immunol 6:1114–1122
157. Gras S, Wilmann PG, Chen Z, Halim H, Liu YC, Kjer-Nielsen L, Purcell AW, Burrows SR, McCluskey J, Rossjohn J (2012) A structural basis for varied αβ TCR usage against an immunodominant EBV antigen restricted to a HLA-B8 molecule. J Immunol 188:311–321
158. Day EB, Guillonneau C, Gras S, La Gruta NL, Vignali DAA, Doherty PC, Purcell AW, Rossjohn J, Turner SJ (2011) Structural basis for enabling T-cell receptor diversity within biased virus-specific CD8+ T-cell responses. Proc Natl Acad Sci USA 108:9536–9541
159. Feng D, Bond CJ, Ely LK, Maynard J, Garcia KC (2007) Structural evidence for a germline-encoded T cell receptor-major histocompatibility complex interaction "codon". Nat Immunol 8:975–983
160. Scott-Browne J, White J, Kappler J, Gapin L, Marrack P (2009) Germline-encoded amino acids in the alphabeta T-cell receptor control thymic selection. Nature 458:1043–1046
161. Manning T, Schlueter C, Brodnicki T, Parke E, Speir J, Garcia K, Teyton L, Wilson I, Kranz D (1998) Alanine scanning mutagenesis of an alphabeta T cell receptor: mapping the energy of antigen recognition. Immunity 8:413–425
162. Jones LL, Colf LA, Stone JD, Garcia KC, Kranz DM (2008) Distinct CDR3 conformations in TCRs determine the level of cross-reactivity for diverse antigens, but not the docking orientation. J Immunol 181:6255–6264
163. Lee P, Churchill H, Daniels M, Jameson S, Kranz D (2000) Role of 2CT cell receptor residues in the binding of self- and allo-major histocompatibility complexes. J Exp Med 191:1355–1364
164. Garcia KC (2012) Reconciling views on T cell receptor germline bias for MHC. Trends Immunol 33:429–436
165. Huseby ES, Stadinski BD, Trenh P, Stern LJ (2012) Response to Garcia et al. Immunity 36:889–890
166. Boniface JJ, Reich Z, Lyons DS, Davis MM (1999) Thermodynamics of T cell receptor binding to peptide-MHC: evidence for a

general mechanism of molecular scanning. Proc Natl Acad Sci USA 28:11446–11451
167. Krogsgaard M, Prado N, Adams EJ, He XL, Chow D-C, Wilson DB, Garcia KC, Davis MM (2003) Evidence that structural rearrangements and/or flexibility during TCR binding can contribute to T cell activation. Mol Cell 12:1367–1378
168. Willcox BE, Gao GF, Wyer JR, Ladbury JE, Bell JI, Jakobsen BK, van der Merwe PA (1999) TCR binding to peptide-MHC stabilizes a flexible recognition interface. Immunity 10:357–365
169. Davis-Harrison RL, Armstrong KM, Baker BM (2005) Two different T cell receptors use different thermodynamic strategies to recognize the same peptide/MHC ligand. J Mol Biol 346:533–550
170. Van Laethem F, Sarafova SD, Park J-H, Tai X, Pobezinsky L, Guinter TI, Adoro S, Adams A, Sharrow SO, Feigenbaum L, Singer A (2007) Deletion of CD4 and CD8 coreceptors permits generation of alphabetaT cells that recognize antigens independently of the MHC. Immunity 27:735–750
171. Tikhonova AN, Van Laethem F, Hanada KI, Lu J, Pobezinsky LA, Hong C, Guinter TI, Jeurling SK, Bernhardt G, Park J-H, Yang JC, Sun PD, Singer A (2012) αβ T cell receptors that do not undergo major histocompatibility complex-specific thymic selection possess antibody-like recognition specificities. Immunity 36:79–91
172. Van Laethem F, Tikhonova AN, Singer A (2012) MHC restriction is imposed on a diverse T cell receptor repertoire by CD4 and CD8 co-receptors during thymic selection. Trends Immunol 33:437–441
173. Barnd DL, Lan MS, Metzgar RS, Finn OJ (1989) Specific, major histocompatibility complex-unrestricted recognition of tumor-associated mucins by human cytotoxic T cells. Proc Natl Acad Sci USA 86:7159–7163
174. Rao A, Ko WW, Faas SJ, Cantor H (1984) Binding of antigen in the absence of histocompatibility proteins by arsonate-reactive T-cell clones. Cell 36:879–888
175. Siliciano RF, Keegan AD, Dintzis RZ, Dintzis HM, Shin HS (1985) The interaction of nominal antigen with T cell antigen receptors. I. Specific binding of multivalent nominal antigen to cytolytic T cell clones. J Immunol 135:906–914
176. Hanada KI, Wang QJ, Inozume T, Yang JC (2011) Molecular identification of an MHC-independent ligand recognized by a human alpha}/{beta T-cell receptor. Blood 117:4816–4825
177. Kim H-J, Guo D, Sant'Angelo DB (2005) Coevolution of TCR-MHC interactions: conserved MHC tertiary structure is not sufficient for interactions with the TCR. Proc Natl Acad Sci USA 102:7263–7267
178. Vidović D, Boulanger N, Kuye O, Toral J, Ito K, Guenot J, Bluethmann H, Nagy ZA (1997) The helper T-cell repertoire of mice expressing class II major histocompatibility complex beta chains in the absence of alpha chains. Immunogenetics 45:325–335
179. Chen J, Eisen HN, Kranz DM (2003) A model T-cell receptor system for studying memory T-cell development. Microbes Infect 5:233–240
180. Kranz DM, Sherman DH, Sitkovsky MV, Pasternack MS, Eisen HN (1984) Immunoprecipitation of cell surface structures of cloned cytotoxic T lymphocytes by clone-specific antisera. Proc Natl Acad Sci USA 81:573–577
181. Udaka K, Tsomides TJ, Walden P, Fukusen N, Eisen HN (1993) A ubiquitous protein is the source of naturally occurring peptides that are recognized by a CD8+ T-cell clone. Proc Natl Acad Sci USA 90:11272–11276
182. Kageyama S, Tsomides TJ, Fukusen N, Papayannopoulos IA, Eisen HN, Sykulev Y (2001) Potent cytolytic response by a CD8+ CTL clone to multiple peptides from the same protein in association with an allogeneic class I MHC molecule. J Immunol 166:3028–3034
183. Sykulev Y, Brunmark A, Jackson M, Cohen RJ, Peterson PA, Eisen HN (1994) Kinetics and affinity of reactions between an antigen-specific T cell receptor and peptide-MHC complexes. Immunity 1:15–22
184. Sha WC, Nelson CA, Newberry RD, Kranz DM, Russell JH, Loh DY (1988) Positive and negative selection of an antigen receptor on T cells in transgenic mice. Nature 336:73–76
185. Sha WC, Nelson CA, Newberry RD, Pullen JK, Pease LR, Russell JH, Loh DY (1990) Positive selection of transgenic receptor-bearing thymocytes by Kb antigen is altered by Kb mutations that involve peptide binding. Proc Natl Acad Sci USA 87:6186–6190
186. Santori FR, Kieper WC, Brown SM, Lu Y, Neubert TA, Johnson KL, Naylor S, Vukmanović S, Hogquist KA, Jameson SC (2002) Rare, structurally homologous self-peptides promote thymocyte positive selection. Immunity 17:131–142
187. Tallquist MD, Weaver AJ, Pease LR (1998) Degenerate recognition of alloantigenic peptides on a positive-selecting class I molecule. J Immunol 160:802–809
188. Nathenson SG, Geliebter J, Pfaffenbach GM, Zeff RA (1986) Murine major histocompatibility complex class-I mutants: molecular analysis and structure-function implications. Annu Rev Immunol 4:471–502

189. Tallquist MD, Pease LR (1995) Alloreactive 2C T cells recognize a self peptide in the context of the mutant Kbm3 molecule. J Immunol 155:2419–2426
190. Tallquist MD, Yun TJ, Pease LR (1996) A single T cell receptor recognizes structurally distinct MHC/peptide complexes with high specificity. J Exp Med 184:1017–1026
191. Udaka, K., Wiesmüller, K.H., Kienle, S., Jung, G., Walden, P. (1996) Self-MHC-restricted peptides recognized by an alloreactive T lymphocyte clone. J immunol Baltimore, Md.:1950. 157:670–8
192. Cho BK, Lian KC, Lee P, Brunmark A, McKinley C, Chen J, Kranz DM, Eisen HN (2001) Differences in antigen recognition and cytolytic activity of CD8(+) and CD8(-) T cells that express the same antigen-specific receptor. Proc Natl Acad Sci USA 98:1723–1727
193. Daniels MA, Jameson SC (2000) Critical role for CD8 in T cell receptor binding and activation by peptide/major histocompatibility complex multimers. J Exp Med 191: 335–346
194. Maurice MM, Gould DS, Carroll J, Vugmeyster Y, Ploegh HL (2001) Positive selection of an MHC class-I restricted TCR in the absence of classical MHC class I molecules. Proc Natl Acad Sci USA 98:7437–7442
195. Ge Q, Holler PD, Mahajan VS, Nuygen T, Eisen HN, Chen J (2006) Development of CD4+ T cells expressing a nominally MHC class I-restricted T cell receptor by two different mechanisms. Proc Natl Acad Sci USA 103:1822–1827
196. Burrows SR, Silins SL, Moss DJ, Khanna R, Misko IS, Argaet VP (1995) T cell receptor repertoire for a viral epitope in humans is diversified by tolerance to a background major histocompatibility complex antigen. J Exp Med 182:1703–1715
197. Argaet VP, Schmidt CW, Burrows SR, Silins SL, Kurilla MG, Doolan DL, Suhrbier A, Moss DJ, Kieff E, Sculley TB, Misko IS (1994) Dominant selection of an invariant T cell antigen receptor in response to persistent infection by Epstein-Barr virus. J Exp Med 180:2335–2340
198. Burrows SR, Sculley TB, Misko IS, Schmidt C, Moss DJ (1990) An Epstein-Barr virus-specific cytotoxic T cell epitope in EBV nuclear antigen 3 (EBNA 3). J Exp Med 171:345–349
199. Burrows SR, Silins SL, Cross SM, Peh CA, Rischmueller M, Burrows JM, Elliott SL, McCluskey J (1997) Human leukocyte antigen phenotype imposes complex constraints on the antigen-specific cytotoxic T lymphocyte repertoire. Eur J Immunol 27:178–182
200. Burrows SR, Khanna R, Burrows JM, Moss DJ (1994) An alloresponse in humans is dominated by cytotoxic T lymphocytes (CTL) cross-reactive with a single Epstein-Barr virus CTL epitope: implications for graft-versus-host disease. J Exp Med 179:1155–1161
201. Gras S, Burrows SR, Kjer-Nielsen L, Clements CS, Liu YC, Sullivan LC, Bell MJ, Brooks AG, Purcell AW, McCluskey J, Rossjohn J (2009) The shaping of T cell receptor recognition by self-tolerance. Immunity 30:193–203
202. Billingham RE, Brent L, Medawar PB (1953) Actively acquired tolerance of foreign cells. Nature 172:603–606
203. Bishop GA, Ierino FL, Sharland AF, Hall BM, Alexander SI, Sandrin MS, Coates PT, McCaughan GW (2011) Approaching the promise of operational tolerance in clinical transplantation. Transplantation 91: 1065–1074
204. Newell KA (2011) Clinical transplantation tolerance. Semin Immunopathol 33:91–104
205. Hennecke J, Wiley DC (2002) Structure of a complex of the human alpha/beta T cell receptor (TCR) HA1.7, influenza hemagglutinin peptide, and major histocompatibility complex class II molecule, HLA-DR4 (DRA*0101 and DRB1*0401): insight into TCR cross-restriction and alloreactivity. J Exp Med 195:571–581
206. Kaas Q, Ehrenmann F, Lefranc M-P (2007) IG, TR and IgSF, MHC and MhcSF: what do we learn from the IMGT Colliers de Perles? Brief Funct Genomic Proteomic 6:253–264
207. Bork P, Holm L, Sander C (1994) The immunoglobulin fold. Structural classification, sequence patterns and common core. J Mol Biol 242:309–320
208. The PyMOL Molecular Graphics System, 1.2r3pre, Schrödinger, LLC
209. Kjer-Nielsen L, Clements CS, Brooks AG, Purcell AW, Fontes MR, McCluskey J, Rossjohn J (2002) The structure of HLA-B8 complexed to an immunodominant viral determinant: peptide-induced conformational changes and a mode of MHC class I dimerization. J Immunol 169:5153–5160

Chapter 2

Antibodies in Transplantation: The Effects of HLA and Non-HLA Antibody Binding and Mechanisms of Injury

Nicole M. Valenzuela and Elaine F. Reed

Abstract

Until recently, allograft rejection was thought to be mediated primarily by alloreactive T cells. Consequently, immunosuppressive approaches focused on inhibition of T cell activation. While short-term graft survival has significantly improved and rejection rates have dropped, acute rejection has not been eliminated and chronic rejection remains the major threat to long-term graft survival. Increased attention to humoral immunity in experimental systems and in the clinic has revealed that donor specific antibodies (DSA) can mediate and promote acute and chronic rejection. Herein, we detail the effects of alloantibody, particularly HLA antibody, binding to graft vascular and other cells, and briefly summarize the experimental methods used to assess such outcomes.

Key words HLA antibodies, Non-HLA antibodies, Donor specific antibodies, Endothelial cell antibodies, Endothelial cell activation, Vascular injury

1 Clinical Frequency and Relevance of Donor Specific Antibodies

1.1 Frequency and Association with Outcome

Sensitization to polymorphic proteins, especially HLA class I and HLA class II molecules, occurs when a patient is exposed to cells from other individuals, via pregnancy, transfusion, or transplantation. Antibodies to donor antigens, called donor specific antibodies (DSA), can be directed against polymorphic HLA class I (HLA I), HLA class II (HLA II), or minor histocompatibility molecules such as MICA and MICB, or against non-HLA antigens expressed on endothelial cells, epithelial cells, or organ specific targets [1]. The frequency of donor specific HLA antibodies among transplant patients ranges greatly, from as low as 4 % to more than 50 % [2]. Based on data from the Organ Procurement and Transplantation Network as of March 2012, 18.7 % of renal transplant recipients had pretransplant antibodies with a calculated panel reactive antibody (cPRA) greater than 10 %, with 5 % of all patients being highly sensitized (>80 % C-PRA). Everly et al. found that 31 % of

Andrea A. Zachary and Mary S. Leffell (eds.), *Transplantation Immunology: Methods and Protocols, Second Edition*, Methods in Molecular Biology, vol. 1034, DOI 10.1007/978-1-62703-493-7_2,

patients developed DSA de novo after transplant [3]. In one study of renal transplant patients, 30 % had HLA antibodies of any specificity, and 30 % of antibody-positive patients had HLA antibodies of donor specificity [4, 5]. Another study found that 35 % of renal patients had donor specific HLA IgG [6], while another report found DSA in as many as 57 % of renal recipients [7–12]. The rates of sensitization are higher in patients awaiting a second renal graft, where only 19.3 % of patients lacked antibody to HLA I (PRA <4 %), with 14.5 % of patients on the waitlist for a second transplant having very high PRA (>60 %). Here, 55 % were also positive for antibodies against HLA II [13].

Despite the variation in reported estimates of DSA prevalence, the literature clearly illustrates that DSA adversely affect the survival of a transplanted organ (Table 1). Numerous studies have linked the presence of preexisting or de novo antibodies to poor graft outcome. For example, renal recipients with positive panel reactive antibodies (PRA recognizing >10 % of HLA alleles) or with DSA have lower graft survival at 3 and 5 years post-transplant [2, 14, 15]. Accordingly, patients diagnosed with antibody mediated rejection are likely to have donor specific HLA antibodies [16], and episodes of AMR predispose recipients to lower renal allograft survival [3], regardless of whether antibodies were preexisting or produced late after transplantation (from 83 % survival without HLA antibodies to 49 % with HLA antibodies) [4]. In a study with more than 1,000 patients, half of those with failed grafts had HLA antibodies, and 21 % had donor specific HLA antibodies [5]. If desensitization or other therapy effectively reduced DSA levels, long-term survival was significantly superior than if the DSA was persistent [17].

The effects of DSA on graft survival are not restricted to renal transplantation. Heart allograft patients with DSA also experience lower graft survival, especially if the antibodies appear after 1 year post-transplant [18]. Further, the presence of HLA specific DSA and the incidence of AMR correlate with chronic rejection in the heart [1, 19]. Even if patients are asymptomatic, HLA-DSA significantly lowers freedom from chronic allograft vasculopathy (CAV) compared to those without DSA [19]. In addition to HLA, DSA to MICA or to non-donor derived endothelial antigens correlate with chronic transplant rejection in the heart (CAV) [1]. Finally, DSA is a strong risk factor for rejection episodes in small bowel transplantation [20–22].

A recent study describes the clinical significance of and risk factors for development of *de novo* donor specific HLA antibody 6 months or later post-transplant. Wiebe et al. found that 15 % of low-risk renal transplant patients without presensitization developed DSA late after transplantation, which reduced graft survival at 10 years. Interestingly, the investigators found that a mismatch at HLA-DRB1 was an independent predictor of the production of

Table 1
Reports of correlation between HLA antibodies and graft outcome

Organ	Time after Tx	Frequency	Correlation with outcome	Number of patients	Assay to Detect DSA	Reference
Heart	Post	75 % of AMR + Px had HLA-DSA (14 % of total patients); 11 % of total had MICA-DSA	HLA or MICA-DSA associated with CAV	43	Luminex	Nath et al. [16]
Heart	Post	35 % developed de novo anti-HLA	Correlated with HLA-A mismatch; CAV correlated with HLA II Ab	71	Flow-PRA	Tambur et al. [155]
Heart	Post	60 % of AMR + Px had HLA-DSA, the remainder had MICA Ab	HLA ± MICA Ab correlates with chronic rejection	168	Luminex	Zhang et al. [1]
Heart	Pre and post	16 % had preexisting anti-HLA, 48 % had post-Tx anti-HLA	Patients with persistent HLA Ab had significantly reduced survival (post ± pre)	950	CDC and solid phase	Ho et al. [18]
Heart	Pre and post	32 % had anti-HLA preTx; 63 % had anti-HLA postTx	preTx anti-HLA correlated with rejection in the first year	219	FC (more sensitive than CDC)	Tambur et al. [59]
Intestine	Pre	12 % had positive PRA, 7 % had HLA-DSA	Correlated with reduced survival	88	CDC and Luminex	Farmer et al. [22]
Intestine	Pre		PRA positivity was risk factor for acute rejection	324	PRA	Gonzalez-Pinto et al. [21]
Intestine	Pre	21 % had positive CM	Correlated with early poor function	28	CDC	Wu et al. [12]

(continued)

Table 1 (continued)

Organ	Time after Tx	Frequency	Correlation with outcome	Number of patients	Assay to Detect DSA	Reference
Islet	Pre		Positive PRA associated with reduced survival	81	CDC	Campbell et al. [11]
Liver	Pre	70 % had anti-HLA I	Lower outcome 1 year, higher rejection rate	80	ELISA	Bishara et al. [8]
Lung	Pre	9 % had positive PRA	PRA positivity increased post-Tx complications	200	CDC	Lau et al. [156]
Lung	Post	HLA ± MICA Ab correlated with BOS incidence		80	Luminex and Flow PRA	Angaswamy et al. [157]
Renal	Post	27 % had anti-HLA		22	ECXM	Canet et al. [53]
Renal	Post	5 % had HLA-DSA, 11 % had non-DSA HLA Ab	Both reduced survival	1,229	CDC and FC	Hourmant et al. [15]
Renal	Post	30 % of Px had anti-HLA, 31 % of those had HLA-DSA	DSA reduced survival	1,014	SAB	Lachmann et al. [5]
Renal	Post	15 % of nonsensitized Px developed de novo HLA-DSA	HLA-DSA reduced 10 year survival	315	Solid phase	Wiebe et al. [23]
Renal	Post (>6 months)	11 % had anti-HLA, 4 % had HLA-DSA	Correlated with reduced function	251	ELISA	Cardarelli et al. [2]
Renal	Post	21 % had anti-HLA I, 10 % had anti-HLA II, 10 % had anti-MICA		191	Luminex	Alvarez-Marquez et al. [144]
Renal	Pre	48 % HLA antibodies, 11 % had HLA-DSA		113	CDC	Aubert et al. [25]

Renal	Pre	80.6 % had PRA positive for HLA I		62	CDC	Barocci et al. [13]
Renal	Pre	17 % had C1q fixing HLA DSA	C4d fixing ability of DSA was not predictive of early rejection	64	SAB with C4d fixation	Hönger et al. [54, 60]
Renal	Pre	22 % were FCXM+, 66 % of those had HLA I-DSA, 34 % had HLA II-DSA	Persistent DSA reduced survival	308	FCXM	Kimball et al. [17]
Renal	Pre		Positive PRA reduced 2 year outcome	154	ELISA	Meng et al. [109]
Renal	Pre	Of those with HLA Ab, 57 % had HLA-DSA	HLA-DSA increased acute rejection incidence, especially HLA II DSA	28 sensitized Px	Luminex	Song et al. [7]
Renal	Pre	11 % had MICA-DSA	MICA Ab correlated with rejection, especially when HLA matching was good	1,910	MICA antigen beads	Zou et al. [136]
Renal	Pre and post	16 % had MICA Ab; 13 % had preTx PRA; 16 % had HLA Ab postTx	HLA ± MICA Ab increased rejection episodes and decreased survival	185	Luminex and ELISA	Panigrahi et al. [135, 158, 159]

anti-HLA HLA Ab of any specificity, *BOS* bronchiolitis obliterans syndrome, *CAV/TCAD* chronic cardiac rejection, *CDC* complement dependent cytotoxicity, *CM* crossmatch, *DSA* donor specific antibodies, *ECXM* endothelial cell crossmatch, *FC* flow cytometric assay, *FCXM* flow crossmatch, *HLA-DSA* donor specific HLA Ab, *Px* patient, *SAB* single antigen beads

de novo DSA, as was recipient nonadherence to immunosuppression [23]. These results and those of Smith et al. [24] point to a model of the "natural history of *de novo* DSA" describing the progressive nature of antibody-mediated rejection leading to graft failure. The authors propose that inflammatory cytokines expressed early after transplant increase HLA expression by the graft, which in turn promotes B cell allorecognition and production of donor specific HLA antibodies. Biopsies may reveal capillaritis with or without C4d staining, but graft function remains stable and any injury is subclinical. Over time in the presence of donor specific HLA antibodies, the graft progresses to clinical dysfunction and ultimately failure due to sustained microvascular injury and cellular infiltration.

While most studies uncovered a correlation of donor specific HLA antibodies with allograft outcome, only a few reports could not find an association. One study found that acute rejection in renal transplants could not be predicted by DSA [25], and in another CAV incidence did not correlate with DSA but rather with T cell alloreactivity [26]. Overall, however, it is well established that preexisting or *de novo* donor specific HLA antibodies have a deleterious effect on graft outcome across solid organ transplants.

1.2 Diagnosis of Antibody-Mediated Rejection

Antibody mediated rejection is a distinct entity from, but can occur concurrently with, T cell-mediated rejection. In kidney and heart transplantation, consensus criteria have been established for the histological characteristics and diagnosis of antibody-mediated rejection. Antibody-mediated rejection in renal transplantation is diagnosed by poor graft function, evidence of complement deposition (C4d) in the peritubules of the graft and/or DSA in the circulation [27]. Intravascular macrophages, endothelial cell swelling, C4d staining and donor specific HLA antibodies indicate antibody-mediated rejection in cardiac transplantation [28]. Similar criteria have been suggested for the diagnosis of antibody-mediated rejection in liver transplantation [29].

2 Experimental Techniques to Measure Effects of Antibodies

Given the strong association of HLA antibodies with inferior graft function and survival, it is crucial to understand the mechanisms of HLA antibody-mediated graft injury. A variety of experimental models are available to test the effects of HLA antibody binding to cells of the graft. The first is a simplified system with cultured graft cells (endothelium, smooth muscle, or airway epithelium), where intracellular signaling and cell–cell interactions can be dissected in detail and specific functional changes can be analyzed. The more complicated but more physiological system utilizes in vivo transplantation into immunodeficient recipients lacking B and T cells, which are passively transferred with DSA to recapitulate antibody-mediated rejection. Finally, the mechanisms uncovered by experimental models can be confirmed in human biopsies. A brief description of methods commonly utilized by our group and others groups follows.

2.1 In Vitro Techniques

Endothelial, smooth muscle, or epithelial cells are cultured and stimulated in vitro with HLA antibodies, and the direct effects can be analyzed in detail. Multiple clones and isotypes of murine or rat origin against human HLA molecules, which recognize monomorphic epitopes on all HLA I, are commercially available from several sources (our lab primarily uses the murine IgG2a clone W6/32). There are also murine anti-HLA antibodies with allele or locus specificity (for example against HLA-A2, A3, or B44) available from Abcam, BioLegend, and other commercial sources. For analysis using human antibodies, polyclonal HLA antibodies can be isolated from the IgG fraction of sensitized patient sera. More recently, human monoclonal antibodies of a single specificity have been developed [30], although these antibodies are only of complement fixing isotypes and are not yet commercially available.

2.1.1 Measurement of HLA Antibody Binding Capacity

Fluorescence intensity in flow cytometry is influenced by a variety of factors, including antibody concentration or titer, the antibody's affinity for its ligand, whether the epitope is monomorphic or polymorphic, and the expression level on the target cell. Further, fluorescence intensity may vary from machine to machine and with changes in machine settings. The actual amount of HLA I antibody on a donor cell can be measured using flow cytometric methods and normalized using fluorescence calibration Molecules of Soluble Fluorochrome (MESF) beads (Simply Cellular). In this way, concentration can be related to target expression and uniformly measured from machine to machine and across acquisition settings. This technique is also useful when comparing two monoclonal antibodies with differing affinity or two targets with differing expression on the cell surface.

2.1.2 Analysis of Intracellular Signaling

HLA I antibody binding to target cells induces a myriad of cell signaling and function events. Intracellular signaling cascades entail sequential phosphorylation of proteins and kinases. These phosphorylation events are monitored in the cells using Western Blotting with phosphorylation site-specific antibodies.

Briefly, endothelial cells are stimulated with HLA I antibody for defined time period (usually between 1 and 30 min depending on the signaling molecule of interest, as phosphorylation events are rapid). Cell lysates are separated by SDS-PAGE, then transferred onto a PVDF membrane, and probed with phosphorylation specific antibodies for Western Blot (Cell Signaling is an excellent source).

2.1.3 Determination of Cell Growth

Cellular proliferation can be measured by several techniques, which involve either radioactive substrates incorporated during division or using flow cytometry. Our lab utilizes a flow cytometric assay exploiting the dilution of fluorescent vital dyes (such as carboxy-fluorescein succinimidyl ester, CFSE) during cell division to measure proliferation. A shift of the histogram to the left (i.e., a decrease in fluorescence intensity) indicates increased cell division due to dilution of the dye, which is analyzed using FlowJo or ModFit (Verity) to calculate the proliferation index. As an alternative approach, cells can be labeled with the pyrimidine nucleotide analog 5-bromo-2′-deoxyuridine (BrdU), which is incorporated into DNA in lieu of thymidine upon cell replication, and which can be detected using antibodies by flow cytometry [31].

2.1.4 Measurement of Leukocyte Adherence

Leukocyte adherence is measured by an adhesion assay in which endothelial monolayers are stimulated and lymphocytes or myeloid cells which are fluorescently labeled with a vital dye such as CFSE are overlaid. Nonadherent cells are washed off and adherent cells are imaged in many fields per sample using fluorescence microscopy. Cells are counted using automated quantification software, such as Image J or CellProfiler (MIT). CellProfiler has excellent counting algorithms that can effectively distinguish single cells even in dense clusters.

2.1.5 Determination of Cytoskeletal Changes and Cell Migration

Migration of cells is assessed by the scratch, or wound healing, assay. Cells are cultured, a wound is introduced by scratching the plate with a pipet tip, and closure of the wound in the absence or presence of stimulants is measured after 24 h using microscopy. Cytoskeletal changes, including stress fiber formation, are monitored by immunofluorescent staining of the actin cytoskeleton using phalloidin, which selectively labels F-actin, and visualized by fluorescent microscopy.

2.1.6 siRNA and Pharmacological Inhibitors

In order to definitively identify a role for proteins in HLA I-mediated intracellular signaling leading to functional changes, it is important to utilize strategies to inhibit the protein's function to verify the upstream and downstream relationship to other proteins in the pathway. Two commonly used methods involve knockdown of expression of the protein of interest by small interfering RNA (siRNA), or pharmacological antagonism of the protein with commercial inhibitors. A variety of inhibitors are available commercially (especially from Tocris, Sigma, or Calbiochem) for the enzymes noted to be crucial to HLA I signaling.

2.2 In Vivo Models of Antibody-Mediated Rejection

Animals deficient in T cells are incapable of mounting a complete humoral response, due to the requirement of antibody-secreting B cells for T cell help during maturation and isotype switching. Therefore, an alternative system was required to assess antibody mediated rejection in the absence of cell-mediated alloimmunity. Murine models are particularly useful because they allow genetic manipulation of putative targets, using knockout or transgenic animals. Russell et al. first described the model in which alloserum alone is sufficient to elicit allograft rejection [32]. In general, a murine or rat immunodeficient recipient, such as severe combined immunodeficiency (SCID) or recombinase activating gene-1 (RAG1) knockout mice, is used, which lacks T cells and B cells, but retains an intact innate immune system, including complement components, monocytes, natural killer (NK) cells, and neutrophils. Recipients transplanted with an MHC mismatched organ are passively transferred with alloantiserum from sensitized animals or with monoclonal DSA. This system has advanced knowledge about antibody-mediated rejection in the physiological setting. Such models have uncovered direct evidence that donor specific MHC antibodies are sufficient to trigger acute and chronic rejection, and yielded some insights into the mechanisms of antibody induced graft injury. Alternatively, human tissue can be transplanted onto an immunodeficient murine recipient, and anti-HLA antibodies or human immune cells are administered [33–35].

There are several important considerations to bear in mind when selecting an animal model of antibody-mediated rejection (reviewed in [36, 37]). The first is the availability of reagents, particularly of donor specific monoclonal antibodies. Secondly, chronic rejection in the mouse varies in location and severity of disease from model to model and from mouse to human. It is likely that monoclonal MHC antibodies are not potent enough to produce fulminant, widespread vascular lesions, as observed with polyclonal MHC alloserum [38]. In designing in vivo experimental systems, one must keep in mind the crucial caveat that the murine and human immune systems differ considerably. For example, the murine system lacks the activating FcγRIIA (CD32A) and FcγRIIC (CD32C) molecules. Inhibitory NK cell receptors are highly divergent between mouse and human—for example, mice do not express KIRs—as are the ligands for the NKG2D molecule (MHC class I chain-related MICA in humans). Further, immunoglobulin isotypes differ between mouse and human, and cytokine regulation of P-selectin expression is distinctive to the mouse. Many chemokines identified in humans are not found in the murine system (extensively reviewed in [39]). Finally, murine anatomical differences result in rejection models that are not always physiologically analogous to the clinical setting—i.e., the location of chronic vascular lesions [37].

2.3 Patient Samples

The final step in translational studies of the effects of HLA antibodies on the graft is to assess changes in transplanted organs during antibody mediated rejection in humans. In vitro findings are confirmed in patient biopsies using immunohistochemical techniques to detect histological changes, complement deposition, cellular infiltration, total protein expression, or phosphorylation status of specific proteins in the graft. RNA from patient biopsies can also be evaluated by microarray and/or sequencing to determine differential expression of proteins of interest and other changes in the transcriptome.

3 Mechanisms of Injury: Fc-Dependent Effects of Antibodies

The effects of HLA antibody binding to graft vascular cells are manifold, and depend on both the canonical antibody functions mediated by the Fc portion of the molecule, and on binding via the Fab fragment, which cross-links the target molecule on donor cells. Fc-dependent functions occur irrespective of the target protein or receptor, but vary depending on the isotype and subclass of the DSA.

3.1 Hyperacute and Acute Rejection

Alloantibody binding to endothelial and smooth muscle cells promotes Fc-dependent functions such as complement cascade activation and antibody-dependent cell-mediated cytotoxicity (ADCC). These effects are particularly relevant in hyperacute and acute humoral rejection.

3.1.1 Complement Activation

The complement cascade is a complex system consisting of proteases that become sequentially activated upon cleavage. There are three pathways of complement, which mediate immunity against different immunologic threats and are activated by different signals. The classical pathway bridges the adaptive and innate immune responses by partnering with substrate bound antibodies. The lectin pathway mediates immunity against bacterial and fungal pathogens by recognizing mannan carbohydrate motifs. The alternative complement pathway is effective against cellular pathogens and facilitates opsonization by phagocytes. For the purposes of this review, we will restrict our discussion to the classical antibody-mediated pathway. In humans, IgM, IgG1, and IgG3 are effective activators of complement. IgG or IgM on the cell surface binds to the low affinity, multivalent C1q molecule, which once "fixed" cleaves C2 and C4. The resultant cleavage products C2a and C4b complex into a protease capable of catalyzing activation of C3, which is a central mediator in all three complement pathways. This event triggers the production of C3b, which in the classical pathway activates C5, yielding the C5a and C5b fragments. C5a is an important inflammatory factor, which acts as a chemoattractant for neutrophils, monocytes and T cells. Local synthesis of C5b at the C1q-antibody site causes complex formation of C5b with C6, C7, C8, and C9 into the macromolecule known as the membrane attack complex (MAC). MAC forms transmembrane pores which cause lysis of the target cell by disrupting the plasma membrane. Cells may resist complement-induced lysis by expressing CD59, which inhibits C5b binding to C9. In addition to forming the MAC, complement split products have a myriad of other functions, including chemoattraction, viral neutralization, opsonization, immune complex clearance, and activation of macrophages and other cells (reviewed in [40]).

Complement fixing ability is particularly relevant to hyperacute and acute rejection. Hyperacute rejection is a predominantly complement-mediated severe injury to the allograft occurring within hours of transplantation. It is caused by high titer of preexisting HLA, or in rare cases non-HLA, antibodies in presensitized patients. The incidence of hyperacute rejection has dropped significantly due to improved detection of DSA and desensitization protocols.

Complement is also an important mediator of acute antibody-mediated rejection. Animal models have demonstrated that donor specific MHC antibodies are sufficient to mediate acute rejection of cardiac and corneal allografts [41, 42]. Histologically, interaction of DSA with the graft is detected by deposition of the complement split product C3d or C4d, which has been shown to associate with diagnosis of antibody-mediated rejection [43]. Allograft bound complement split products are only found in murine models of rejection when DSA is also present [44], and donor specific HLA antibodies correlate with C4d deposition [2, 45], which associated with inferior graft survival. However, C4d may not be a sensitive marker, as several reports suggest that C4d deposition may not have sufficiently reliable predictive value for diagnosis of antibody mediated rejection or graft outcome [46–51].

Antibody subclass and isotype define the effector functions of the molecule, including complement fixation. The literature on the pathogenicity of an antibody with respect to its isotype is conflicting. In murine models, immunoglobulin knockout (IgKO) allograft recipients have significantly longer graft survival than their wild-type counterparts. Acute rejection could be restored by passive transfer of donor MHC antibodies of the complement fixing isotype murine IgG2b but not the noncomplement fixing isotype murine IgG1 [52]. HLA I antibodies in patients reportedly are predominantly IgG1 [53], but can be of any of the four IgG isotypes [54]. Recently, it has been reported that skewing of DSA to complement fixing IgG3 predisposes the recipient to rejection [55]. An assay has been developed that can identify both the specificity and the complement fixing ability of HLA antibodies by binding of C1q on single antigen beads. The specificity of a patient's HLA antibodies can be determined using single antigen luminex beads that consist of fluorescent microbeads conjugated to single recombinant HLA class I and class II molecules. Complement fixing ability is assessed by the binding of C1q to

HLA antibodies present in the serum, which are bound to the HLA antigen coated microbeads. In several studies, C1q positive DSA associate with antibody mediated rejection in cardiac and renal transplantation when compared with antibodies identified only by IgG [56]. C1q positive antibodies had a positive predictive value for early episodes of antibody-mediated rejection [57]. It is postulated that noncomplement fixing antibodies will have a lower pathogenicity; indeed, three patients who were transplanted across high titer anti-donor HLA II antibodies had long-term AMR-free survival, possibly because the preexisting antibodies were of non-complement fixing isotypes IgG2 and IgG4 [58]. In contrast, another group reported that, while IgG-DSA positive patients had a significantly lower graft survival, there was no significant difference when groups with C1q-fixing and non-C1q fixing DSA were compared [6]. Similarly, antibodies detected using solid phase flow cytometry detection of DSAa flow PRA could predict early rejection episodes, while CDC-identified antibodies could not [59]. Particularly when DSA was at lower titers, complement fixing ability could not predict early antibody-mediated rejection [54, 60]. Therefore, the clinical data regarding the relationship between antibody isotype and its pathogenicity is conflicting.

Moreover, the clinical relevance of an HLA antibody's capacity to fix complement in chronic rejection is less well defined. Murine models of AMR have demonstrated that chronic rejection lesions can develop in response to MHC antibodies that are not complement fixing, or in complement deficient allograft recipients [61]. Taken together, the literature suggests that complement fixation, while important, may not be the only factor influencing the pathogenesis of a donor specific HLA antibody.

3.1.2 Antibody-Dependent Cell-Mediated Cytotoxicity

Antibodies bridge the innate and adaptive arms of the immune system by interacting with natural killer (NK) cells through their FcγRIII (CD16), which binds the constant Fc region of the antibody. NK cells recognize antibody-coated cells and cause cell lysis. Although the general mechanism of antibody-dependent cell-mediated cytotoxicity is understood, there is limited evidence about ADCC in alloimmune responses. Antibodies from sensitized patients increased the lytic capacity of CD3−CD16+ (NK) peripheral blood mononuclear cells against renal epithelium [62]. Long ago it was recognized that a positive ex vivo ADCC reaction using patient sera containing alloantibody bound to target endothelial cells was a risk factor for transplant rejection [63, 64]. NK cell cytotoxicity against human umbilical vein endothelial cells (HUVEC) could also be facilitated by IgG1 non-HLA anti-endothelial cell antibodies [65]. Although this topic has received less priority over the last decade, recent reports implicating NK cells in MHC antibody-mediated chronic rejection in the mouse [66, 67] and in human antibody-mediated rejection [68] will likely excite more interest in this area.

4 Mechanisms of Injury: Target Cell Signaling Induced by HLA I Antibodies

HLA I ligation directly induces intracellular signaling cascades which have important implications for cell functional changes, especially cellular proliferation which is central to the pathogenesis of chronic rejection.

4.1 Survival and Accommodation

The presence of circulating donor specific HLA antibodies may not always indicate ongoing rejection. Some patients, as many as 24 %, maintain good graft function despite detectable titers of HLA-DSA, in a poorly defined state thought to represent transplant accommodation [5]. Little is understood about accommodation, but it is expected that antibody titer may be an important factor. For example, a high titer of antibody in renal patients (cutoff of 4,487 MFI for class II) correlated with and accurately predicted AMR incidence [7], suggesting that symptomatic rejection has a threshold for the amount of antibody to which the graft is exposed. However, the persistence of DSA on its own is a strong predictor of late graft loss independently of AMR episodes; thus, accommodation does not indicate indefinite graft survival, and likely there are ongoing subclinical events in response to alloantibody that damage the graft and result in chronic rejection. For example, cardiac transplant recipients with asymptomatic AMR had a lower 5 year freedom from chronic rejection than those without any AMR [19], suggesting that accommodation is better defined as clinically silent antibody-mediated graft damage that slowly causes failure.

Several in vitro studies indicate a possible mechanism for HLA I antibody-mediated transplant accommodation, where the graft is resistant to acute antibody-induced damage, such as complement activation and apoptosis. One group reported that while HLA I antibodies from patient sera or monoclonal antibodies trigger endothelial cell death at high concentrations, at low concentrations HLA I antibodies confer resistance to complement induced cell death by inducing heme oxygenase (HO-1) and activating cyclic AMP-dependent protein kinase A (PKA) [69, 70]. HLA I antibodies also increase endothelial Nrf-2 mediated antioxidant responses, which provide protection of endothelial cells from complement induced death via HO-1 and ferritin H [71]. Additionally, treatment with HLA I antibody at low doses increases PI3K/Akt signaling, which results in inactivation of the proapoptotic factor Bad and increased expression of apoptosis inhibitors Bcl-2 and Bcl-xL in vitro [72]. These observations were confirmed in a murine transplant model, where Bcl-2 and HO-1 were upregulated in an HLA-A*02 transgenic allograft by pretreatment with low titer of HLA I antibodies, which prevented subsequent rejection by high titers of HLA I antibodies [73]. Further, biopsies from patients with AMR have elevated Bcl-2 expression [72], demonstrating that donor specific HLA antibodies activate these pathways in the clinical setting.

4.2 Cell Proliferation

Chronic rejection, or transplant vasculopathy, is a predominantly proliferative disease, in which the vessels of the graft become occluded by a severely thickened intima invaded by smooth muscle cells. Donor specific HLA antibodies are strongly associated with vasculopathy in heart and kidney transplantation [1]. There is strong evidence that ligation of HLA I by antibodies triggers proliferation and cytoskeletal changes in vascular cells.

4.2.1 In Vitro Evidence

We and others found that, rapidly following HLA I ligation by antibodies, Rho-GTP, Src and focal adhesion kinase (FAK) become activated [74, 75]. Src activation triggers the PI3K/Akt signaling axis, which is a key regulator of survival and cell cycle progression. Akt promotes the activity of mammalian target of rapamycin (mTOR), a serine/threonine kinase which exists in two complexes. mTOR complex 1, composed of raptor, mTOR, and GβL, targets S6 kinase (S6K), S6 ribosomal protein and 4EBP1, molecules involved in protein synthesis which become phosphorylated after HLA I ligation [76]. mTORC2, which contains rictor, mTOR, GβL, is a central regulator of the cytoskeleton as well as of extracellular regulated kinases (ERK1/2) [77, 78]. HLA I cross-linking activates the mitogen-activated protein kinases ERK1/2, which promote cell proliferation through a parallel pathway. Consequently, stimulation of endothelial cells and smooth muscle cells with HLA I antibody directly increases cellular proliferation in the absence of exogenous growth factors [31, 79, 80]. Interestingly, HLA I antibody stimulation of smooth muscle cell growth was dependent on the activation of matrix metalloproteases/sphingolipid signaling, a stress-induced pathway [81], illustrating the pleiotropic effects of HLA I ligation leading to cellular proliferation.

Because HLA I molecule has no known signaling motif, we postulated that HLA I associated with a coreceptor to carry out its proximal signaling requirements. Using immunoprecipitation, we discovered a molecular association between HLA I and integrin β4 which was required to activate downstream signaling and cell proliferation [31]. These results demonstrated for the first time the mechanism by which HLA I molecules transduce signals into the cell.

In addition to regulating signaling molecules central to cell cycle progression and proliferation, HLA I ligation causes dramatic reorganization of the actin cytoskeleton. Cytoskeletal rearrangements are relevant to cell migration and proliferation, as well as endothelial cell permeability. FAK mediates cytoskeletal changes by acting on paxillin. We observe increased stress fiber formation and association of several unique proteins with the cytoskeleton after treatment of endothelial cells and smooth muscle cells with HLA I antibody [79, 82, 83]. Further, HLA I antibody increases cell migration and wound healing [79].

These observations of the direct effects of HLA I antibody are not restricted to vascular cells. Stimulation of lung epithelial carcinoma with HLA sera from patients increases proliferation and tyrosine phosphorylation [84], pointing to a mechanism by which HLA antibodies may provoke bronchiolitis obliterans syndrome (BOS).

4.2.2 In Vivo Evidence

The experimental evidence linking MHC I antibodies and cellular proliferation in vivo is emerging. Initially the proliferative changes observed in chronic rejection were thought to be T cell mediated [38]. However, when murine cardiac allograft recipients were depleted of T cells after generation of MHC alloantibodies, the grafts still developed arteriosclerosis to a greater extent than those without DSA [32]. Further, in murine recipients deficient in B cells, but with an intact T cell immune response, the allograft did not progress to vasculopathy [32]. These data suggest that the humoral response is required for full chronic rejection. In a seminal study, transfer of allosera to SCID allograft recipients reproduced these obstructive lesions [32], results which have been confirmed more recently using donor specific MHC I monoclonal antibodies [61, 67]. Further, vasculopathy is elicited by human antibodies in human grafts. SCID mice were transplanted with human mesenteric arteries and passively transferred with HLA I antibody. The investigators observed increased neointimal thickening in response to HLA I antibody in this study [81]. These data demonstrate that humoral immunity is sufficient to produce vasculopathy.

Importantly, MHC I antibodies elicited vascular lesions in RAG1 knockout recipients of cardiac allografts even when the antibodies were of noncomplement fixing isotypes or allograft recipients were deficient in complement [61, 66]. These results strongly indicate that MHC I antibodies mediate chronic rejection via a complement-independent mechanism and are consistent with the in vitro work demonstrating that HLA I cross-linking directly triggers proliferation and cell signaling.

We confirmed HLA I-induced cell signaling in vivo. Allografts from RAG1 knockout mice reconstituted with anti-donor MHC I antibody had significantly increased phosphorylated Akt, mTOR and S6K compared with the control group [85]. Further, our group investigated endothelial cell signaling downstream of HLA I cross-linking in patient cardiac allograft biopsies. We found that phosphorylated S6 ribosomal protein (S6RP) was increased in AMR patients and was a more sensitive marker of AMR than C4d [86]. Therefore, activation of signaling molecules which promote proliferation occurs in both animal models of antibody-mediated rejection and in the clinical setting.

4.3 Induction of Secondary Factors

In addition to direct activation of intracellular signaling cascades, in vitro experiments have revealed that HLA I antibodies increase sensitivity to and production of soluble mediators which promote autocrine proliferative signaling. HLA I cross-linking rapidly increases cell surface expression of fibroblast growth factor receptor (FGFR) on endothelial cells. The proliferative response to bFGF is thus significantly enhanced by sensitization with HLA I antibodies [87–89]. Stimulation of HLA I also triggers endothelial cell production of cytokines which may have a secondary effect on cell growth. For example, HLA I antibodies increase endothelial production of vascular endothelial growth factor (VEGF), which activates cells in an autocrine manner via its receptor VEGFR2 [90]. Treatment of lung airway epithelial cells with HLA I antibodies increased platelet-derived growth factor (PDGF), insulin-like growth factor 1 (IGF-1), and fibroblast growth factor (bFGF) production, which promoted paracrine proliferation of fibroblasts [91]. Therefore, HLA I activation of endothelial cells increases sensitivity to bFGF and production of other soluble mediators which trigger autocrine and paracrine cell proliferation.

4.4 Leukocyte Recruitment

4.4.1 Infiltration in Antibody-Mediated Rejection

In addition to antibody-induced complement deposition, antibody mediated rejection is frequently characterized by intravascular macrophages [92], which can promote both acute and chronic rejection [93, 94]. Further, NK cells were required for neointimal thickening in a murine AMR model [66]. Thus, recruitment of immune cells into the allograft facilitates innate cell-mediated injury.

4.4.2 HLA I Antibody-Induced Leukocyte Recruitment

Endothelial cells contain intracellular rod-shaped vesicles called Weibel–Palade bodies, which contain preformed von Willebrand Factor (vWF), P-selectin, and other vascular mediators. Release of these vesicles, which fuse with the cell membrane and secrete contents into the extracellular space, is regulated by calcium or cAMP-dependent secretagogues, such as thrombin, histamine, or forskolin (reviewed in [95]). Recently, it has been reported that HLA I ligation by monoclonal murine antibody triggers exocytosis of these vesicles, externalizing vWF and increasing cell surface P-selectin. HLA I antibody-induced P-selectin mediated increased adherence of the promyelocytic cell line HL60 in vitro. Further, treatment of SCID mice engrafted with human skin with the monoclonal HLA I antibody in vivo also triggered vWF externalization and neutrophil influx [96]. In a similar study, wild-type murine cardiac recipients had evidence of vWF release and P-selectin expression by allograft endothelium during acute rejection, which was absent in IgKO recipients [52]. In a murine lung transplant model, treatment with MHC antibodies increased neutrophil infiltration and inflammation [97]. Thus, MHC or HLA I antibody binding to endothelial cells causes rapid endothelial cell activation, promoting recruitment of leukocytes.

The clinical relevance of this pathway to AMR has not been definitively elucidated; however, in human cardiac biopsies, capillary endothelium displayed increased expression of vWF during rejection [98, 99]. In a variety of murine allograft models, selectin deficiency in the donor graft prolongs graft survival and reduces cellular infiltration [100–102], suggesting that HLA I antibody-induced P-selectin and/or vWF may be a rational therapeutic target to decrease immune cell recruitment.

4.5 Therapies Suggested from Experimental Evidence

The knowledge gained from the experimental systems described above reveals potential therapeutic targets to alleviate the proliferative and inflammatory effects of HLA I antibodies. For example, we and others found that HLA I cross-linking on endothelial cells activated RhoA, which was necessary for proliferation in vitro [74, 83]. Inactivation of Rho and Rho kinase (ROCK) by pharmacological inhibitors in animal models reduces neointimal thickening: in a rabbit vein graft model, intimal thickening was inhibited by fasudil (ROCK inhibitor) [103]; in a murine model of chronic cardiac rejection, intimal thickening was suppressed by fasudil [104], while another Rho kinase inhibitor, Y-27632, prolonged survival, reduced immune cell infiltration, and prevented intimal thickening [105].

We also reported that mTOR is a central signaling molecule in HLA I-induced cellular proliferation [77]. Pretreatment of endothelial cells with rapamycin, an mTOR inhibitor, reduced HLA I Ab-triggered endothelial proliferation, Akt phosphorylation, and Bcl-2 expression [77]. Recent reports suggest that rapamycin and its analogs (everolimus, sirolimus) may have clinical therapeutic potential. For example, everolimus therapy prevented remodeling after heart transplantation in human patients [106]. The exact mechanism of protection from rejection conferred by rapamycin is not understood, but mTOR inhibition in endothelial and smooth muscle cells may prevent HLA I antibody-induced proliferation.

Other potential therapies for antibody mediated rejection include adhesion molecule antagonists to reduce leukocyte infiltration and complement inhibitors to prevent complement-mediated tissue injury. In a presensitized primate renal allograft model, complement inhibition reduced AMR and prolonged allograft survival [107]. Use of eculizimab, a monoclonal antibody which blocks activation of C5, reduced antibody-mediated rejection incidence in patients with DSA [108]. Therefore, the progress which has been made in understanding the mechanisms of HLA I antibody-mediated graft injury has suggested rational clinical therapies in the treatment and prevention of AMR.

5 HLA II Antibodies

Although the mechanism by which HLA I antibodies promote inflammation and proliferation has been revealed by experimental models, the pathogenesis of HLA II antibodies is less defined.

5.1 Association with Outcome

Antibodies to HLA II frequently accompany chronic rejection in renal transplants [43] and correlate with AMR incidence in the absence of a positive T cell crossmatch [7, 109]. The presence of antibody to HLA II significantly correlates with worse graft outcome, in addition to antibody to HLA I [90].

5.2 Limitations to Studying HLA II in Model Systems

Investigation of the effects of HLA II antibodies on graft cells has been limited by its restricted expression pattern and by constraints in experimental systems. HLA II is not expressed on endothelial cells of most vascular beds, with the possible exception of renal microvasculature [110, 111], but it can be upregulated after inflammatory insult [112–115]. Indeed, several reports have demonstrated HLA II expression on endothelia in grafts [99, 116], which suggests that allogeneic attack or transplantation itself may upregulate MHC II expression as reported in murine cardiac allografts [117–119].

In vivo studies on MHC II are constrained by the different expression pattern of MHC II in mice, where normal cardiac tissue does not express MHC II molecules. In the mouse, MHC II may be upregulated after transplantation [118, 119], similar to reports in human cardiac allografts, where HLA-DR was increased during rejection [99]. Human microvascular endothelia have been found to express HLA II, but cultured endothelial cells rapidly lose constitutive expression. HLA II can be reinduced by treatment of endothelium with cytokines such as TNFα or IFNγ. However, cytokine treatment introduces a layer of complexity with respect to cell activation that masks many intracellular signals, upregulates a variety of other factors, and thus obscures analysis and conclusions. There is, therefore, a need for an in vitro system in which the effects of HLA II antibodies on vascular cells can be investigated without additional confounding factors.

5.3 Mechanisms

Due to the limitations discussed above, the consequences of cross-linking of HLA II on vascular cells are not well defined. Some insights may be inferred from data regarding HLA II engagement on other cell types. In B lymphocytes and antigen presenting cells, HLA II ligation triggers an increase in intracellular calcium and tyrosine phosphorylation, with varying functional effects. Cells become activated and proliferate or undergo apoptosis depending on which intracellular pathway is predominantly activated [120–122]. Fibroblasts stimulated through HLA II increase production of prostaglandin E [123], RANTES, interleukin (IL)-6, monocyte chemoattractant protein (MCP)-1, and GROα [124, 125], through Janus kinase (JNK) and FAK signaling [126]. These HLA II-induced soluble factors produced by fibroblasts could promote proliferation of endothelial cells [124]. However, little to no data is available to establish how HLA II cross-linking on endothelial or smooth muscle cells might trigger functional changes leading to rejection.

6 Non-HLA Antibodies

A new appreciation of non-HLA antibodies has arisen due to reports of antibody-mediated rejection or C4d deposition in the absence of circulating donor specific HLA antibodies. Non-HLA antibodies in transplantation can be directed against either polymorphic or nonallelic proteins. The development of antibodies against nonpolymorphic targets may be due to upregulation during inflammation, in response to transplantation, or when proteins are exposed to the immune system during injury. It is thought that the intragraft microenvironment or rejection may break humoral tolerance to autoantigens [127]. Moreover, the indication for renal transplantation is often autoimmunity, where patients may be predisposed to humoral responses against self antigens.

6.1 Frequency and Outcome

Non-HLA antibodies are commonly found in transplant recipients. Le Bas-Bernadet et al. reported that nearly half of renal patients who had DSA to HLA also had non-HLA anti-endothelial cell antibodies (AECA) [128]. Another study found anti-endothelial cell antibodies in 23 % of renal patients, which associated with a greater rate of cellular rejection and lower graft function [129]. Similarly, a significantly higher rate of AECA positivity was found in patients with failed renal transplants compared to those with functioning grafts [130]. Non-HLA antibodies binding to airway epithelial cells were detected in lung transplant patients with chronic rejection, bronchiolitis obliterans syndrome (BOS), but not in patients without BOS [131]. One group identified endothelial cell-binding IgM and IgG using flow cytometry in about half of cardiac transplant patients with transplant coronary artery disease (TCAD) and in patients with failed renal allografts. Interestingly, they did not find such antibodies in pretransplant patients or controls [132]. Another group reported that non-HLA antibodies were found at a higher rate in cardiac and renal transplant recipients with or without rejection than in normal or wait-listed subjects [133], suggesting that these antigens become immunogenic during transplantation. Also remarkable is the observation that the array of non-HLA antigens recognized by the alloimmune response varies from patient to patient, with only a few markers overlapping [134].

Several of the ligands for non-HLA antibodies have been identified. Nonclassical histocompatibility antigens are frequent targets of the alloimmune humoral response. The major histocompatibility class I related chain (MIC) genes are non-HLA proteins with some homology to HLA class I molecules. MICA and MICB do not associate with β2 microglobulin and function as ligands for the NK cell receptor NKG2D rather than the T cell receptor. Although not nearly as polymorphic as HLA molecules, MICA and MICB have more than 30 alleles each. Antibodies to MICA and MICB are found in renal [135, 136], as well as cardiac transplant recipients, where they associate with chronic rejection [1, 16, 137].

Other targets of antibodies in transplantation include vascular receptors, adhesion molecules, and intermediate filaments (reviewed in [1, 138]). Using immunoprecipitation and mass spectrometry, Qin et al. revealed the nucleolar protein nucleolin as a target of non-HLA antibodies in transplant patients [133]. Further, neuropilin, a cell surface coreceptor for VEGFR; heterogenous nuclear ribonucleoprotein K; an intermediate filament protein; ribosomal protein L7; and CD36, a scavenger receptor for oxidized LDL and other lipoproteins, have all been identified as ligands for non-HLA endothelial cell antibodies in patients with chronic cardiac allograft rejection [134, 139–141]. Antibodies to nondonor derived antigens, particularly vimentin and cardiac myosin [137, 142], are present in a majority (65 %) of cardiac transplant patients with chronic rejection and correlate with CAV incidence [1, 143]. In renal transplantation, antibodies recognizing glutathione-*S*-transferase (GST), a cytosolic enzyme which metabolizes toxins, were found in patients experiencing antibody-mediated rejection [144, 145].

6.2 Experimental Models

Not much is known about the mechanism of graft injury by non-HLA antibodies. The clinical relevance and pathogenic mechanism of antibodies to intracellular proteins, such as glutathione-S-transferase (GST), vimentin, and ribonucleoprotein, is unclear. Such antibodies may represent a marker for injury or bystander humoral activation rather than having independent pathogenic potential. Non-HLA antibodies against cell surface markers may fix complement or mediate ADCC. Considering the agonistic function of an antibody when it cross-links its target, the mechanism of action may depend on the signaling capacity and biological function of the ligand as with HLA I molecules. For example, angiotensin II receptor AT1 autoantibodies are well-established agonists, which promote hypertension and may contribute to renal allograft rejection [146–148]. Antibodies from autoimmune sera upregulate adhesion molecules and cytokines on endothelial cells [149–151], but when the target is unknown the precise mechanism remains elusive. To date, little has been studied on the actions of non-HLA antibodies during the humoral alloimmune response.

In some experimental studies, non-HLA antibodies do not cause injury. For example, rat allosera lacking MHC antibodies caused only minor complement-mediated cytotoxicity against rat endothelial cells when compared with MHC specific allosera [152, 153]. Further, C3 deposition was only observed in the cardiac allograft vasculature of an MHC-mismatched rat model but not in a rejection model with non-MHC alloserum production [153]. A possible explanation may be that the isotype of non-HLA antibodies is different from that of HLA antibodies. One clinical study found non-HLA antibodies predominantly of the noncomplement fixing isotypes IgG2 and IgG4 [129]. Further, as mentioned above, the signaling capacity of the target molecule may shape the effect of antibody binding. For example, anti-MICA antibodies did not increase neointimal thickening of human mesenteric arteries grafted in SCID mice, while HLA I antibody was sufficient to elicit lesions [80].

In contrast, other studies have suggested that non-HLA antibodies have pathogenic potential. Anti-airway epithelial cell antibodies isolated from patients induced intracellular calcium increase, proliferation, and tyrosine phosphorylation in airway epithelium, although the cell surface ligands remain unknown [131]. Anti-donor antibodies produced by rat cardiac recipients could induce apoptosis of rat vascular endothelial cells [19]. Antibodies to nucleolin or unidentified endothelial targets also caused apoptosis of human endothelial cells [128, 133]. Although nucleolin is primary localized to the nucleus, this protein was detected on the cell surface in proliferating tumor and endothelial cells [133], suggesting that intracellular targets of the humoral response may be exposed under certain conditions. Moreover, mice sensitized against vimentin experienced rejection, C3d deposition and P-selectin expression in cardiac allografts, effects which were specifically mediated by antibodies to vimentin [154].

Therefore, antibodies to donor antigens correlate with rejection and may promote graft injury. More work is needed to understand whether non-HLA antibodies are relevant only as a marker of humoral activation and graft injury, or whether they also function as independent actors of alloreactivity.

7 Conclusions

Alloantibody binding to donor cells injures the graft by a myriad of mechanisms (Fig. 1). Complement cascade activation by alloantibody results in inflammation and destruction of the graft vasculature. Agonistic stimulation of HLA I, HLA II, endothelial or epithelial cell surface markers may induce intracellular signaling leading to recruitment of immune cells, apoptosis, survival or proliferation. Thus, alloantibody can elicit complement deposition and neutrophil infiltration, features of acute rejection, as well as cellular proliferation and vascular lesion formation, characteristic of chronic rejection.

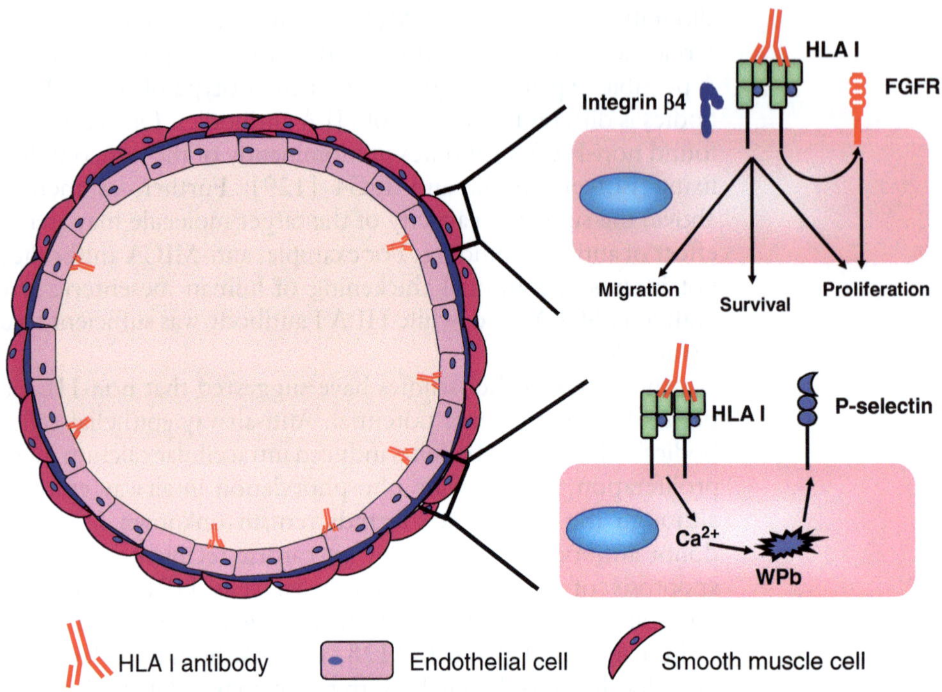

Fig. 1 The pleiotropic effects of HLA I antibody binding to graft vascular cells. Donor specific HLA I antibodies bind to HLA I molecules expressed on the surface of endothelial cells lining the vasculature of the transplanted organ. In addition to triggering complement activation through their Fcγ fragment, antibodies recognizing HLA I molecules cross-link these receptors at the cell surface, inducing intracellular signaling. HLA I-mediated cell signaling results in increased FGFR at the endothelial cell surface, migration, proliferation, and resistance to apoptosis and complement-induced death. Cellular proliferation requires a molecular association between HLA I molecules and integrin β4. HLA I cross-linking also increases cytosolic calcium (Ca^{2+}), which triggers mobilization of Weibel–Palade bodies and increased cell surface P-selectin, leading to adherence of selectin-ligand bearing immune cells

References

1. Zhang Q, Cecka JM, Gjertson DW, Ge P, Rose ML, Patel JK et al (2011) HLA and MICA: targets of antibody-mediated rejection in heart transplantation. Transplantation 91: 1153–1158
2. Cardarelli F, Pascual M, Tolkoff-Rubin N, Delmonico FL, Wong W, Schoenfeld DA et al (2005) Prevalence and significance of anti-HLA and donor-specific antibodies long-term after renal transplantation. Transpl Int 18: 532–540
3. Everly MJ, Everly JJ, Arend LJ, Brailey P, Susskind B, Govil A et al (2009) Reducing de novo donor-specific antibody levels during acute rejection diminishes renal allograft loss. Am J Transplant 9:1063–1071
4. Lachmann N, Terasaki PI, Schonemann C (2006) Donor-specific HLA antibodies in chronic renal allograft rejection: a prospective trial with a four-year follow-up. Clin Transpl 171–199
5. Lachmann N, Terasaki PI, Budde K, Liefeldt L, Kahl A, Reinke P et al (2009) Anti-human leukocyte antigen and donor-specific antibodies detected by luminex posttransplant serve as biomarkers for chronic rejection of renal allografts. Transplantation 87:1505–1513
6. Otten HG, Verhaar MC, Borst HP, Hene RJ, Zuilen AD (2012) Pretransplant donor-specific HLA class-I and -II antibodies are associated with an increased risk for kidney graft failure. Am J Transplant 12(6): 1618–1623
7. Song EY, Lee YJ, Hyun J, Kim YS, Ahn C, Ha J et al (2012) Clinical relevance of pretransplant HLA class II donor-specific antibodies

in renal transplantation patients with negative T-cell cytotoxicity crossmatches. Ann Lab Med 32:139–144
8. Bishara A, Brautbar C, Eid A, Scherman L, Ilan Y, Safadi R (2002) Is presensitization relevant to liver transplantation outcome? Hum Immunol 63:742–750
9. Appel JZ III, Hartwig MG, Davis RD, Reinsmoen NL (2005) Utility of peritransplant and rescue intravenous immunoglobulin and extracorporeal immunoadsorption in lung transplant recipients sensitized to HLA antigens. Hum Immunol 66:378–386
10. Bond G, Reyes J, Mazariegos G, Wu T, Schaefer N, Demetris J et al (2000) The impact of positive T-cell lymphocytotoxic crossmatch on intestinal allograft rejection and survival. Transplant Proc 32:1197–1198
11. Campbell PM, Salam A, Ryan EA, Senior P, Paty BW, Bigam D et al (2007) Pretransplant HLA antibodies are associated with reduced graft survival after clinical islet transplantation. Am J Transplant 7:1242–1248
12. Wu T, Abu-Elmagd K, Bond G, Demetris AJ (2004) A clinicopathologic study of isolated intestinal allografts with preformed IgG lymphocytotoxic antibodies. Hum Pathol 35:1332–1339
13. Barocci S, Valente U, Nocera A (2007) Detection and analysis of HLA class I and class II specific alloantibodies in the sera of dialysis recipients waiting for a renal retransplantation. Clin Transplant 21:47–56
14. OPTN 2004 Annual Report of the U.S. Organ Procurement and Transplantation Network and the Scientific Registry of Transplant Recipients: Transplant Data 1994–2003. Department of Health and Human Services, Health Resources and Services Administration, Healthcare Systems Bureau, Division of Transplantation, Rockville, MD; United Network for Organ Sharing, Richmond, VA; University Renal Research and Education Association, Ann Arbor, MI
15. Hourmant M, Cesbron-Gautier A, Terasaki PI, Mizutani K, Moreau A, Meurette A et al (2005) Frequency and clinical implications of development of donor-specific and non-donor-specific HLA antibodies after kidney transplantation. J Am Soc Nephrol 16:2804–2812
16. Nath DS, Angaswamy N, Basha HI, Phelan D, Moazami N, Ewald GA et al (2010) Donor-specific antibodies to human leukocyte antigens are associated with and precede antibodies to major histocompatibility complex class I-related chain A in antibody-mediated rejection and cardiac allograft vasculopathy after human cardiac transplantation. Hum Immunol 71:1191–1196
17. Kimball PM, Baker MA, Wagner MB, King A (2011) Surveillance of alloantibodies after transplantation identifies the risk of chronic rejection. Kidney Int 79:1131–1137
18. Ho EK, Vlad G, Vasilescu ER, de la Torre L, Colovai AI, Burke E et al (2010) Pre- and posttransplantation allosensitization in heart allograft recipients: major impact of de novo alloantibody production on allograft survival. Hum Immunol 72:5–10
19. Wu GW, Kobashigawa JA, Fishbein MC, Patel JK, Kittleson MM, Reed EF et al (2009) Asymptomatic antibody-mediated rejection after heart transplantation predicts poor outcomes. J Heart Lung Transplant 28:417–422
20. Tsai HL, Island ER, Chang JW, Gonzalez-Pinto I, Tryphonopoulos P, Nishida S et al (2011) Association between donor-specific antibodies and acute rejection and resolution in small bowel and multivisceral transplantation. Transplantation 92:709–715
21. Gonzalez-Pinto IM, Tzakis AG, Tsai HL, Chang JW, Tryphonopoulos P, Nishida S et al (2010) Association between panel reactive antibodies and acute small bowel rejection: analysis of a series of 324 intestinal transplants. Transplant Proc 42:4269–4271
22. Farmer DG, Venick RS, Colangelo J, Esmailian Y, Yersiz H, Duffy JP et al (2010) Pretransplant predictors of survival after intestinal transplantation: analysis of a single-center experience of more than 100 transplants. Transplantation 90:1574–1580
23. Wiebe C, Gibson IW, Blydt-Hansen TD, Karpinski M, Ho J, Storsley LJ et al (2012) Evolution and clinical pathologic correlations of de novo donor-specific HLA antibody post kidney transplant. Am J Transplant 12: 1157–1167
24. Smith RN, Kawai T, Boskovic S, Nadazdin O, Sachs DH, Cosimi AB et al (2008) Four stages and lack of stable accommodation in chronic alloantibody-mediated renal allograft rejection in Cynomolgus monkeys. Am J Transplant 8:1662–1672
25. Aubert V, Venetz JP, Pantaleo G, Pascual M (2009) Low levels of human leukocyte antigen donor-specific antibodies detected by solid phase assay before transplantation are frequently clinically irrelevant. Hum Immunol 70:580–583
26. Hosenpud JD, Everett JP, Morris TE, Mauck KA, Shipley GD, Wagner CR (1995) Cardiac allograft vasculopathy. Association with cell-mediated but not humoral alloimmunity to donor-specific vascular endothelium. Circulation 92:205–211
27. Solez K, Colvin RB, Racusen LC, Sis B, Halloran PF, Birk PE et al (2007) Banff '05

Meeting Report: differential diagnosis of chronic allograft injury and elimination of chronic allograft nephropathy ('CAN'). Am J Transplant 7:518–526

28. Berry GJ, Angelini A, Burke MM, Bruneval P, Fishbein MC, Hammond E et al (2011) The ISHLT working formulation for pathologic diagnosis of antibody-mediated rejection in heart transplantation: evolution and current status (2005–2011). J Heart Lung Transplant 30:601–611
29. Kozlowski T, Rubinas T, Nickeleit V, Woosley J, Schmitz J, Collins D et al (2011) Liver allograft antibody-mediated rejection with demonstration of sinusoidal C4d staining and circulating donor-specific antibodies. Liver Transpl 17:357–368
30. Mulder A, Kardol MJ, Arn JS, Eijsink C, Franke ME, Schreuder GM et al (2010) Human monoclonal HLA antibodies reveal interspecies crossreactive swine MHC class I epitopes relevant for xenotransplantation. Mol Immunol 47:809–815
31. Zhang X, Rozengurt E, Reed EF (2010) HLA class I molecules partner with integrin beta4 to stimulate endothelial cell proliferation and migration. Sci Signal 3:ra85
32. Russell PS, Chase CM, Winn HJ, Colvin RB (1994) Coronary atherosclerosis in transplanted mouse hearts. II. Importance of humoral immunity. J Immunol 152:5135–5141
33. Yacoub-Youssef H, Marcheix B, Calise D, Thiers JC, Benoist H, Blaes N et al (2005) Use of human mesenteric arteries to study chronic vascular rejection in SCID/beige mice reconstituted with human spleen cells. Transplant Proc 37:75–76
34. Marcheix B, Yacoub-Youssef H, Calise D, Thiers JC, Therville N, Benoist H et al (2006) Multiple human mesenteric arterial grafts from the same donor to study human chronic vascular rejection in humanized SCID/beige mice. J Heart Lung Transplant 25:675–682
35. Lorber MI, Wilson JH, Robert ME, Schechner JS, Kirkiles N, Qian HY et al (1999) Human allogeneic vascular rejection after arterial transplantation and peripheral lymphoid reconstitution in severe combined immunodeficient mice. Transplantation 67:897–903
36. Baldwin WM III, Valujskikh A, Fairchild RL (2010) Antibody-mediated rejection: emergence of animal models to answer clinical questions. Am J Transplant 10:1135–1142
37. Wehner JR, Morrell CN, Rodriguez ER, Fairchild RL, Baldwin WM III (2009) Immunological challenges of cardiac transplantation: the need for better animal models to answer current clinical questions. J Clin Immunol 29:722–729
38. Russell PS, Chase CM, Colvin RB (1997) Alloantibody- and T cell-mediated immunity in the pathogenesis of transplant arteriosclerosis: lack of progression to sclerotic lesions in B cell-deficient mice. Transplantation 64:1531–1536
39. Mestas J, Hughes CC (2004) Of mice and not men: differences between mouse and human immunology. J Immunol 172: 2731–2738
40. Hughes PD, Cohney SJ (2011) Modifiers of complement activation for prevention of antibody-mediated injury to allografts. Curr Opin Organ Transplant 16:425–433
41. Hegde S, Mellon JK, Hargrave SL, Niederkorn JY (2002) Effect of alloantibodies on corneal allograft survival. Invest Ophthalmol Vis Sci 43:1012–1018
42. Nozaki T, Amano H, Bickerstaff A, Orosz CG, Novick AC, Tanabe K et al (2007) Antibody-mediated rejection of cardiac allografts in CCR5-deficient recipients. J Immunol 179:5238–5245
43. Colvin RB (2007) Antibody-mediated renal allograft rejection: diagnosis and pathogenesis. J Am Soc Nephrol 18:1046–1056
44. Murata K, Fox-Talbot K, Qian Z, Takahashi K, Stahl GL, Baldwin WM III et al (2007) Synergistic deposition of C4d by complement-activating and non-activating antibodies in cardiac transplants. Am J Transplant 7:2605–2614
45. Mauiyyedi S, Pelle PD, Saidman S, Collins AB, Pascual M, Tolkoff-Rubin NE et al (2001) Chronic humoral rejection: identification of antibody-mediated chronic renal allograft rejection by C4d deposits in peritubular capillaries. J Am Soc Nephrol 12:574–582
46. Satoskar AA, Lehman AM, Nadasdy GM, Sedmak DD, Pesavento TE, Henry ML et al (2008) Peritubular capillary C4d staining in late acute renal allograft rejection—is it relevant? Clin Transplant 22:61–67
47. Sis B, Grynoch R, Murray AG, Campbell P, Solez K (2008) Antibody-mediated rejection with a striking interstitial monocyte/macrophage infiltration in a renal allograft under FTY720 treatment. Am J Kidney Dis 51:127–130
48. Fedson SE, Daniel SS, Husain AN (2008) Immunohistochemistry staining of C4d to diagnose antibody-mediated rejection in cardiac transplantation. J Heart Lung Transplant 27:372–379
49. Ionescu DN, Girnita AL, Zeevi A, Duquesnoy R, Pilewski J, Johnson B et al (2005) C4d deposition in lung allografts is associated with

circulating anti-HLA alloantibody. Transpl Immunol 15:63–68
50. Arias LF, Fernandez R, Fernandez D, Jaramillo JC, Gil M, Lopez Garcia-Asenjo JA (2010) C4D immunostaining in surveillance endomyocardial biopsies from well-functioning heart allografts. Transplant Proc 42:1793–1796
51. Troxell ML, Higgins JP, Kambham N (2006) Evaluation of C4d staining in liver and small intestine allografts. Arch Pathol Lab Med 130:1489–1496
52. Wasowska BA, Qian Z, Cangello DL, Behrens E, Van Tran K, Layton J et al (2001) Passive transfer of alloantibodies restores acute cardiac rejection in IgKO mice. Transplantation 71:727–736
53. Canet E, Devalliere J, Gerard N, Karam G, Giral M, Charreau B et al (2012) Profiling posttransplant circulating antibodies in kidney transplantation using donor endothelial cells. Transplantation 93:257–264
54. Honger G, Hopfer H, Arnold ML, Spriewald BM, Schaub S, Amico P (2011) Pretransplant IgG subclasses of donor-specific human leukocyte antigen antibodies and development of antibody-mediated rejection. Transplantation 92:41–47
55. Kaneku H, O'Leary JG, Taniguchi M, Susskind BM, Terasaki PI, Klintmalm GB (2012) Donor-specific HLA antibodies of IgG3 subclass are associated with chronic rejection and graft loss after liver transplantation. Liver Transpl 18(8):984–992
56. Chen G, Sequeira F, Tyan DB (2011) Novel C1q assay reveals a clinically relevant subset of human leukocyte antigen antibodies independent of immunoglobulin G strength on single antigen beads. Hum Immunol 72:849–858
57. Chin C, Chen G, Sequeria F, Berry G, Siehr S, Bernstein D et al (2011) Clinical usefulness of a novel C1q assay to detect immunoglobulin G antibodies capable of fixing complement in sensitized pediatric heart transplant patients. J Heart Lung Transplant 30:158–163
58. Lobashevsky A, Rosner K, Goggins W, Higgins N (2010) Subtypes of immunoglobulin (Ig)-G antibodies against donor class II HLA and cross-match results in three kidney transplant candidates. Transpl Immunol 23:81–85
59. Tambur AR, Bray RA, Takemoto SK, Mancini M, Costanzo MR, Kobashigawa JA et al (2000) Flow cytometric detection of HLA-specific antibodies as a predictor of heart allograft rejection. Transplantation 70:1055–1059
60. Honger G, Wahrmann M, Amico P, Hopfer H, Bohmig GA, Schaub S (2010) C4d-fixing capability of low-level donor-specific HLA antibodies is not predictive for early antibody-mediated rejection. Transplantation 89:1471–1475
61. Hirohashi T, Uehara S, Chase CM, DellaPelle P, Madsen JC, Russell PS et al (2010) Complement independent antibody-mediated endarteritis and transplant arteriopathy in mice. Am J Transplant 10:510–517
62. Kirby JA, Givan AL, Shenton BK, Talbot D, Forsythe JL, Lennard TW et al (1990) Renal allograft rejection. Possible involvement of antibody-dependent cell-mediated cytotoxicity. Transplantation 50:225–229
63. Yard B, Spruyt-Gerritse M, Claas F, Thorogood J, Bruijn JA, Paape ME et al (1993) The clinical significance of allospecific antibodies against endothelial cells detected with an antibody-dependent cellular cytotoxicity assay for vascular rejection and graft loss after renal transplantation. Transplantation 55:1287–1293
64. Wasik M, Gradowska L, Lao M, Rowinska D, Orlowski T (1978) Study of antibody dependent cellular cytotoxicity (ADCC). II. ADCC activity in renal graft recipients and acute accelerated graft rejection. Arch Immunol Ther Exp (Warsz) 26:311–314
65. Miltenburg AM, Meijer-Paape ME, Weening JJ, Daha MR, van Es LA, van der Woude FJ (1989) Induction of antibody-dependent cellular cytotoxicity against endothelial cells by renal transplantation. Transplantation 48:681–688
66. Hirohashi T, Chase CM, Della Pelle P, Sebastian D, Alessandrini A, Madsen JC et al (2012) A novel pathway of chronic allograft rejection mediated by NK cells and alloantibody. Am J Transplant 12:313–321
67. Uehara S, Chase CM, Cornell LD, Madsen JC, Russell PS, Colvin RB (2007) Chronic cardiac transplant arteriopathy in mice: relationship of alloantibody, C4d deposition and neointimal fibrosis. Am J Transplant 7:57–65
68. Hidalgo LG, Sis B, Sellares J, Campbell PM, Mengel M, Einecke G et al (2010) NK cell transcripts and NK cells in kidney biopsies from patients with donor-specific antibodies: evidence for NK cell involvement in antibody-mediated rejection. Am J Transplant 10: 1812–1822
69. Narayanan K, Jaramillo A, Phelan DL, Mohanakumar T (2004) Pre-exposure to sub-saturating concentrations of HLA class I antibodies confers resistance to endothelial cells against antibody complement-mediated lysis by regulating Bad through the phosphatidylinositol 3-kinase/Akt pathway. Eur J Immunol 34:2303–2312
70. Narayanan K, Jendrisak MD, Phelan DL, Mohanakumar T (2006) HLA class I anti-

body mediated accommodation of endothelial cells via the activation of PI3K/cAMP dependent PKA pathway. Transpl Immunol 15:187–197

71. Iwasaki K, Miwa Y, Haneda M, Uchida K, Nakao A, Kobayashi T (2010) Significance of HLA class I antibody-induced antioxidant gene expression for endothelial cell protection against complement attack. Biochem Biophys Res Commun 391:1210–1215
72. Jin YP, Fishbein MC, Said JW, Jindra PT, Rajalingam R, Rozengurt E et al (2004) Anti-HLA class I antibody-mediated activation of the PI3K/Akt signaling pathway and induction of Bcl-2 and Bcl-xL expression in endothelial cells. Hum Immunol 65:291–302
73. Fukami N, Ramachandran S, Narayanan K, Liu W, Nath DS, Jendrisak M et al (2012) Mechanism of accommodation in a sensitized human leukocyte antigen transgenic murine cardiac transplant model. Transplantation 93:364–372
74. Coupel S, Leboeuf F, Boulday G, Soulillou JP, Charreau B (2004) RhoA activation mediates phosphatidylinositol 3-kinase-dependent proliferation of human vascular endothelial cells: an alloimmune mechanism of chronic allograft nephropathy. J Am Soc Nephrol 15:2429–2439
75. Jin YP, Korin Y, Zhang X, Jindra PT, Rozengurt E, Reed EF (2007) RNA interference elucidates the role of focal adhesion kinase in HLA class I-mediated focal adhesion complex formation and proliferation in human endothelial cells. J Immunol 178:7911–7922
76. Jin YP, Jindra PT, Gong KW, Lepin EJ, Reed EF (2005) Anti-HLA class I antibodies activate endothelial cells and promote chronic rejection. Transplantation 79:S19–S21
77. Jindra PT, Jin YP, Rozengurt E, Reed EF (2008) HLA class I antibody-mediated endothelial cell proliferation via the mTOR pathway. J Immunol 180:2357–2366
78. Jin YP, Singh RP, Du ZY, Rajasekaran AK, Rozengurt E, Reed EF (2002) Ligation of HLA class I molecules on endothelial cells induces phosphorylation of Src, paxillin, and focal adhesion kinase in an actin-dependent manner. J Immunol 168:5415–5423
79. Li F, Zhang X, Jin YP, Mulder A, Reed EF (2011) Antibody ligation of human leukocyte antigen class I molecules stimulates migration and proliferation of smooth muscle cells in a focal adhesion kinase-dependent manner. Hum Immunol 72:1150–1159
80. Galvani S, Auge N, Calise D, Thiers JC, Canivet C, Kamar N et al (2009) HLA class I antibodies provoke graft arteriosclerosis in human arteries transplanted into SCID/beige mice. Am J Transplant 9:2607–2614
81. Galvani S, Trayssac M, Auge N, Thiers JC, Calise D, Krell HW et al (2011) A key role for matrix metalloproteinases and neutral sphingomyelinase-2 in transplant vasculopathy triggered by anti-HLA antibody. Circulation 124:2725–2734
82. Ziegler ME, Souda P, Jin YP, Whitelegge JP, Reed EF (2012) Characterization of the endothelial cell cytoskeleton following HLA class I ligation. PLoS One 7:e29472
83. Lepin EJ, Jin YP, Barwe SP, Rozengurt E, Reed EF (2004) HLA class I signal transduction is dependent on Rho GTPase and ROK. Biochem Biophys Res Commun 323:213–217
84. Reznik SI, Jaramillo A, Zhang L, Patterson GA, Cooper JD, Mohanakumar T (2000) Anti-HLA antibody binding to HLA class I molecules induces proliferation of airway epithelial cells: a potential mechanism for bronchiolitis obliterans syndrome. J Thorac Cardiovasc Surg 119:39–45
85. Jindra PT, Hsueh A, Hong L, Gjertson D, Shen XD, Gao F et al (2008) Anti-MHC class I antibody activation of proliferation and survival signaling in murine cardiac allografts. J Immunol 180:2214–2224
86. Lepin EJ, Zhang Q, Zhang X, Jindra PT, Hong LS, Ayele P et al (2006) Phosphorylated S6 ribosomal protein: a novel biomarker of antibody-mediated rejection in heart allografts. Am J Transplant 6:1560–1571
87. Bian H, Harris PE, Mulder A, Reed EF (1997) Anti-HLA antibody ligation to HLA class I molecules expressed by endothelial cells stimulates tyrosine phosphorylation, inositol phosphate generation, and proliferation. Hum Immunol 53:90–97
88. Bian H, Harris PE, Reed EF (1998) Ligation of HLA class I molecules on smooth muscle cells with anti-HLA antibodies induces tyrosine phosphorylation, fibroblast growth factor receptor expression and cell proliferation. Int Immunol 10:1315–1323
89. Bian H, Reed EF (1999) Alloantibody-mediated class I signal transduction in endothelial cells and smooth muscle cells: enhancement by IFN-gamma and TNF-alpha. J Immunol 163:1010–1018
90. Bieri M, Oroszlan M, Farkas A, Ligeti N, Bieri J, Mohacsi P (2009) Anti-HLA I antibodies induce VEGF production by endothelial cells, which increases proliferation and paracellular permeability. Int J Biochem Cell Biol 41:2422–2430
91. Jaramillo A, Zhang L, Mohanakumar T (2001) Binding of anti-HLA class I antibodies to airway epithelial cells induces activation and growth factor production and indirectly upregulates lung fibroblast proliferation. J Heart Lung Transplant 20:166

92. Fishbein MC, Kobashigawa J (2004) Biopsy-negative cardiac transplant rejection: etiology, diagnosis, and therapy. Curr Opin Cardiol 19:166–169
93. Kitchens WH, Chase CM, Uehara S, Cornell LD, Colvin RB, Russell PS et al (2007) Macrophage depletion suppresses cardiac allograft vasculopathy in mice. Am J Transplant 7:2675–2682
94. Liu W, Xiao X, Demirci G, Madsen J, Li XC (2012) Innate NK cells and macrophages recognize and reject allogeneic nonself in vivo via different mechanisms. J Immunol 188:2703–2711
95. Lowenstein CJ, Morrell CN, Yamakuchi M (2005) Regulation of Weibel-Palade body exocytosis. Trends Cardiovasc Med 15:302–308
96. Yamakuchi M, Kirkiles-Smith NC, Ferlito M, Cameron SJ, Bao C, Fox-Talbot K et al (2007) Antibody to human leukocyte antigen triggers endothelial exocytosis. Proc Natl Acad Sci USA 104:1301–1306
97. Saini D, Angaswamy N, Tiriveedhi V, Fukami N, Ramachandran S, Hachem R et al (2012) Synergistic effect of antibodies to human leukocyte antigens and defensins in pathogenesis of bronchiolitis obliterans syndrome after human lung transplantation. J Heart Lung Transplant 29:1330–1336
98. Taylor PM, Rose ML, Yacoub MH (1989) Expression of MHC antigens in normal human lungs and transplanted lungs with obliterative bronchiolitis. Transplantation 48:506–510
99. Taylor PM, Rose ML, Yacoub MH, Pigott R (1992) Induction of vascular adhesion molecules during rejection of human cardiac allografts. Transplantation 54:451–457
100. Yamazaki S, Isobe M, Suzuki J, Tojo S, Horie S, Okubo Y et al (1998) Role of selectin-dependent adhesion in cardiac allograft rejection. J Heart Lung Transplant 17:1007–1016
101. Shi C, Feinberg MW, Zhang D, Patel A, Sim CU, Dong ZM et al (1999) Donor MHC and adhesion molecules in transplant arteriosclerosis. J Clin Invest 103:469–474
102. Raisky O, Morrison KJ, Obadia JF, McGregor J, Yacoub MH, Rose ML (2001) Acute rejection and cardiac graft vasculopathy in the absence of donor-derived ICAM-1 or P-selectin. J Heart Lung Transplant 20:340–349
103. Furuyama T, Komori K, Shimokawa H, Matsumoto Y, Uwatoku T, Hirano K et al (2006) Long-term inhibition of Rho kinase suppresses intimal thickening in autologous vein grafts in rabbits. J Vasc Surg 43:1249–1256
104. Hattori T, Shimokawa H, Higashi M, Hiroki J, Mukai Y, Kaibuchi K et al (2004) Long-term treatment with a specific Rho-kinase inhibitor suppresses cardiac allograft vasculopathy in mice. Circ Res 94:46–52
105. Ohki S, Iizuka K, Ishikawa S, Kano M, Dobashi K, Yoshii A et al (2001) A highly selective inhibitor of Rho-associated coiled-coil forming protein kinase, Y-27632, prolongs cardiac allograft survival of the BALB/c-to-C3H/He mouse model. J Heart Lung Transplant 20:956–963
106. Hiemann NE, Wellnhofer E, Lehmkuhl HB, Knosalla C, Hetzer R, Meyer R (2011) Everolimus prevents endomyocardial remodeling after heart transplantation. Transplantation 92:1165–1172
107. Chen Song S, Zhong S, Xiang Y, Li JH, Guo H, Wang WY et al (2011) Complement inhibition enables renal allograft accommodation and long-term engraftment in presensitized nonhuman primates. Am J Transplant 11:2057–2066
108. Stegall MD, Diwan T, Raghavaiah S, Cornell LD, Burns J, Dean PG et al (2011) Terminal complement inhibition decreases antibody-mediated rejection in sensitized renal transplant recipients. Am J Transplant 11: 2405–2413
109. Meng HL, Jin XB, Li XT, Wang HW, Lu JJ (2009) Impact of human leukocyte antigen matching and recipients' panel reactive antibodies on two-year outcome in presensitized renal allograft recipients. Chin Med J (Engl) 122:420–426
110. Muczynski KA, Ekle DM, Coder DM, Anderson SK (2003) Normal human kidney HLA-DR-expressing renal microvascular endothelial cells: characterization, isolation, and regulation of MHC class II expression. J Am Soc Nephrol 14:1336–1348
111. Muczynski KA, Cotner T, Anderson SK (2001) Unusual expression of human lymphocyte antigen class II in normal renal microvascular endothelium. Kidney Int 59:488–497
112. Geppert TD, Lipsky PE (1985) Antigen presentation by interferon-gamma-treated endothelial cells and fibroblasts: differential ability to function as antigen-presenting cells despite comparable Ia expression. J Immunol 135:3750–3762
113. McDouall RM, Yacoub M, Rose ML (1996) Isolation, culture, and characterisation of MHC class II-positive microvascular endothelial cells from the human heart. Microvasc Res 51:137–152
114. McDouall RM, Batten P, McCormack A, Yacoub MH, Rose ML (1997) MHC class II

expression on human heart microvascular endothelial cells: exquisite sensitivity to interferon-gamma and natural killer cells. Transplantation 64:1175–1180
115. Salom RN, Maguire JA, Hancock WW (1998) Endothelial activation and cytokine expression in human acute cardiac allograft rejection. Pathology 30:24–29
116. Deng MC, Bell S, Huie P, Pinto F, Hunt SA, Stinson EB et al (1995) Cardiac allograft vascular disease. Relationship to microvascular cell surface markers and inflammatory cell phenotypes on endomyocardial biopsy. Circulation 91:1647–1654
117. Hasegawa S, Becker G, Nagano H, Libby P, Mitchell RN (1998) Pattern of graft- and host-specific MHC class II expression in long-term murine cardiac allografts: origin of inflammatory and vascular wall cells. Am J Pathol 153:69–79
118. Wang YC, Mayne A, Sell KW, Ahmed-Ansari A (1990) The influence of MHC and non-MHC genes on the nature of murine cardiac allograft rejection. I. Kinetic analysis of mononuclear cell infiltrate and MHC-class I/ class II expression in donor tissue. Transplantation 50:313–324
119. Xu R, Burdick JF, Scott A, Beschorner WE, Adler W, Kittur DS (1992) Graft-specific MHC class II gene expression in response to allogeneic stimulus in heterotopic murine cardiac allografts. Immunology 75:361–365
120. Truman JP, Garban F, Choqueux C, Charron D, Mooney N (1996) HLA class II signaling mediates cellular activation and programmed cell death. Exp Hematol 24:1409–1415
121. Truman JP, Choqueux C, Charron D, Mooney N (1996) HLA class II molecule signal transduction leads to either apoptosis or activation via two different pathways. Cell Immunol 172:149–157
122. Truman JP, Ericson ML, Choqueux-Seebold CJ, Charron DJ, Mooney NA (1994) Lymphocyte programmed cell death is mediated via HLA class II DR. Int Immunol 6:887–896
123. Kato-Kogoe N, Ohyama H, Nishimura F, Meguro M, Yoshizawa S, Okada Y et al (2010) Fibroblasts stimulated via HLA-II molecules produce prostaglandin E(2) and regulate cytokine production from helper T cells. Lab Invest 90:1747–1756
124. Okada Y, Meguro M, Ohyama H, Yoshizawa S, Takeuchi-Hatanaka K, Kato N et al (2009) Human leukocyte histocompatibility antigen class II-induced cytokines from human gingival fibroblasts promote proliferation of human umbilical vein endothelial cells: potential association with enhanced angiogenesis in chronic periodontal inflammation. J Periodontal Res 44:103–109
125. Meguro M, Nishimura F, Ohyama H, Takashiba S, Murayama Y, Matsushita S (2003) Ligation of IFN-gamma-induced HLA-DR molecules on fibroblasts induces RANTES expression via c-Jun N-terminal kinase (JNK) pathway. Cytokine 22:107–115
126. Yoshizawa S, Meguro M, Ohyama H, Takeuchi-Hatanaka K, Matsushita S, Takashiba S et al (2007) Focal adhesion kinase mediates human leukocyte histocompatibility antigen class II-induced signaling in gingival fibroblasts. J Periodontal Res 42:572–579
127. Thaunat O, Graff-Dubois S, Fabien N, Duthey A, Attuil-Audenis V, Nicoletti A et al (2012) A stepwise breakdown of B-cell tolerance occurs within renal allografts during chronic rejection. Kidney Int 81: 207–219
128. Le Bas-Bernardet S, Hourmant M, Coupel S, Bignon JD, Soulillou JP, Charreau B (2003) Non-HLA-type endothelial cell reactive alloantibodies in pre-transplant sera of kidney recipients trigger apoptosis. Am J Transplant 3:167–177
129. Jackson AM, Lucas DP, Melancon JK, Desai NM (2011) Clinical relevance and IgG subclass determination of non-HLA antibodies identified using endothelial cell precursors isolated from donor blood. Transplantation 92:54–60
130. Perrey C, Brenchley PE, Johnson RW, Martin S (1998) An association between antibodies specific for endothelial cells and renal transplant failure. Transpl Immunol 6:101–106
131. Jaramillo A, Naziruddin B, Zhang L, Reznik SI, Smith MA, Aloush AA et al (2001) Activation of human airway epithelial cells by non-HLA antibodies developed after lung transplantation: a potential etiological factor for bronchiolitis obliterans syndrome. Transplantation 71:966–976
132. Ferry BL, Welsh KI, Dunn MJ, Law D, Proctor J, Chapel H et al (1997) Anti-cell surface endothelial antibodies in sera from cardiac and kidney transplant recipients: association with chronic rejection. Transpl Immunol 5:17–24
133. Qin Z, Lavingia B, Zou Y, Stastny P (2011) Antibodies against nucleolin in recipients of organ transplants. Transplantation 92:829–835
134. Bates RL, Frampton G, Rose ML, Murphy JJ (2003) High diversity of non-human leukocyte antigens in transplant-associated coronary artery disease. Transplantation 75: 1347–1350

135. Panigrahi A, Gupta N, Siddiqui JA, Margoob A, Bhowmik D, Guleria S et al (2007) Post transplant development of MICA and anti-HLA antibodies is associated with acute rejection episodes and renal allograft loss. Hum Immunol 68:362–367
136. Zou Y, Stastny P, Susal C, Dohler B, Opelz G (2007) Antibodies against MICA antigens and kidney-transplant rejection. N Engl J Med 357:1293–1300
137. Nath DS, Ilias Basha H, Tiriveedhi V, Alur C, Phelan D, Ewald GA et al (2010) Characterization of immune responses to cardiac self-antigens myosin and vimentin in human cardiac allograft recipients with antibody-mediated rejection and cardiac allograft vasculopathy. J Heart Lung Transplant 29:1277–1285
138. Dragun D (2008) Humoral responses directed against non-human leukocyte antigens in solid-organ transplantation. Transplantation 86:1019–1025
139. Acevedo LM, Barillas S, Weis SM, Gothert JR, Cheresh DA (2008) Semaphorin 3A suppresses VEGF-mediated angiogenesis yet acts as a vascular permeability factor. Blood 111:2674–2680
140. Ationu A (1998) Identification of endothelial antigens relevant to transplant coronary artery disease from a human endothelial cell cDNA expression library. Int J Mol Med 1:1007–1010
141. Linke AT, Marchant B, Marsh P, Frampton G, Murphy J, Rose ML (2001) Screening of a HUVEC cDNA library with transplant-associated coronary artery disease sera identifies RPL7 as a candidate autoantigen associated with this disease. Clin Exp Immunol 126:173–179
142. Kalache S, Dinavahi R, Pinney S, Mehrotra A, Cunningham MW, Heeger PS (2011) Anticardiac myosin immunity and chronic allograft vasculopathy in heart transplant recipients. J Immunol 187:1023–1030
143. Jurcevic S, Ainsworth ME, Pomerance A, Smith JD, Robinson DR, Dunn MJ et al (2001) Antivimentin antibodies are an independent predictor of transplant-associated coronary artery disease after cardiac transplantation. Transplantation 71:886–892
144. Alvarez-Marquez A, Aguilera I, Gentil MA, Caro JL, Bernal G, Fernandez Alonso J et al (2009) Donor-specific antibodies against HLA, MICA, and GSTT1 in patients with allograft rejection and C4d deposition in renal biopsies. Transplantation 87:94–99
145. Alvarez-Marquez A, Aguilera I, Blanco RM, Pascual D, Encarnacion-Carrizosa M, Alvarez-Lopez MR et al (2008) Positive association of anticytoskeletal endothelial cell antibodies and cardiac allograft rejection. Hum Immunol 69:143–148
146. Dragun D, Muller DN, Brasen JH, Fritsche L, Nieminen-Kelha M, Dechend R et al (2005) Angiotensin II type 1-receptor activating antibodies in renal-allograft rejection. N Engl J Med 352:558–569
147. Walther T, Jank A, Heringer-Walther S, Horn LC, Stepan H (2008) Angiotensin II type 1 receptor has impact on murine placentation. Placenta 29:905–909
148. Walther T, Stepan H (2007) Agonist autoantibodies against the angiotensin AT1 receptor in renal and hypertensive disorders. Curr Hypertens Rep 9:128–132
149. Papa ND, Raschi E, Moroni G, Panzeri P, Borghi MO, Ponticelli C et al (1999) Anti-endothelial cell IgG fractions from systemic lupus erythematosus patients bind to human endothelial cells and induce a pro-adhesive and a pro-inflammatory phenotype in vitro. Lupus 8:423–429
150. Muller Kobold AC, van Wijk RT, Franssen CF, Molema G, Kallenberg CG, Tervaert JW (1999) In vitro up-regulation of E-selectin and induction of interleukin-6 in endothelial cells by autoantibodies in Wegener's granulomatosis and microscopic polyangiitis. Clin Exp Rheumatol 17:433–440
151. Del Papa N, Guidali L, Sironi M, Shoenfeld Y, Mantovani A, Tincani A et al (1996) Anti-endothelial cell IgG antibodies from patients with Wegener's granulomatosis bind to human endothelial cells in vitro and induce adhesion molecule expression and cytokine secretion. Arthritis Rheum 39:758–766
152. Derhaag JG, Duijvestijn AM, Damoiseaux JG, van Breda Vriesman PJ (2000) Effects of antibody reactivity to major histocompatibility complex (MHC) and non-MHC alloantigens on graft endothelial cells in heart allograft rejection. Transplantation 69:1899–1906
153. Diujvestijn AM, Derhaag JG, van Breda Vriesman PJ (2000) Complement activation by anti-endothelial cell antibodies in MHC-mismatched and MHC-matched heart allograft rejection: anti-MHC-, but not anti non-MHC alloantibodies are effective in complement activation. Transpl Int 13:363–371
154. Mahesh B, Leong HS, McCormack A, Sarathchandra P, Holder A, Rose ML (2007) Autoantibodies to vimentin cause accelerated rejection of cardiac allografts. Am J Pathol 170:1415–1427
155. Tambur AR, Pamboukian SV, Costanzo MR, Herrera ND, Dunlap S, Montpetit M et al (2005) The presence of HLA-directed antibodies after heart transplantation is

associated with poor allograft outcome. Transplantation 80:1019–1025
156. Lau CL, Palmer SM, Posther KE, Howell DN, Reinsmoen NL, Massey HT et al (2000) Influence of panel-reactive antibodies on posttransplant outcomes in lung transplant recipients. Ann Thorac Surg 69:1520–1524
157. Angaswamy N, Saini D, Ramachandran S, Nath DS, Phelan D, Hachem R et al (2010) Development of antibodies to human leukocyte antigen precedes development of antibodies to major histocompatibility class I-related chain A and are significantly associated with development of chronic rejection after human lung transplantation. Hum Immunol 71:560–565
158. Panigrahi A, Siddiqui JA, Rai A, Margoob A, Khaira A, Bhowmik D et al (2007) Allosensitization to HLA and MICA is an important measure of renal graft outcome. Clin Transpl 211–217
159. Panigrahi A, Gupta N, Siddiqui JA, Margoob A, Bhowmik D, Guleria S et al (2007) Monitoring of anti-HLA and anti-Major histocompatibility complex class I related chain A antibodies in living related renal donor transplantation. Transplant Proc 39: 759–760

Chapter 3

Cell Mediated Rejection

Kathryn J. Wood, Masaaki Zaitsu, and Ryoichi Goto

Abstract

Rejection is the major barrier to successful transplantation and usually results from the integration of multiple mechanisms. Activation of elements of the innate immune system, triggered as a consequence of tissue injury sustained during cell isolation or organ retrieval as well as ischemia–reperfusion, will initiate and amplify the adaptive response. For cell mediated rejection, T cells require multiple signals for activation, the minimum being two signals; antigen recognition and costimulation. The majority of B cells require help from T cells to initiate alloantibody production. Antibodies reactive to donor HLA molecules, minor histocompatibility antigens, endothelial cells, red blood cells, or autoantigens can trigger or contribute to rejection early as well as late after transplantation.

Key words Transplantation, Allograft, T cell, B cell, Alloantibody, Cytotoxicity, Innate, Adaptive

1 Tissue Injury

The physical process of removing, transplanting, and reperfusing tissue or organs initiates injury and stress responses that inevitably lead to changes in gene and protein expression [1–3] that impact the immunological response [4]. In the case of deceased organ donors some of these changes are also a direct consequence of brain or cardiac death [5].

Tissue injury results in the expression of damage associated molecular patterns (DAMPS) by cells within the transplanted organ or tissue. DAMPS can be detected by cells of the innate immune system as they express invariant pathogen associated pattern recognition receptors (PRRs) enabling them to respond to injured tissues. Examples of DAMPS include reactive oxygen species, heat shock proteins, heparin sulfate, high mobility group box (HMBG)-1. When DAMPS bind to PRRs it results in the potent activation of the inflammasome [6], upregulating gene transcription and the production of inflammatory mediators that stimulate adaptive immunity. It is important to remember that activation of the innate immune system in the early phase post-transplant is

Andrea A. Zachary and Mary S. Leffell (eds.), *Transplantation Immunology: Methods and Protocols, Second Edition*, Methods in Molecular Biology, vol. 1034, DOI 10.1007/978-1-62703-493-7_3, © Springer Science+Business Media, LLC 2013

largely in response to tissue damage irrespective of whether or not there is a genetic difference between the donor and recipient [7]. Obviously, the majority of donors and recipients are mismatched for major and/or minor histocompatibility antigens; thus, the response to tissue injury and the attendant inflammation will stimulate the migration of donor derived antigen presenting cells (APCs), dendritic cells (DCs) from the transplant to recipient lymphoid tissue where they will encounter T cells [8, 9].

2 Allorecognition and T Cell Activation

Recognition of alloantigen by T cells is the first step in the adaptive immune response to a transplant in a recipient receiving a mismatched cell or solid organ graft who does not have preformed anti-donor antibodies. A high precursor frequency of T cells able to respond to mismatched major histocompatibility complex (MHC) molecules exists in every individual. This results from a combination of specific recognition of alloantigens or alloantigenic peptides by T cells as well as through cross-reactivity of T cells specific for other peptide–MHC complexes with alloantigen. miH antigens are peptides derived from a wide variety of proteins from genes encoded throughout the genome. They can be presented as peptides by either host or recipient derived MHC molecules. miH antigens are not necessarily expressed by cells of the immune system, in other words they can be tissue derived [10].

Recipient T cells can respond to donor alloantigen via three distinct pathways [11]. Direct allorecognition is the interaction of the T cell receptor (TCR) with intact allogeneic MHC–peptide complexes presented by donor derived APCs. Indirect allorecognition occurs when peptides derived from donor MHC or miH antigen are degraded by antigen processing pathways and presented by recipient APCs to T cells. Semi-direct allorecognition is the capture of donor MHC–peptide complexes by host APCs as a consequence of the exchange of fragments of cell membrane containing donor MHC molecules between cells that contact each other.

Antigen presentation via the direct pathway of allorecognition plays a dominant role in initiating the adaptive immune response to an MHC mismatched transplant. This pathway is triggered predominantly by the migration of donor derived passenger leukocytes as mentioned above. However, since a finite number of passenger leukocytes are usually present in a transplanted organ or tissue, the role of the direct pathway in allograft rejection is thought to diminish with time. Other types of donor cells, such as endothelial cells, can also stimulate direct pathway T cells under some conditions. Donor endothelial cells can persist long term after transplantation thereby stimulating direct allorecognition in the longer term. The indirect pathway of allorecognition is available for antigen presentation for as long as the graft continues to function and therefore is thought to become the dominant mode of allorecognition in the longer term after transplantation. The significance of the semi-direct pathway of allorecognition in the context of cellular rejection remains to be elucidated.

2.1 Costimulation

When a T cell recognizes alloantigen by any of the three pathways outlined above, antigen specific signals are delivered via the TCR-CD3 complex—often referred to collectively as signal 1. On their own, these signals are not sufficient to activate naïve T cells; second signals are also required and are provided by the interaction of costimulatory molecules with their ligands on both the T cell and APC. Costimulatory molecules can be divided into families [12]: immunoglobulin superfamily members that include B7 molecules and the T cell costimulatory molecule CD28 [13], and the tumor necrosis factor (TNF)/tumor necrosis factor receptor (TNFR) family that includes CD40 expressed by APC and CD154 (CD40L) expressed by T cells [14].

CD28 is expressed by T cells and binds members of the B7 family, CD80 and CD86 on APCs. CD86 is constitutively expressed at low levels and rapidly upregulated in response to cytokines. Signaling via CD28 lowers the threshold for T cell activation, increases the stability of IL-2 mRNA and therefore the expression of IL-2 protein. In this way costimulation through CD28 promotes T cell proliferation and the resistance of T cells to activation induced cell death. During an immune response, activated T cells upregulate expression of CD152 (CTLA-4), a molecule that has close homology to CD28, that can also bind to CD80 and CD86. The difference between CD152 and CD28 is the affinity with which each molecule binds B7 family members. CD152 has a binding affinity 10–20 times greater than that of CD28. Upregulation of CD152 results in the attenuation, rather than amplification, of an immune response. This feature of CD152 was demonstrated in CD152 knockout mice that when exposed to a wide range of environmental antigens developed a fatal disorder characterized by massive proliferation of lymphocytes [15].

Another effect of CD28 signaling during T cell activation is to upregulate expression of other costimulatory molecules that can deliver additional signals to the responding T cell. For example, CD154 (CD40L) is the ligand for CD40 expressed by APCs, including B cells. In addition to delivering a positive signal to the T cell, CD40–CD154 ligation activates APCs leading to increased expression of B7 family molecules. In this way it acts as an amplification mechanism for T cell activation.

The outcome of T cell–APC interaction is determined by integrating information from many pathways, including the avidity of the cognate TCR–MHC–peptide interaction and the balance of positive (CD28; CD154) and negative signals (CD152, PD1) delivered by the costimulatory molecules present on the surface of the participating cells, as well as the small soluble molecules, cytokines that result from tissue injury, antigen presenting cells, and T cells.

3 T Cell Differentiation

Following activation, depending on the microenvironment and additional signals T cells receive, they will be driven to differentiate into cells that have different cytokine signatures and functional capabilities. $CD4^+$ class II restricted T cells usually acquire helper function (Th). Different Th subsets exist, each with a unique transcription factor and cytokine signature referred to as Th1, Th2, Th17, Th9, and Tfh (follicular helper) populations. $CD8^+$ class I restricted T cells are usually cytotoxic and can also be divided into subsets with Tc1 and Tc2 being the best described, although IL-17 producing $CD8^+$ cells have been reported [16].

Multiple factors influence T cell differentiation following activation and costimulation, including the immune status of the recipient at the time of transplantation, the degree of ischemia–reperfusion injury, the degree of donor recipient mismatch or antigen load and the immunosuppressive drug regimen being used. All of these elements will impact the combination of chemokines and cytokines released by the transplanted tissue, the migration of donor derived passenger leukocytes to the secondary lymphoid tissues and the recruitment of recipient leukocytes. For example, DAMPS produced as a result of ischemia-reperfusion injury will trigger TLR signaling stimulating APCs to secrete IL-12 which drives the differentiation of Th1 cells that express the transcription factor Tbet and secrete IFNγ, as well as activating other cell populations, including NK cells. For the differentiation of Th2 cells, IL-4 is required in the microenvironment at the time of T cell activation. This leads to the development of T cells that express the transcription factor GATA-3^+ T cells that secrete IL-4 themselves and attract eosinophils to the graft. Th2 cells have been shown to be capable of initiating rejection in their own right [17]. Th17 cells are a relatively recently described subset of T cells. TGFβ, IL-6, IL1β, and IL-23 have been implicated in Th17 differentiation, although the precise influence of each mediator is both species and concentration dependent [18, 19]. IL-23 and IL-21 signaling upregulates the transcription factor *RORγT* that directs IL-17 transcription by the T cell. IL-17 is pro-inflammatory in vivo, predominantly stimulating granulopoiesis and neutrophil migration to the inflammatory site [20]. There is evidence that Th17 cells and IL-17 producing $CD8^+$ T cells have the capacity to play a role in rejection, particularly in the absence of a Th1 response [21–23].

Th9 differentiation requires TGFβ and IL-4 to present in the microenvironment during activation. As their name suggests Th9 cells secrete IL-9 and they recruit mast cells. Tfh cells are found in lymph nodes and are important for B cell maturation, most likely contributing to the process of antibody mediated rejection. Tfh require IL-21 for differentiation and express the transcription factor bcl-6.

In addition to T cells that promote rejection or GvHD, there are also populations of T cells that regulate or control immune responsiveness, so-called regulatory or suppressor T cells (Treg) [24–26]. Treg are either selected in the thymus, so-called naturally occurring or thymus derived Treg or can be induced in the presence of antigen and a permissive microenvironment in the periphery, so-called induced or adaptive Treg. Treg exhibit sustained expression of the transcription factor Foxp3 [27]. Thymus derived Treg are present in all individuals at the time of transplantation, but in the face of responses to donor major and minor histocompatibility antigens are not sufficient in number or potency to control the response in their own right. As the immune system responds to antigen, induced Treg will be generated. The quantity and quality of Treg induced will depend on many variables including the antigen load and immunosuppression.

4 B Cell Activation and Function

B cells are generally thought of as antibody secreting cells, but it is important to remember that they are a multifunctional leukocyte population that can play different roles in the cellular immune response to an allograft. B cells can act as antigen presenting cells as they express MHC and costimulatory molecules including CD40 [28]. As APC, B cells engage T cells via their TCR and costimulatory molecules, creating a cell cluster that enables cytokines secreted by the T cell to influence B cell activation, differentiation, and antibody production. B cells also express complement receptors and can therefore interact with complement coated damaged cells, facilitating antigen presentation and therefore regulation of adaptive immunity [29].

The majority of B cells are dependent on T cell help for activation and antibody production and encounter antigen in the secondary lymphoid tissue [30]. Antibody mediated rejection is now well recognized in clinical transplantation. Interestingly, B cells themselves may be able to contribute to the rejection process as B cells, B cell clusters, and B cell transcripts have been found in rejecting allografts [31–35]. However, the presence of intragraft B cells may not always be harmful [36] and B cells have been described as being present in immunosuppression free transplant recipients that exhibit operational tolerance to donor alloantigens

[37–39]. Thus, B cells may also have the ability to regulate the alloimmune response depending on the specific circumstances in individual transplant recipients.

5 Mechanisms of Graft Destruction

Although the initiation of the adaptive immune response that results in allograft rejection is critically dependent on T cell recognition of alloantigen (see above), many components of the immune system can subsequently contribute to the destruction of the transplanted tissue. Additional factors, including many already mentioned, modify the character of the immune response to an individual allograft, including the ischemia–reperfusion injury, the organ or tissue transplanted, the site of transplantation, the histocompatibility match/mismatch, the immune status of the recipient at the time of transplantation, and of course, a topic not covered in this review, immunosuppression.

5.1 A Role for the Innate Immune System in Mediating Graft Damage

As well as creating an environment that facilitates activation of the adaptive immune system, the innate immune system represents a "preformed" set of mechanisms that can mediate some graft damage in their own right [40]. While in most cases, these mechanisms will not be sufficient to elicit rejection in the absence of adaptive immunity, they will contribute to the overall process and importantly the activity of the components of the innate immunity will be augmented in the presence of an adaptive immune response.

Initially, macrophages and other phagocytic cells when activated by recognizing DAMPS through PRRs, will contribute to the local inflammatory environment. One way of thinking of this is that these processes light up the graft as available for immune attack or destruction.

Macrophages are present in inflammatory infiltrates following transplantation as they are recruited to the graft in response to proinflammatory cytokines such as IL-1 and IL-6. Macrophages can produce both reactive oxygen species and potent degradative enzymes that have the potential to cause injury to the vascular endothelium and parenchyma. They can produce growth factors such as transforming growth factor beta (TGF-β), platelet-derived growth factor (PDGF), and insulin-like growth factor-1 (IGF-1), and chemokines such as MIG/CXCL9 and RANTES/CCL5. Macrophages have been shown to contribute to acute and chronic allograft rejection [41].

Neutrophils are widely implicated in tissue injury, particularly when homeostasis is perturbed by stress or ischemia [42]. Neutrophils are short-lived cells, circulating half-life 6–8 h, and are produced in large numbers every day—of the order of up to 10^{11} cells/day. Neutrophils circulate in the blood as dormant cells, but at sites of infection or in the case of a transplant, endothelial cells capture bypassing neutrophils and guide them through the endothelial cell lining whereby they are activated. Tight regulation of neutrophils is vital as they have the ability to damage cells and are widely implicated in tissue injury, including damage to the graft. Neutrophils are recruited to a graft as part of the innate response early post-transplant as well as following T cell activation, particularly in response to IL-17 production. Once involved, neutrophils mediate tissue injury in part by secreting chemokines CXCL1, 2, 3, and 8, binding to other cells, including endothelial cells as a consequence of adhesion molecules, β_2 integrins, interacting with endothelial cell ICAM-1, and through degranulation and secretion of heparin-binding protein. Neutrophils also generate reactive oxygen species that induce vascular leakage.

Later in the rejection process, these innate cells have the capacity to act as antigen presenting cells augmenting T cell activation. They can bind alloantibody secreted by activated B cells via Fc receptors expressed at the cell surface that will either further augment cellular activation or trigger antibody dependent cellular cytotoxicity (ADCC), or bind immune complexes or cells coated with complement via complement receptors (CR), a process known as opsonization. This results in the ingestion of damaged or necrotic donor tissue that removes antigen but also augments antigen presentation. Each of these functions acts to amplify the response or clear antigen from the system.

Activated complement components constitute a proteolytic cascade present in the plasma. This generates a range of effector molecules that can damage the graft in their own right, facilitate antigen presentation and integrate the innate and adaptive immune response [43]. Interestingly, some complement components are synthesized by the kidney and the liver; thus, for some types of transplant the donor tissue will produce complement components locally in the graft potentially amplifying the early response to the transplant.

Natural killer (NK) cells are large granular lymphocytes that are able to kill virus infected or mutated host cells in an identical manner to cytotoxic $CD8^+$ lymphocytes (see below) and release proinflammatory mediators. They express a unique recognition system that involves activating and inhibitory receptors that enables them to detect and respond to nonself [44]. The inhibitory NK cell receptors include killer-cell immunoglobulin-like receptors (KIRs) and NKG2A/CD94 whose ligands are self MHC class I molecules. Thus, NK cells can recognize when self MHC class I molecules are absent, so-called “missing self”, triggering NK cell activation. NK cells have been shown to be capable of rejecting bone marrow cells that express very low levels of MHC class I molecules, and NK cells with the ability to kill target cells ex vivo can be found in rejecting allografts, with evidence that they can play a critical role in acute and chronic rejection [40, 45].

5.2 Leukocyte Recruitment to the Graft

The inflammatory processes at the site of transplantation result in the production of chemokines and upregulation of chemokine receptor expression by activated leukocytes, including macrophages, neutrophils, NK cells (mentioned above) as well as T cells and B cells, enabling them to migrate along the chemoattractant gradient to reach the graft tissue [46]. Traffic of naïve lymphocytes is usually restricted to recirculation between the blood and lymphatic systems, but, once primed in the secondary lymphoid tissues (see above), activated T and B cells can migrate into tissues, in this case the transplanted tissue.

Inflammatory signals, including cytokines, chemokines, and complement components, produced locally within the graft in the early post-transplant period affect blood vessels in the transplant causing vasodilation and endothelial activation. Activated endothelial cells rapidly externalize preformed granules called Weibel–Palade bodies that contain the adhesion molecule P-selectin. At the same time chemokines released from the graft become tethered to the endothelium. These alterations in endothelial surface markers advertise to passing leukocytes that an inflammatory process is occurring in the neighboring tissue. Leukocytes are usually conveyed within the fast laminar flow at the center of blood vessels, but once activated leukocytes reach post-capillary venules in proximity to the graft, they are able to leave this rapid flow and move towards the edge of the vessel. This occurs in response to the local chemokine gradient and is assisted by the slower blood flow in the vasodilated blood vessels near the graft. Leukocyte extravasation is a multistep process. Initially, low affinity interactions develop between endothelial P-selectin and sialyl-Lewis^X moieties that are present on the surface of activated leukocytes. These interactions continually form and break down and the leukocyte "rolls" along the endothelial surface. If chemokines are present on the endothelial surface, conformational changes in leukocyte integrin molecules occur that allow them to bind other endothelial adhesion molecules such as ICAM-1. These higher affinity interactions cause arrest of the leukocyte on the endothelial surface allowing it to commence extravasation. Having entered the tissues the activated leukocytes continue to migrate along chemokine gradients in order to invade the graft.

5.3 Cytotoxic T Cells

Naïve MHC class I restricted CD8$^+$ cytotoxic T cells (CTLs) are activated either as a result of the formation of a three cell cluster with the helper cell and the antigen presenting cell, or as a result of an activated CD4$^+$ T helper cell "licensing" the antigen presenting cell to activate CTLs. CD40/CD154 costimulatory signals play an important role in this process. Activated CTLs migrate to the graft site where they are able to identify their target cells by recognition of allogeneic class I MHC molecules. Once they have located their target cell they release granules containing cytotoxic molecules such as perforin and granzyme B, as well as upregulating cell surface expression of Fas ligand (FasL) and secreting soluble mediators such as TNFα. In kidney transplant recipients experiencing rejection, increased levels of perforin and granzyme B mRNA have been found in the urine [47]. Target cell killing by CTLs is achieved by the induction of apoptosis. Perforins polymerize and insert into the target cell membrane, forming a pore that facilitates the entry of granzyme B and other compounds into the cell. Granzyme B is a protease that is able to initiate apoptosis by several mechanisms including activation of caspase cascades. Binding of FasL to Fas on the target cell surface is also able to trigger apoptosis by activating caspases.

6 B Cells and Antibody Mediated Rejection

The antigenic targets of alloantibodies are mismatched MHC molecules, but antibodies that recognize miH, endothelial cell, blood group antigens, and autoantigens also contribute to rejection [48]. Antibody mediated rejection is demonstrated most dramatically if patients have preformed alloantibodies at the time of transplantation, where hyperacute rejection frequently results in graft destruction within minutes of organ reperfusion. In this situation the antibodies (which are usually directed at allogeneic MHC molecules, ABO blood group antigens or antigens expressed on graft endothelium, that include the angiotensin type 1 receptor) cause local activation of the coagulation and complement cascades resulting in extensive thrombosis within the vascular supply to the graft culminating in infarction. Although modern crossmatch techniques have made hyperacute rejection through HLA reactive antibodies extremely rare, the humoral arm of the immune system is increasingly being implicated in the pathogenesis of acute rejection episodes as well as chronic allograft damage [34, 48].

Anti-donor antibodies that form after transplantation can trigger rejection within days after transplantation but they can also contribute to late graft loss [49]. The mechanism of antibody-mediated damage is most likely primarily, but not exclusively, via complement fixation. Antibodies can also elicit damage to the graft through other mechanisms. For example, NK cells and macrophages express receptors that bind to the Fc region of antibodies. This stimulates these cells to kill target cells through ADCC providing a second mechanism by which alloantibodies can induce donor cell death.

7 Immunological Memory and Its Impact on Cell Mediated Rejection

Following primary antigen exposure, long lived antigen-specific memory T and B cells are generated that are able to deliver a more rapid and higher magnitude immune response if the same antigen is encountered on a subsequent occasion. Memory cells have a reduced activation threshold and are less dependent on costimulation [50]. As a result they are able to upregulate effector function and cytokine secretion more rapidly than naïve lymphocytes. With increasing age the proportion of memory T cells within an individual's peripheral T cell pool increases reflecting cumulative antigen exposure and can be as high as 50 % in adult humans.

While the generation of immunological memory is beneficial for protection against infectious pathogens, in transplantation the presence of allospecific memory produces an accelerated or "second-set" rejection response. In clinical transplantation, evidence of prior sensitization to donor antigens is associated with increased risk of acute rejection episodes and premature graft failure. Memory-type responses towards alloantigens are frequently a result of exposure to alloantigens at the time of a previous blood transfusion, pregnancy or transplant. However, it is now recognized that memory-type responses may also be generated as a consequence of antigen receptor cross-reactivity (heterologous immunity) or by homeostatic proliferation of lymphocytes following an episode of lymphopenia such as are induced in transplant recipients by administration of leukocyte depleting agents.

Sequential viral infections in mice were found to generate populations of alloreactive memory-phenotype T cells [51]. Thus, heterologous immunity will result in some recipients, maybe the majority, having populations of memory T cells that can cross-react with donor alloantigen resulting in memory-phenotype responses towards the graft without prior sensitization to donor alloantigen.

The size of the peripheral T cell pool, as well as the relative ratios of $CD4^+$:$CD8^+$ and naïve:memory cells, are tightly regulated in vivo by homeostatic mechanisms. A consequence of this is that reduction of the overall T cell population, either during illness or following induction therapy in transplantation, induces the residual T cells to proliferate, whether or not cognate antigen is present. A proportion of T cells undergoing homeostatic proliferation in response to lymphopenia differentiate into a phenotype that resembles that of antigen-experienced or memory T cells. This includes downregulation of CD62L (L-selectin), an adhesion molecule that is highly expressed on naïve T cells and is necessary for entry into lymph nodes via high endothelial venules, and upregulation of CD44, an adhesion molecule that binds to hyaluronic acid and enables activated or memory-phenotype T cells to leave the vascular system and enter peripheral tissues. These T cells also exhibit memory T cell-like behavior as they are less dependent on costimulation via CD28 and, as a result have a reduced activation threshold. Moreover, following activation their capacity to secrete cytokines, proliferate, and manifest effector functions is enhanced compared to naïve T cells.

Acknowledgments

The work from the authors' own laboratory described in this review was supported by grants from The Wellcome Trust, Medical Research Council, British Heart Foundation, Kidney Research UK, Garfield Weston Trust, and European Union through the Indices of Tolerance, RISET, OPTISTEM, TRIAD, and BioDRIM projects.

References

1. Pallet N, Fougeray S, Beaune P, Legendre C, Thervet E, Anglicheau D (2009) Endoplasmic reticulum stress: an unrecognized actor in solid organ transplantation. Transplantation 88(5):605–613. doi:10.1097/TP.0b013e3181b22cec
2. Mühlberger I, Perco P, Fechete R, Mayer B, Oberbauer R (2009) Biomarkers in renal transplantation ischemia reperfusion injury. Transplantation 88(3S):S14–S19. doi:10.1097/TP.0b013e3181af65b5
3. Famulski KS, Broderick G, Einecke G, Hay K, Cruz J, Sis B et al (2007) Transcriptome analysis reveals heterogeneity in the injury response of kidney transplants. Am J Transplant 7(11):2483–2495
4. Kim IK, Bedi DS, Denecke C, Ge X, Tullius SG (2008) Impact of innate and adaptive immunity on rejection and tolerance. Transplantation 86(7):889–894. doi:10.1097/TP.0b013e318186ac4a
5. Wilhelm MJ, Pratschke J, Beato F, Taal M, Kusaka M, Hancock WW et al (2000) Activation of the heart by donor brain death accelerates acute rejection after transplantation. Circulation 102(19):2426–2433
6. Ogura Y, Sutterwala FS, Flavell RA (2006) The inflammasome: first line of the immune response to cell stress. Cell 126(4):659–662
7. Carvalho-Gaspar M, Billing JS, Spriewald BM, Wood KJ (2005) Chemokine gene expression during allograft rejection: comparison of two quantitative PCR techniques. J Immunol Methods 301(1–2):41–52
8. Larsen C, Morris P, Austyn J (1990) Migration of dendritic leukocytes form cardiac allografts into host spleens: a novel pathway for initiation of rejection. J Exp Med 171:307–314
9. van Kooten C, Lombardi G, Gelderman KA, Sagoo P, Buckland M, Lechler R et al (2011) Dendritic cells as a tool to induce transplantation tolerance: obstacles and opportunities. Transplantation 91(1):2–7. doi:10.1097/TP.0b013e31820263b3
10. Dierselhuis M, Goulmy E (2009) The relevance of minor histocompatibility antigens in solid organ transplantation. Curr Opin Organ Transplant 14(4):419–425. doi:10.1097/MOT.0b013e32832d399c
11. Afzali B, Lombardi G, Lechler RI (2008) Pathways of major histocompatibility complex allorecognition. Curr Opin Organ Transplant 13(4):438–444. doi:10.1097/MOT.0b013e328309ee31
12. Kinnear G, Jones ND, Wood KJ (2013) Costimulation blockade: current perspectives and implications for therapy. Transplantation 95(4):527–535
13. Greenwald RJ, Freeman GJ, Sharpe AH (2005) The B7 family revisited. Annu Rev Immunol 23(1):515–548
14. Li XC, Rothstein DM, Sayegh MH (2009) Costimulatory pathways in transplantation: challenges and new developments. Immunol Rev 229(1):271–293
15. Walunas T, Lenschow D, Bakker C, Linsley P, Freeman G, Green J et al (1994) CTLA-4 can function as a negative regulator of T cell activation. Immunity 1:405–413
16. Burrell BE, Bishop DK (2010) Th17 cells and transplant acceptance. Transplantation 90(9):945–948. doi:10.1097/TP.0b013e3181f5c3de

17. Barbara J, Turvery S, Kingsley C, Spriewald B, Hara M, Witzke O et al (2000) Islet allograft rejection can be mediated by CD4+, alloantigen experienced direct pathway T cells or TH1 and TH2 cytokine phenotype. Transplantation 70:1641–1649
18. Chen Y, Wood KJ (2007) Interleukin-23 and TH17 cells in transplantation immunity: does 23+17 equal rejection? Transplantation 84: 1071–1074
19. Heidt S, San Segundo D, Chadha R, Wood KJ (2010) The impact of Th17 cells on transplant rejection and the induction of tolerance. Curr Opin Organ Transplant 15(4):456–461. doi:10.1097/MOT.0b013e32833b9bfb
20. Chadha R, Heidt S, Wood KJ (2011) Th17: contributors to allograft rejection and a barrier to the induction of transplantation tolerance? Transplantation 91(9):939–945
21. Yuan X, Paez-Cortez J, Schmitt-Knosalla I, D'Addio F, Mfarrej B, Donnarumma M et al (2008) A novel role of CD4 Th17 cells in mediating cardiac allograft rejection and vasculopathy. J Exp Med 205(13):3133–3144
22. Faust SM, Lu G, Marini BL, Zou W, Gordon D, Iwakura Y et al (2009) Role of T cell TGFβ signaling and IL-17 in allograft acceptance and fibrosis associated with chronic rejection. J Immunol 183(11):7297–7306
23. Chadha R, Heidt S, Jones ND, Wood KJ (2011) Th17: contributors to allograft rejection and a barrier to the induction of transplantation tolerance? Transplantation 91(9):939–945. doi:10.1097/TP.0b013e3182126eeb
24. Long E, Wood KJ (2009) Regulatory T cells in transplantation: transferring mouse studies to the clinic. Transplantation 88(9):1050–1056
25. Wood KJ, Sakaguchi S (2003) Regulatory T cells in transplantation tolerance. Nat Rev Immunol 3:199–210
26. Wood KJ, Bushell A, Hester J (2012) Regulatory immune cells in transplantation. Nat Rev Immunol 12(6):417–430
27. Long E, Wood KJ (2007) Understanding FOXP3: progress towards achieving transplantation tolerance. Transplantation 84:459–461
28. Tarlinton DM, Batista F, Smith KGC (2008) The B-cell response to protein antigens in immunity and transplantation. Transplantation 85(12):1698–1704. doi:10.097/TP.0b013e3181777a39
29. Carroll MC (2004) The complement system in regulation of adaptive immunity. Nat Immunol 5(10):981–986
30. Cyster JG (2010) B cell follicles and antigen encounters of the third kind. Nat Immunol 11(11):989–996
31. Sarwal M, Chua M, Kambham N (2003) Molecular heterogeneity in acute renal allograft rejection identified by DNA microarray profiling. N Engl J Med 349:125
32. Naesens M, Zarkhin V, Kambham N, Li L, Kwok S, Hsieh S et al (2008) Evaluation of intra-graft B-cell subsets in renal allograft rejection: 664. Transplantation 86(2S):233–234. doi:10.1097/01.tp.0000332191.92932.c7
33. Zarkhin V, Li L, Sarwal M (2008) To B or not to B? B-cells and graft rejection. Transplantation 85(12):1705–1714. doi:10.097/TP.0b013e318177793e
34. Kwun J, Knechtle SJ (2009) Overcoming chronic rejection-can it B? Transplantation 88(8):955–961. doi:10.1097/TP.0b013e3181b96646
35. Thaunat O (2011) Pathophysiologic significance of B-cell clusters in chronically rejected grafts. Transplantation 92(2):121–126. doi:10.1097/TP.0b013e31821f74fe
36. Scheepstra C, Bemelman FJ, van der Loos C, Rowshani AT, van Donselaar-Van der Pant KA, Idu MM et al (2008) B cells in cluster or in a scattered pattern do not correlate with clinical outcome of renal allograft rejection. Transplantation 86(6):772–778. doi:10.1097/TP.0b013e3181860a74
37. Sagoo P, Perucha E, Sawitzki B, Tomiuk S, Stephens DA, Miqueu P et al (2010) Development of a cross-platform biomarker signature to detect renal transplant tolerance in humans. J Clin Invest 120(6):1848–1861
38. Newell KA, Asare A, Kirk AD, Gisler TD, Bourcier K, Suthanthiran M et al (2010) Identification of a B cell signature associated with renal transplant tolerance in humans. J Clin Invest 120(6):1836–1847
39. Le Texier L, Thebault P, Lavault A, Usal C, Merieau E, Quillard T et al (2011) Long-term allograft tolerance is characterized by the accumulation of B cells exhibiting an inhibited profile. Am J Transplant 11(3):429–438
40. Li XC (2010) The significance of non-T-cell pathways in graft rejection: implications for transplant tolerance. Transplantation 90(10):1043–1047. doi:10.97/TP.0b013e3181efcfe9
41. Kitchens WH et al (2007) Macrophage depletion suppresses cardiac allograft vasculopathy in mice. Am J Transplant 7:2675–2682
42. Summers C, Rankin SM, Condliffe AM, Singh N, Peters AM, Chilvers ER (2010) Neutrophil kinetics in health and disease. Trends Immunol 31(8):318–324
43. Asgari E, Zhou W, Sacks S (2010) Complement in organ transplantation. Curr Opin Organ Transplant 15(4):486–491. doi:10.1097/MOT.0b013e32833b9cb7
44. Lanier LL (2008) Up on the tightrope: natural killer cell activation and inhibition. Nat Immunol 9(5):495–502

45. Kitchens WH, Uehara S, Chase CM, Colvin RB, Russell PS, Madsen JC (2006) The changing role of natural killer cells in solid organ rejection and tolerance. Transplantation 81(6):811–817. doi:10.1097/01.tp.0000202844.33794.0e
46. Luster AD, Alon R, von Andrian UH (2005) Immune cell migration in inflammation: present and future therapeutic targets. Nat Immunol 6(12):1182–1190
47. Anglicheau D, Suthanthiran M (2008) Noninvasive prediction of organ graft rejection and outcome using gene expression patterns. Transplantation 86(2):192–199. doi:10.1097/TP.0b013e31817eef7b
48. Win TS, Pettigrew GJ (2010) Humoral autoimmunity and transplant vasculopathy: when allo is not enough. Transplantation 90(2):113–120. doi:10.1097/TP.0b013e3181e25a59
49. Terasaki PI, Cai J (2008) Human leukocyte antigen antibodies and chronic rejection: from association to causation. Transplantation 86(3):377–383. doi:10.1097/TP.0b013e31817c4cb8
50. Brook M, Wood K, Jones N (2006) The impact of memory T cells on rejection and tolerance. Transplantation 82:1–9
51. Adams A, Williams MA, Jones T, Shiasugi N, Durham MM, Kaech S et al (2003) Heterologous immunity provides a potent barrier to transplantation tolerance. J Clin Invest 111:1887–1895

Chapter 4

Transplantation Tolerance

Colin Brinkman, Bryna Burrell, Joseph Scalea, and Jonathan S. Bromberg

Abstract

Tolerance has been defined as graft-specific survival in the absence of continued immunosuppression. The mechanisms of central and peripheral tolerance are discussed in this review, as well as the barriers and limitations in achieving graft-specific tolerance. The need remains for definitive laboratory assays to determine the presence of a tolerant state. Genetic biomarker analysis pre-transplant may allow for better donor: recipient matching, lessening the need for immunosuppression, while post-transplant analysis of biomarkers, certain cytokines, and regulatory leukocytes may permit minimally invasive assessment of graft function and potentially, of graft-specific tolerance.

Key words Transplantation, Tolerance, Suppression

1 Tolerance Definition

Since the first successful human transplant in 1954 [1], inducing long-term recipient tolerance to grafted tissue has remained an intangible goal. Over the past five decades, improved surgical and immunosuppressive techniques, and comprehension of underlying immune responses, have improved graft survival time dramatically. However, the Holy Grail of transplant tolerance (described by the "Father of Transplantation," Peter Medawar in 1953 as graft-specific tolerance in the absence of continued immunotherapy [2]) remains elusive. The current definition has been updated to "the specific absence of a destructive immune response to transplanted tissue in the absence of immunosuppression" [3].

Tolerance can mechanistically be divided between two categories: central and peripheral tolerance. Central tolerance refers to the process by which self-antigen reactive lymphocytes are deleted at the site of lymphocyte development; in the bone marrow for B cells and in the thymus for T cells [4]. In contrast, peripheral tolerance refers to the deletion or anergy of lymphocytes activated in a

Andrea A. Zachary and Mary S. Leffell (eds.), *Transplantation Immunology: Methods and Protocols, Second Edition*, Methods in Molecular Biology, vol. 1034, DOI 10.1007/978-1-62703-493-7_4, © Springer Science+Business Media, LLC 2013

noninflammatory setting, outside of these primary lymphoid tissues [5]. Transplant tolerance is concerned almost exclusively with peripheral tolerance, as this form of tolerance can be induced at the time of transplantation. In the periphery, graft-reactive cells can be deleted, become anergic or ignorant (fail to respond to restimulation), become suppressive regulatory cells, and/or undergo clonal exhaustion (due to either chronic or suboptimal stimulation) [6].

2 Barriers and Limitations to Tolerance

Immunosuppressive drugs have dramatically reduced the instances of acute graft rejection yet chronic graft rejection remains a significant issue. Further, these drugs need to be continuously administered for the remainder of the patient's life and expose the patient to other infections and malignancies [7]. Hence, the generation of specific immunosuppression, aimed solely at potential or active graft-reactive cells, would comprise a major advance in transplantation.

In terms of the recipient immune response, the largest barrier to transplant tolerance is the pool of preformed, recipient cells that cross-react with donor alloantigen. Between 1 and 10 % of recipient T cells can recognize donor cells as foreign, a very large percentage of endogenous T cells [8]. A second major barrier to transplant tolerance includes memory T cells, as cross-reactivity and molecular mimicry occur between viral and transplanted antigens (reviewed in [9]). Anti-rejection therapies are less effective in older individuals, and one possible explanation is their larger population of experienced memory T cells [10].

3 Assays for Transplant Tolerance and What They Tell Us About the Immune Response

The most overarching theme that can be gleaned from the multiple assays performed to assess the function and prognosis of the transplanted organ is that transplant tolerance is a beast with many heads. Inhibition of one pathway of rejection is often met with the induction of another. Assays can generally be split into two broad categories; those performed before transplant to measure the potential reactivity of the recipient towards the donor graft, and those performed after transplant to evaluate the active reactivity of the donor towards the graft.

Some assays seek to minimize the amount of difference between the recipient and donor, hence limiting the anti-graft response. For example, cross-match HLA testing assesses the levels of preformed, donor-reactive antibody in the recipient serum [11, 12]. Mixed lymphocyte reactions (MLR) are also useful in determining the amount of cross-reactivity between donor lymphocytes and recipient T cells; however, this test requires a living donor and at least 72 h to perform [13, 14]. Other assays, such as testing for C4d deposition [15] and antibodies against normally cryptic cellular and structural proteins (i.e., myosin [16] and collagen [17]) measure the current state of donor reactivity. However, current assays only measure anti-donor responses (or lack thereof) and fail to differentiate between immune ignorance and immune tolerance. Generation of assays that directly assess levels of immune tolerance would be helpful from a clinical standpoint, as they could provide a more concrete indication as to when and if it is safe to begin withdrawing recipients from immunosuppressive therapy.

4 Gene Arrays

Pre-transplant genetic biomarker analysis of both donors and recipients may allow for better matching, lessening the need for immunosuppression and minimizing the potential for future chronic rejection [18]. In kidney transplant patients, 15 single nucleotide polymorphisms (SNPs), detected before transplant, have been associated with episodes of acute rejection [19].

Post-transplant genetic biomarker analysis may allow for minimally invasive analysis of graft function. In renal transplantation, expression of perforin, granzyme B, and granulysin RNA by urinary cells correlates with acute rejection episodes, confirmed by tissue biopsy [18]. Tribbles-1 expression in peripheral blood cells predicts chronic graft dysfunction, again confirmed by biopsy [18]. In cardiac transplant patients, peripheral blood gene expression profiles can assess the absence of graft rejection [18].

Gene arrays may also identify patients that would benefit from adjustment or withdrawal from immunosuppressive protocols. Operationally tolerant kidney recipients (individuals free of both immunosuppression and rejection instances for at least 1 year) have a unique, ten gene lymphocytic cell signature in their peripheral blood [20]. Similarly, a study of noncompliant kidney transplant recipients that maintained graft tolerance revealed an increase in the number, differentiation, and activation of B cells within the graft [21]. This signature is unique to tolerant recipients when compared both to those stable on immunosuppression and healthy controls [21]. Importantly, these signatures comprised a few genes and were observed in peripheral blood RNA samples, making this test simple and minimally invasive to the recipient. For liver transplant recipients, approximately 30 genes in the peripheral blood are indicative of operational tolerance and hence individuals that would be eligible to discontinue immunosuppressive therapy without the risk of rejection incidents [22].

5 Urine Biomarkers

Use of urine biomarkers is an attractive strategy for post-transplant monitoring of allograft health because urine can be obtained non-invasively, and in the case of kidney transplants, its production is intimately tied to the target organ's function. Urine can be used to monitor creatinine clearance as a measure of kidney function, but this method requires 24 h urine collection, is not exclusively indicative of kidney function, and provides no information about the immune status of the subject. Recently, it has been reported that mRNA transcripts for various immune cell associated molecules can be assayed in human urine [23]. One study reported that mRNAs encoding OX40, OX40L, and PD-1, costimulatory molecules that can be expressed on immune cells, can be found in the urine of kidney transplant recipients, and that higher levels of these mRNAs correlated with graft dysfunction and acute rejection [24]. Another study has suggested that granzyme A mRNA levels in urine can be used to detect renal injury and predict impending acute rejection [25]. It has also been argued that urine levels of Foxp3 mRNA, a transcription factor that specifies regulatory T cells, are predictive of certain outcomes in kidney transplant recipients [26]; however, this assertion has been challenged [27]. Other groups have measured chemokines in the urine of human kidney transplant patients and have found evidence that CXCL9, CXCL10, and CXCL11 were associated with acute kidney graft failure [28, 29], while CCL2 was associated with late graft failure [30].

One limitation of urine biomarkers is that they tend to be weighted toward assessing kidney health and are of more limited utility in monitoring liver, cardiac, or other allografts. A further disadvantage of using urine is that its production can be impaired and hamper collection, particularly if the kidneys are under stress. Furthermore, all of the markers discussed are measures of organ health or indicators of impending rejection. The absence of rejection markers is not a robust criterion to declare tolerance has been achieved, though a positive result is useful in indicating that tolerance has not been achieved and may allow for timely intervention to prevent the loss of the organ. Nevertheless, all current assays of urine biomarkers currently fall short of being able to indicate if a tolerant state has been reached, though urinary mRNA measurements show promise and may 1 day be useful in assaying tolerance if the right combination of markers is found.

6 ImmunKnow® Assay

The ImmunKnow® assay, produced by Cylex, Inc. (Columbia, MD), is designed to detect "cell-mediated immunity (CMI) by measuring the concentration of adenosine triphosphate (ATP) from CD4 cells following stimulation." In large part, this test measures a nonspecific marker indirectly attributed to the inflammatory state. Peripheral blood samples (whole blood) are diluted 1:4 and stimulated with phytohemagglutinin-L (PHA) for 15–18 h. Thereafter, magnetic beads coated with anti-CD4 antibody are added to the stimulated whole-blood sample. After a series of washes, the cells are lysed and a luminescence agent (Luciferin) added. The level of ATP in the lysate is then compared with an ATP calibration curve. The data are then interpreted based on stimulation. Thus, if the ATP index from stimulated cells is <225, circulating immune cells have a "low" response to PHA. A level of 226–524 implies "moderate" response, and a level of 525 or greater is interpreted to be a "high" response.

7 B Cells

Recent reports in both kidney and liver transplant literature have suggested that B cell biomarkers may provide a useful signature for patients that are operationally tolerant of their allografts [21, 31].

7.1 Urine Biomarkers

In a study published in the AJT in 2010, authors compared 25 patients with "operational tolerance," or stable renal function for greater than 1 year, despite withdrawal from immunosuppression with both stably chemically immunosuppressed and non-transplanted patients. In that study, authors analyzed urine sediment pellets taken from both the tolerant and non-tolerant groups and found that, of 18 candidate genes, the only difference between the groups was the CD20 RNA transcript, as determined by quantitative reverse transcription polymerase chain reaction (RT-PCR) [21].

7.2 Gene Arrays and PCR

In the same 2010 AJT study evaluating differences in patients with and without operational tolerance of renal grafts, genetic microarrays were performed on samples of whole-blood total RNA [21]. The authors identified five unique genes (TUBB2A, TCL1A, BRDG1, HTPAP, and PPPAPDC1B) which correlated with clinical differences between the groups. Interestingly, of the 30 genes that demonstrated a 2-fold or greater increase in expression in the tolerant group, 22 were B cell specific [21]. Further, Newell et al. used multiplex real-time PCR to evaluate 228 additional genes and found 31 unique genes that were different between tolerant patients and patients on stable immunosuppression. These differences were largely not observed between the healthy comparator group and the tolerant group [21].

7.3 Flow Cytometry

Using 5-color flow cytometry, it has been shown that, of 32 different cell surface marker combinations, patients tolerant of their renal allografts had significantly higher numbers of total B cells (CD19+) and naive B cells (CD19 + CD27 − IgM + IgD+) when compared with the stably immunosuppressed group, but not the healthy non-transplanted control group [21].

8 T Cells

Although the authors' primary conclusion in the 2010 AJT comparison of operationally tolerant and non-tolerant (healthy controls in addition to transplanted patients with stable renal function on immunosuppression) was that a distinct B cell signature may be found in patients that are tolerant of their renal allografts, this study and others have shown that both gamma-delta T cells and T regulatory cells may be upregulated in tolerant transplant recipients [21]. In contrast to renal transplantation, as many as 20 % of liver transplant recipients may become tolerant, or operationally tolerant, of their allograft [32]. In a study similar to Newell et al., a group from Spain compared a cohort of operationally tolerant liver transplant recipients to patients that were either healthy non-transplanted, or transplanted with stable graft function on immunosuppression, and found a significant difference in the T cell and natural killer (NK) cell populations between the two groups [32].

8.1 Urine Biomarkers

When cells in urine sediment from healthy volunteers were compared with those from tolerant patients, Newell et al. observed that FOXP3 was expressed to a significantly lower degree when compared with patients that were tolerant of their grafts [21]. The authors also noted significantly lower expression of CD3 and Perforin in healthy patients when compared to tolerant patients [21].

8.2 Gene Arrays and PCR

By using genetic microarrays, Martínez-Llordella et al. were able to determine, with a high degree of reliability (99.5 %), genes relating to T cells were more likely to be upregulated in patients tolerant of their hepatic allografts. These results were validated using RT-PCR. The investigators evaluated 462 candidate genes and found the most significant correlations with tolerance were observed with T cell specific transcripts. There was also a strong correlation with NK cells [32]. Similar results were shown in a French study of operationally tolerant renal transplant patients, suggesting that using a genetic footprint of 33 genes predicts tolerance versus chronic rejection phenotype with 99 and 86 % specificity [33]. These data, and others presented herein, have led some groups to advocate for transcriptional profiling of peripheral blood to identify liver transplant recipients who may be candidates for withdrawal of immunosuppression [22, 34].

8.3 Flow Cytometry

Also in the Spanish study conducted by Martínez-Llordella et al., the authors assessed differences in populations of circulating peripheral lymphocytes. The investigators showed that tolerant patients have a significantly greater percentage of gamma-delta T cells, when compared with both healthy non-transplanted controls, and transplanted patients on stable immunosuppression [32]. Although there was no difference in effector memory cells between the tolerant and non-tolerant live transplant groups, there were higher percentages of CD4+/CD25 + hi/CD62L + hi in tolerant patients [32]. These data are supported by a Japanese study performed in operationally tolerant liver transplant recipients, in which CD4 + CD25+ peripheral blood lymphocytes, in addition to gamma-delta T cells, were noted to be elevated in tolerant versus non-tolerant patients [31].

9 Treg

T cells with regulatory capacity (regulatory T cells, or Treg) suppress the reactivity of other immune cells and are divided into two categories, dependent upon their development. Natural Treg (nTreg) contribute heavily to central tolerance. These cells dampen responses against autologous antigens and develop in the thymus [35]. Treg that are educated in the periphery against antigens in a tolerant environment are adaptive or inducible Treg (iTreg [35]). iTreg are potentially more important in controlling anti-graft responses [36]. For example, recipient Treg can be educated with donor APC, hence becoming allospecific iTreg [37]. In humanized mouse experiments, expansion and transfer of these cells prolongs the survival of skin grafts [38]. However, a potential major pitfall of these therapies is that the iTreg may not stably hold their suppressive phenotype, and may revert to effector T cells in an inflammatory environment [36]. In monkey studies, when donor bone marrow cells are administered in combination with an immunosuppressive protocol peritransplant, intragraft Foxp3 levels are elevated [39]. This protocol has been adapted to human clinical trials, and in haematopoietic stem cell transplantation co-transfer of donor Treg, along with conventional T cells and hematopoietic stem cells, prevented graft-vs-host disease (GVHD) and resulted in lymphoid reconstitution without immunosuppression [40]. Lastly, Treg can be found within the graft following transplantation [6]. Indeed, in liver transplantation, donor Treg can be transferred with the graft itself and migrate from the tissue into the recipient following transplantation, and these cells are allosuppressive [41].

Potential assays for quantifying Treg presence include detection of intragraft Foxp3 by performing RT-PCR on graft biopsy tissue [39]. The presence of this transcription factor can be extrapolated to indicate the presence of Treg, although human effector T cells have been shown to upregulate Foxp3 [42], and human T cells with suppressive function do not necessarily express Foxp3 [43]. A more operative method of assessing functional tolerance may be a post-transplant MLR, in which peripheral lymphocytes from the recipient are cultured with unresponsive (usually irradiated) donor cells, and anti-donor responses are quantified in terms of cytokine production and/or proliferation [39]. However, this assay requires a living donor as a source of cells.

10 Myeloid-Derived Suppressor Cells

Myeloid-derived suppressor cells (MDSC) are composed of a heterogeneous population that may include myeloid precursor cells, immature macrophages, immature granulocytes, and immature dendritic cells. MDSC were initially described in cancer patients and are thought to negatively regulate the immune response to tumors by a variety of mechanisms. In mice, MDSC accumulate in blood and lymphoid organs in response to a number of immunological insults [44–51]. In many cases these cells are associated with impaired immune reactivity [52]. MDSC mediate immune suppression via multiple pathways, including the activities of inducible nitric oxidase synthase (iNOS) and arginase (Arg-1) [53], as well as production of reactive oxygen species [54, 55].

There is some indication that these cells are also associated with tolerance to transplanted tissues in rodent models of tissue tolerance [56, 57]. In one study, MDSC protected islet transplants in mice by inducing Treg in a B7-H1 (also called programmed death ligand 1(PD-L1))-dependent manner [58]. Induction of MDSC in concert with Treg also prolonged skin allograft survival in mice in another study [59]. Adoptive transfer of MDSC prevented GVHD [60], and these cells accumulated in the blood and kidneys of rats that displayed long-term tolerance of kidney allografts [61]. In this model, the suppressive activity depended upon iNOS in the MDSC. Finally, the monocytic subset of MDSC is important in graft survival in an allogeneic cardiac transplantation model [62].

So far, there are no data on MDSC in human transplant patients, but given the seeming importance of these cells in regulating the immune response to a variety of human tumors, and the work on allograft tolerance in mice, it would not be surprising to find that MDSC can play a role in transplant tolerance in humans. As the surface molecules that define MDSC differ between mouse and human [63], there is a need for better means of identifying and phenotyping MDSC in humans. The requirements for location, number, percentage, phenotype, and functionality of MDSC in mediating human allograft tolerance also need to be defined. Given such information, interrogation of MDSC or MDSC-related genes such as iNOS and Arg-1 in tissue biopsies, blood, urine, or combinations thereof may be useful in defining a tolerant state in human transplant patients.

11 Immature Dendritic Cells

Dendritic cells (DC) fall into one of two categories, depending upon their maturation status. Immature dendritic cells (iDC) are antigen-capture specialized cells that express low levels of costimulatory molecules, whereas mature DC are specialized to present antigen, in the presence of costimulation, to T cells [64]. In contrast to mature DC, repetitive stimulation with iDC induces suppressive CD4+ T cells [65]. This CD4+ T cell phenotype is irreversible, and these cells to not proliferate or produce cytokines, even after stimulation with mature DC [65]. Indeed, iDC of donor origin induce a state of graft tolerance [66]. When engaged by T cells with a cognate T cell receptor (TCR), these iDC induce cell death via apoptosis in the graft reactive T cell, hence controlling the donor-reactive T cell population. iDC also express surface-bound transforming growth factor beta (TGF-β) associated with the latency associated peptide and inducible T cell costimulator (ICOS), two T cell activation inhibitory molecules [67, 68]. Following the apoptosis of graft-reactive CD4+ T cells, the resulting apoptotic bodies are taken up by the iDC and re-presented to potentially alloreactive cytotoxic lymphocytes, still in the absence of costimulation [66, 69]. Hence, both CD4+ and CD8+ alloreactive T cells can be controlled by iDC. Donor-derived iDC can also promote allospecific iTreg development [65]. Activated iTreg in turn prevent DC maturation, hence inhibiting upregulation of the costimulatory molecules CD80 and CD86 [70]. A variety of immunosuppressive drugs maintain DC in their immature state, including cyclosporine A (CsA), tacrolimus, and glucocorticoids [71]. One potential pitfall of using iDC to promote transplant tolerance clinically is that if these donor-derived iDC are phagocytized by recipient APC, donor antigen can be cross-presented to recipient T cells, resulting in stimulation instead of suppression of the alloresponse [72].

12 IL-10

Interleukin 10 (IL-10) consistently arises as a mediator of immune suppression associated with both induced and self-tolerance. While the detection of IL-10 serum levels cannot be used as a surrogate for tolerance, it may indicate tissues or states predisposed to a tolerant state.

12.1 Urine Biomarkers

IL-10 can be measured using ELISA and flow-cytometry. Additionally, IL-10, or markers of IL-10 activity, may be detectable in urine. Mice deficient in IL-10 (IL-10−/−) develop colitis and are used as a model for Crohn's disease. Interestingly, these mice have reduced urinary markers of inflammation [73]. In this model, urinary levels of xanthurenic acid in knock-out mice were significantly higher than in controls. The implication of this work is that urinary biomarkers may help to elucidate patterns of immunologic tolerance.

12.2 Flow Cytometry

Based on the findings that B cells may provide a signature to determine if patients are tolerant of renal allografts, Newell et al. stained peripheral blood mononuclear cells (PBMCs) from tolerant and non-tolerant patients for intracellular IL-10 and found increased levels of IL-10 in the tolerant, but neither non-transplanted nor stably immunosuppressed comparator groups [21].

13 Transforming Growth Factor Beta

The transforming growth factor beta (TGF-β) family is made of up three isoforms encoded by three different genes: TGF-β1, TGF-β2, and TGF-β3. TGF-β1 is the dominant isoform in the mammalian immune system, and is required for maintenance of self-tolerance [74, 75]. The complex role of TGF-β1 in transplantation tolerance has been well reviewed by others [76]. One of the best-described activities of TGF-β1 in transplant tolerance is its role in inducing so-called adaptive or inducible Treg in both mice and humans [77, 78]. As reviewed here and elsewhere, Treg are important in inducing and maintaining tolerance to transplanted tissues [36]. However, TGF-β1 has pleiotropic effects on T cells that depend upon other contextual signals. For example, IL-4 and IFN-γ inhibit TGF-β1-induced Treg development [79, 80], and TGF-β1 can also induce pathogenic TH17 in conjunction with IL-6 [81, 82]. ATP; the transcription factor, RORα; aryl hydrocarbon receptor; the transcription factor, Batf; interferon-regulatory factor 4; tumor necrosis factor alpha, TNFα; and interleukin 1, IL-1, have all been shown to promote Th17 differentiation even in the presence of TGF-β1 [83–85]. The complicated interplay among TGF-β1 and other factors makes TGF-β1 by itself an insufficient marker for the development of tolerance, however, assays that detect TGF-β1 as well as molecules that both synergize and antagonize its anti-inflammatory effects could have value. Possible strategies for detection include urine or serum protein or mRNA, gene arrays on tissue biopsies, or flow cytometry for TGF-β1 on particular cells of interest.

14 IDO-Positive Cells

Indoleamine 2,3-dioxygenase (IDO) is an enzyme responsible for catalyzing the metabolism of tryptophan to *N*-formyl-kynurenine, and has been implicated in immune regulation [86, 87]. Recent reports have suggested that IDO-expressing cells may recruit Treg in addition to controlling immunologic responses associated with pregnancy and malignancy [86, 88]. When pregnant mice were administered IDO inhibitors, concepti were uniformly rejected; subsequently the authors showed that IDO activity suppressed T cell mediated responses to alloantigens. Testing for the presence of IDO is not necessarily a surrogate for the detection of tolerance, but may indirectly highlight tissues which are tolerogenic.

14.1 Gene Arrays and PCR

IDO, encoded by INDO, is present on chromosome 8, and has been studied at the genetic level. Using gene array chips, the presence of INDO has been used to evaluate the immunologic response to neoplasia in human tissue samples [89]. After gene array analysis revealed an increase in IDO in human CD14+ decidual (immunoregulatory uterine) cells, IDO expression detected by RT-PCR confirmed differential genetic regulation of IDO in experimental cells when compared with CD14+ peripheral blood cells [90]. This study confirmed that IDO cells are present and functional at the maternal-fetal barrier, and that they likely act in an immunoregulatory capacity.

14.2 Flow Cytometry

In studies using human recipients, the presence of IDO cells has been measured using flow cytometry. IDO is an intracellular protein, and cells must be permeabilized prior to IDO detection. Isolation and identification of IDO-expressing cells has been successful using sheep anti-human IDO [91]. In a study of human patients with autoimmune disorders (arthritis and lupus), authors showed that peripheral IDO cells were down-regulated in these disease states, and that IDO may play a crucial role in the loss of self-tolerance [91].

14.3 Protein Arrays and ELISA

ELISA can be utilized to determine IDO activity. In a study of gliomas, levels of the IDO metabolites tryptophan and kynurenine were measured in the supernatant of IDO-containing cell populations to evaluate enzyme activity [92, 93]. Authors used these techniques to show that IDO, in addition to PD-L1, was immunosuppressive, and that blocking both IDO and PDL-1 may prove fruitful in patients that have glioblastoma multiforme [92].

14.4 Immunohistochemistry

IDO is detectable by immunohistochemistry. In a study of human malignancy, investigators observed a strong correlation between stromal or epithelial IDO positivity and the burden of lymphocyte infiltration [89]. These findings support a role for IDO in immune regulation and tolerance.

14.5 Other Studies for IDO

In a study aimed at investigating the regulation of T cell activation, IDO enzyme presence and expression were measured using chemiluminescence [94], which evaluates enzymatic activity via high-pressure liquid chromatography and spectrophotometry. Using these techniques the authors concluded that (1) prostaglandin E2 (PGE-2) induces mRNA expression of IDO, but that (2) a second signal [via tumor necrosis factor receptor (TNFR) or Toll-like receptor (TLR)] is required for enzyme activation. These data suggest that T cell regulation of PGE-2 may be, at least in part, due to effects of IDO [94].

15 Chimerism

Chimerism has been used to induce tolerance in both experimental models and humans. In protocols for transplantation, chimerism is generally induced after brief non-myeloablative preconditioning followed by bone marrow transplantation [39, 95]. Chimerism can be detected with any means capable of distinguishing between donor and recipient cells. Macrochimersim, or detectable donor cells in the peripheral blood (typically using flow cytometry), implies a greater percentage of chimerism in comparison to microchimerism wherein donor cells are only detectable at the genetic level (PCR, CFU following expansion, etc.). Techniques for detecting chimerism include: karyotyping, restriction fragment length polymorphism, fluorescent in situ hybridization, fluorescence resonance energy transfer, in situ fluorescence resonance energy transfer, and PCR [96, 97]. In a non-human primate (NHP) model of chimerism, quantitative PCR of bone marrow or peripheral blood cells directed at identifying the sex determining region (SRY) was reported as successfully detecting chimerism [98].

PCR-Southern blot analysis, flow-cytometry, short tandem repeats (STR), or variable number of tandem repeats (VNTRs), have also been successful in differentiating donor from recipient [99]. In a recent study of same-sex NHP tolerance induction using chimerism, investigators showed that of the available modalities for testing chimerism, real-time quantitative PCR was capable of detecting donor-specific DNA with high sensitivity. However, the authors concluded that still more sensitive assays are needed [97].

16 Conclusion

An ever-expanding pool of assays exist that serve to quantify and characterize the anti-donor response, or lack thereof, in transplant recipients. While these assays are instrumental in managing the continued survival and function of the graft, they are unable to differentiate between true immune tolerance and immune ignorance. The development of a method by which immune tolerance could be generated, followed by a noninvasive method by which immune tolerance could be monitored, would serve to not only widen the pool of potential transplant donor–recipient pairs, but also identify patients for whom immunosuppressive therapy withdrawal may be feasible and prudent.

References

1. Murray JE, Tilney NL, Wilson RE (1976) Renal transplantation: a twenty-five year experience. Ann Surg 184(5):565–573
2. Billingham RE, Brent L, Medawar PB (1953) Actively acquired tolerance of foreign cells. Nature 172(4379):603–606
3. Sachs DH (2011) Transplant tolerance: bench to bedside–26th annual Samuel Jason Mixter Lecture. Arch Surg 146(5):501–505
4. Hogquist KA, Baldwin TA, Jameson SC (2005) Central tolerance: learning self-control in the thymus. Nat Rev Immunol 5(10):772–782
5. Mueller DL (2010) Mechanisms maintaining peripheral tolerance. Nat Immunol 11(1): 21–27
6. Wood KJ, Sakaguchi S (2003) Regulatory T cells in transplantation tolerance. Nat Rev Immunol 3(3):199–210
7. Sayegh MH, Remuzzi G (2007) Clinical update: immunosuppression minimisation. Lancet 369(9574):1676–1678
8. Suchin EJ, Langmuir PB, Palmer E et al (2001) Quantifying the frequency of alloreactive T cells in vivo: new answers to an old question. J Immunol 166(2):973–981
9. Ford ML, Larsen CP (2011) Overcoming the memory barrier in tolerance induction: molecular mimicry and functional heterogeneity among pathogen-specific T-cell populations. Curr Opin Organ Transplant 15(4):405–410
10. Du W, Shen H, Galan A et al (2011) An age-specific CD8+ T cell pathway that impairs the effectiveness of strategies to prolong allograft survival. J Immunol 187(7):3631–3640
11. Mulley WR, Kanellis J (2011) Understanding crossmatch testing in organ transplantation: a case-based guide for the general nephrologist. Nephrology (Carlton) 16(2):125–133
12. Karpinski M, Rush D, Jeffery J et al (2001) Flow cytometric crossmatching in primary renal transplant recipients with a negative anti-human globulin enhanced cytotoxicity crossmatch. J Am Soc Nephrol 12(12): 2807–2814
13. Fanning LR, Hegerfeldt Y, Tary-Lehmann M et al (2008) Allogeneic transplantation of multiple umbilical cord blood units in adults: role of pretransplant-mixed lymphocyte reaction to predict host-vs-graft rejection. Leukemia 22(9):1786–1790
14. Ashokkumar C, Talukdar A, Sun Q et al (2009) Allospecific CD154+ T cells associate with rejection risk after pediatric liver transplantation. Am J Transplant 9(1): 179–191
15. Takeda A, Horike K, Ohtsuka Y et al (2011) Current problems of chronic active antibody-mediated rejection. Clin Transplant 25(Suppl 23):2–5
16. Schutz A, Breuer M, Kemkes BM (1997) Antimyosin antibodies in cardiac rejection. Ann Thorac Surg 63(2):578–581

17. Zhang Q, Reed EF (2010) Non-MHC antigenic targets of the humoral immune response in transplantation. Curr Opin Immunol 22(5):682–688
18. Roedder S, Vitalone M, Khatri P et al (2011) Biomarkers in solid organ transplantation: establishing personalized transplantation medicine. Genome Med 3(6):37
19. Israni A, Leduc R, Holmes J et al (2010) Single-nucleotide polymorphisms, acute rejection, and severity of tubulitis in kidney transplantation, accounting for center-to-center variation. Transplantation 90(12):1401–1408
20. Sagoo P, Perucha E, Sawitzki B et al (2010) Development of a cross-platform biomarker signature to detect renal transplant tolerance in humans. J Clin Invest 120(6):1848–1861
21. Newell KA, Asare A, Kirk AD et al (2010) Identification of a B cell signature associated with renal transplant tolerance in humans. J Clin Invest 120(6):1836–1847
22. Martinez-Llordella M, Lozano JJ, Puig-Pey I et al (2008) Using transcriptional profiling to develop a diagnostic test of operational tolerance in liver transplant recipients. J Clin Invest 118(8):2845–2857
23. Hartono C, Muthukumar T, Suthanthiran M (2010) Noninvasive diagnosis of acute rejection of renal allografts. Curr Opin Organ Transplant 15(1):35–41
24. Afaneh C, Muthukumar T, Lubetzky M et al (2010) Urinary cell levels of mRNA for OX40, OX40L, PD-1, PD-L1, or PD-L2 and acute rejection of human renal allografts. Transplantation 90(12):1381–1387
25. van Ham SM, Heutinck KM, Jorritsma T et al (2010) Urinary granzyme A mRNA is a biomarker to diagnose subclinical and acute cellular rejection in kidney transplant recipients. Kidney Int 78(10):1033–1040
26. Muthukumar T, Dadhania D, Ding R et al (2005) Messenger RNA for FOXP3 in the urine of renal-allograft recipients. N Engl J Med 353(22):2342–2351
27. Kamoun M, Boyd JC (2006) Urinary FOXP3 messenger RNA and renal-allograft rejection. N Engl J Med 354(21):2291–2293, author reply 2291-2293
28. Hu H, Aizenstein BD, Puchalski A et al (2004) Elevation of CXCR3-binding chemokines in urine indicates acute renal-allograft dysfunction. Am J Transplant 4(3):432–437
29. Jackson JA, Kim EJ, Begley B et al (2011) Urinary chemokines CXCL9 and CXCL10 are noninvasive markers of renal allograft rejection and BK viral infection. Am J Transplant 11(10):2228–2234
30. Ho J, Rush DN, Gibson IW et al (2010) Early urinary CCL2 is associated with the later development of interstitial fibrosis and tubular atrophy in renal allografts. Transplantation 90(4):394–400
31. Li Y, Koshiba T, Yoshizawa A et al (2004) Analyses of peripheral blood mononuclear cells in operational tolerance after pediatric living donor liver transplantation. Am J Transplant 4(12):2118–2125
32. Martinez-Llordella M, Puig-Pey I, Orlando G et al (2007) Multiparameter immune profiling of operational tolerance in liver transplantation. Am J Transplant 7(2):309–319
33. Brouard S, Mansfield E, Braud C et al (2007) Identification of a peripheral blood transcriptional biomarker panel associated with operational renal allograft tolerance. Proc Natl Acad Sci USA 104(39):15448–15453
34. Benitez C, Lozano JJ, Fueyo AS (2009) Gene expression profiling and transplantation tolerance in the clinic. Transplantation 88(3 Suppl):S50–S53
35. Curotto de Lafaille MA, Lafaille JJ (2009) Natural and adaptive foxp3+ regulatory T cells: more of the same or a division of labor? Immunity 30(5):626–635
36. Schliesser U, Streitz M, Sawitzki B (2012) Tregs: application for solid-organ transplantation. Curr Opin Organ Transplant 17(1): 34–41
37. Peters JH, Hilbrands LB, Koenen HJ et al (2008) Ex vivo generation of human alloantigen-specific regulatory T cells from CD4(pos)CD25(high) T cells for immunotherapy. PLoS One 3(5):e2233
38. Sagoo P, Ali N, Garg G et al (2011) Human regulatory T cells with alloantigen specificity are more potent inhibitors of alloimmune skin graft damage than polyclonal regulatory T cells. Sci Transl Med 3(83):83ra42
39. Kawai T, Cosimi AB, Spitzer TR et al (2008) HLA-mismatched renal transplantation without maintenance immunosuppression. N Engl J Med 358(4):353–361
40. Di Ianni M, Falzetti F, Carotti A et al (2011) Tregs prevent GVHD and promote immune reconstitution in HLA-haploidentical transplantation. Blood 117(14):3921–3928
41. Demirkiran A, Bosma BM, Kok A et al (2007) Allosuppressive donor CD4+CD25+ regulatory T cells detach from the graft and circulate in recipients after liver transplantation. J Immunol 178(10):6066–6072
42. Kmieciak M, Gowda M, Graham L et al (2009) Human T cells express CD25 and Foxp3 upon activation and exhibit effector/memory phenotypes without any regulatory/suppressor function. J Transl Med 7:89
43. Zheng Y, Manzotti CN, Burke F et al (2008) Acquisition of suppressive function by activated human CD4+ CD25- T cells is associated with the expression of CTLA-4 not FoxP3. J Immunol 181(3):1683–1691

44. Goni O, Alcaide P, Fresno M (2002) Immunosuppression during acute Trypanosoma cruzi infection: involvement of Ly6G (Grl(+))CD11b(+)immature myeloid suppressor cells. Int Immunol 14(10):1125–1134
45. Giordanengo L, Guinazu N, Stempin C et al (2002) Cruzipain, a major Trypanosoma cruzi antigen, conditions the host immune response in favor of parasite. Eur J Immunol 32(4):1003–1011
46. Voisin MB, Buzoni-Gatel D, Bout D et al (2004) Both expansion of regulatory GR1+ CD11b+myeloid cells and anergy of T lymphocytes participate in hyporesponsiveness of the lung-associated immune system during acute toxoplasmosis. Infect Immun 72(9):5487–5492
47. Mencacci A, Montagnoli C, Bacci A et al (2002) CD80+Gr-1+ myeloid cells inhibit development of antifungal Th1 immunity in mice with candidiasis. J Immunol 169(6):3180–3190
48. Kerr EC, Raveney BJ, Copland DA et al (2008) Analysis of retinal cellular infiltrate in experimental autoimmune uveoretinitis reveals multiple regulatory cell populations. J Autoimmun 31(4):354–361
49. Nicholson LB, Raveney BJ, Munder M (2009) Monocyte dependent regulation of autoimmune inflammation. Curr Mol Med 9(1):23–29
50. Haile LA, von Wasielewski R, Gamrekelashvili J et al (2008) Myeloid-derived suppressor cells in inflammatory bowel disease: a new immunoregulatory pathway. Gastroenterology 135(3):871–881, 881 e871–875
51. Llopiz D, Dotor J, Casares N et al (2009) Peptide inhibitors of transforming growth factor-beta enhance the efficacy of antitumor immunotherapy. Int J Cancer 125(11):2614–2623
52. Serafini P, De Santo C, Marigo I et al (2004) Derangement of immune responses by myeloid suppressor cells. Cancer Immunol Immunother 53(2):64–72
53. Rodriguez PC, Ochoa AC (2008) Arginine regulation by myeloid derived suppressor cells and tolerance in cancer: mechanisms and therapeutic perspectives. Immunol Rev 222:180–191
54. Sauer H, Wartenberg M, Hescheler J (2001) Reactive oxygen species as intracellular messengers during cell growth and differentiation. Cell Physiol Biochem 11(4):173–186
55. Szuster-Ciesielska A, Hryciuk-Umer E, Stepulak A et al (2004) Reactive oxygen species production by blood neutrophils of patients with laryngeal carcinoma and antioxidative enzyme activity in their blood. Acta Oncol 43(3):252–258
56. Boros P, Ochando JC, Chen SH et al (2010) Myeloid-derived suppressor cells: natural regulators for transplant tolerance. Hum Immunol 71(11):1061–1066
57. Dilek N, van Rompaey N, Le Moine A et al (2010) Myeloid-derived suppressor cells in transplantation. Curr Opin Organ Transplant 15:765–768
58. Chou HS, Hsieh CC, Charles R et al (2011) Myeloid-derived suppressor cells protect islet transplants by B7-H1 mediated enhancement of T regulatory cells. Transplantation 93(3):272–282
59. Adeegbe D, Serafini P, Bronte V et al (2010) In vivo induction of myeloid suppressor cells and CD4(+)Foxp3(+) T regulatory cells prolongs skin allograft survival in mice. Cell Transplant 20(6):941–954
60. Zhou Z, French DL, Ma G et al (2010) Development and function of myeloid-derived suppressor cells generated from mouse embryonic and hematopoietic stem cells. Stem Cells 28(3):620–632
61. Dugast AS, Haudebourg T, Coulon F et al (2008) Myeloid-derived suppressor cells accumulate in kidney allograft tolerance and specifically suppress effector T cell expansion. J Immunol 180(12):7898–7906
62. Garcia MR, Ledgerwood L, Yang Y et al (2010) Monocytic suppressive cells mediate cardiovascular transplantation tolerance in mice. J Clin Invest 120(7):2486–2496
63. Gabrilovich DI, Nagaraj S (2009) Myeloid-derived suppressor cells as regulators of the immune system. Nat Rev Immunol 9(3):162–174
64. Banchereau J, Steinman RM (1998) Dendritic cells and the control of immunity. Nature 392(6673):245–252
65. Jonuleit H, Schmitt E, Schuler G et al (2000) Induction of interleukin 10-producing, non-proliferating CD4(+) T cells with regulatory properties by repetitive stimulation with allogeneic immature human dendritic cells. J Exp Med 192(9):1213–1222
66. Olszewski WL (2003) Tolerogenic properties of dendritic cells in allografting. Ann Transplant 8(4):5–9
67. Gandhi R, Anderson DE, Weiner HL (2007) Cutting edge: immature human dendritic cells express latency-associated peptide and inhibit T cell activation in a TGF-beta-dependent manner. J Immunol 178(7):4017–4021
68. Tuettenberg A, Huter E, Hubo M et al (2009) The role of ICOS in directing T cell responses: ICOS-dependent induction of T cell anergy by tolerogenic dendritic cells. J Immunol 182(6):3349–3356
69. Steinman RM, Turley S, Mellman I et al (2000) The induction of tolerance by dendritic

cells that have captured apoptotic cells. J Exp Med 191(3):411–416
70. Misra N, Bayry J, Lacroix-Desmazes S et al (2004) Cutting edge: human CD4+CD25+ T cells restrain the maturation and antigen-presenting function of dendritic cells. J Immunol 172(8):4676–4680
71. Thomson AW, Robbins PD (2008) Tolerogenic dendritic cells for autoimmune disease and transplantation. Ann Rheum Dis 67(Suppl 3):iii90–iii96
72. van Kooten C, Lombardi G, Gelderman KA et al (2011) Dendritic cells as a tool to induce transplantation tolerance: obstacles and opportunities. Transplantation 91(1):2–7
73. Otter D, Cao M, Lin HM et al (2011) Identification of urinary biomarkers of colon inflammation in IL10-/- mice using Short-Column LCMS metabolomics. J Biomed Biotechnol 2011:974701
74. Shull MM, Ormsby I, Kier AB et al (1992) Targeted disruption of the mouse transforming growth factor-beta 1 gene results in multifocal inflammatory disease. Nature 359(6397):693–699
75. Kulkarni AB, Huh CG, Becker D et al (1993) Transforming growth factor beta 1 null mutation in mice causes excessive inflammatory response and early death. Proc Natl Acad Sci USA 90(2):770–774
76. Regateiro FS, Howie D, Cobbold SP et al (2011) TGF-beta in transplantation tolerance. Curr Opin Immunol 23(5):660–669
77. Chen W, Jin W, Hardegen N et al (2003) Conversion of peripheral CD4+CD25- naive T cells to CD4+CD25+ regulatory T cells by TGF-beta induction of transcription factor Foxp3. J Exp Med 198(12):1875–1886
78. Zheng SG, Wang JH, Gray JD et al (2004) Natural and induced CD4+CD25+ cells educate CD4+CD25- cells to develop suppressive activity: the role of IL-2, TGF-beta, and IL-10. J Immunol 172(9):5213–5221
79. Takaki H, Ichiyama K, Koga K et al (2008) STAT6 Inhibits TGF-beta1-mediated Foxp3 induction through direct binding to the Foxp3 promoter, which is reverted by retinoic acid receptor. J Biol Chem 283(22):14955–14962
80. Fragale A, Gabriele L, Stellacci E et al (2008) IFN regulatory factor-1 negatively regulates CD4+ CD25+ regulatory T cell differentiation by repressing Foxp3 expression. J Immunol 181(3):1673–1682
81. Bader BL, Rayburn H, Crowley D et al (1998) Extensive vasculogenesis, angiogenesis, and organogenesis precede lethality in mice lacking all alpha v integrins. Cell 95(4):507–519
82. Veldhoen M, Hocking RJ, Atkins CJ et al (2006) TGFbeta in the context of an inflammatory cytokine milieu supports de novo differentiation of IL-17-producing T cells. Immunity 24(2):179–189
83. Atarashi K, Nishimura J, Shima T et al (2008) ATP drives lamina propria T(H)17 cell differentiation. Nature 455(7214):808–812
84. Brustle A, Heink S, Huber M et al (2007) The development of inflammatory T(H)-17 cells requires interferon-regulatory factor 4. Nat Immunol 8(9):958–966
85. Chen Q, Yang W, Gupta S et al (2008) IRF-4-binding protein inhibits interleukin-17 and interleukin-21 production by controlling the activity of IRF-4 transcription factor. Immunity 29(6):899–911
86. Mellor AL, Sivakumar J, Chandler P et al (2001) Prevention of T cell-driven complement activation and inflammation by tryptophan catabolism during pregnancy. Nat Immunol 2(1):64–68
87. Baban B, Chandler PR, Sharma MD et al (2009) IDO activates regulatory T cells and blocks their conversion into Th17-like T cells. J Immunol 183(4):2475–2483
88. Prendergast GC, Metz R, Muller AJ (2009) IDO recruits Tregs in melanoma. Cell Cycle 8(12):1818–1819
89. Jacquemier J, Bertucci F, Finetti P et al (2012) High expression of indoleamine 2,3-dioxygenase in the tumour is associated with medullary features and favourable outcome in basal-like breast carcinoma. Int J Cancer 130(1):96–104
90. Gustafsson C, Mjosberg J, Matussek A et al (2008) Gene expression profiling of human decidual macrophages: evidence for immunosuppressive phenotype. PLoS One 3(4):e2078
91. Furuzawa-Carballeda J, Lima G, Jakez-Ocampo J et al (2011) Indoleamine 2,3-dioxygenase-expressing peripheral cells in rheumatoid arthritis and systemic lupus erythematosus: a cross-sectional study. Eur J Clin Invest 41(10):1037–1046
92. Avril T, Saikali S, Vauleon E et al (2010) Distinct effects of human glioblastoma immunoregulatory molecules programmed cell death ligand-1 (PDL-1) and indoleamine 2,3-dioxygenase (IDO) on tumour-specific T cell functions. J Neuroimmunol 225(1–2):22–33
93. Widner B, Werner ER, Schennach H et al (1997) Simultaneous measurement of serum tryptophan and kynurenine by HPLC. Clin Chem 43(12):2424–2426
94. Braun D, Longman RS, Albert ML (2005) A two-step induction of indoleamine 2,3 dioxygenase (IDO) activity during dendritic-cell maturation. Blood 106(7):2375–2381

95. Nadazdin O, Abrahamian G, Boskovic S et al (2011) Stem cell mobilization and collection for induction of mixed chimerism and renal allograft tolerance in cynomolgus monkeys. J Surg Res 168(2):294–300
96. Lobashevsky AL, Jiang XL, Thomas JM (2002) Allele-specific in situ analysis of microchimerism by fluorescence resonance energy transfer (FRET) in nonhuman primate tissues. Hum Immunol 63(2):108–120
97. Han D, Berman DM, Kenyon NS (2007) Sequence-specific analysis of microchimerism by real-time quantitative polymerase chain reaction in same-sex nonhuman primates after islet and bone marrow transplantation. Transplantation 84(12):1677–1685
98. Reitsma MJ, Harrison MR, Pallavicini MG (1993) Detection of a male-specific sequence in nonhuman primates through use of the polymerase chain reaction. Cytogenet Cell Genet 64(3–4):213–216
99. Kawai T, Sogawa H, Boskovic S et al (2004) CD154 blockade for induction of mixed chimerism and prolonged renal allograft survival in nonhuman primates. Am J Transplant 4(9):1391–1398

Chapter 5

Composite Tissue Transplantation

Gerald Brandacher

Abstract

Composite tissue transplantation is an emerging new era in transplant medicine and has become a viable reconstructive option for patients with large and devastating tissue defects. Advances in microsurgical techniques, transplant immunology and the development of potent immunosuppressive agents have enabled the realization of such types of transplants. Over the past decade, a rapidly growing number of face and upper extremity transplantations have been performed worldwide with highly encouraging outcomes. However, despite the fact that surgical, immunological and functional results are highly encouraging, the need for long-term and high-dose immunosuppression to enable graft survival and to treat/reverse acute skin rejection episodes remains a pace-limiting obstacle towards wide spread application. In this chapter we review the history and development of this novel field, the functional and immunological outcomes based on the world experience, unique biological features of such transplants, mechanisms and treatment protocols for acute skin rejection, as well as novel concepts for immune modulation and tolerance induction.

Key words Composite tissue transplantation, Hand, Face, Immunosuppression, Acute rejection, Tolerance induction

1 Introduction

Composite tissue transplantation has become a clinical reality over the past decade with globally more than 200 procedures of different types of composite allografts successfully performed including hand, forearm, arm, partial facial tissue and full face, abdominal wall, larynx, trachea, vascularized bone and joint, tongue or even uterus and penis [1, 2]. The cumulative world record substantiates the fact that vascularized composite allotransplantation (VCA) or reconstructive transplantation as we refer to such type of transplants today has become a valuable treatment option for those many patients in need suffering from complex tissue injuries and devastating defects where conventional reconstructive approaches and techniques are not available or feasible.

However, the idea of transplanting extremities or other body parts from one individual to another actually is not new and seems to have always been a dream of mankind. One of the earliest and

Andrea A. Zachary and Mary S. Leffell (eds.), *Transplantation Immunology: Methods and Protocols, Second Edition*, Methods in Molecular Biology, vol. 1034, DOI 10.1007/978-1-62703-493-7_5, © Springer Science+Business Media, LLC 2013

most cited reports dating back to the ancient times of human history is the myth of the two Arabian saints Cosmos and Damian who attempted in the early third-century to replace the amputated gangrenous leg of a monk with the limb of an Ethiopian Moor [3]. Inspired by the seminal achievements in solid organ transplantation in the late 1950s, the world's first attempt to transplant a human hand in more recent history was performed in 1964 by Roberto Gilbert Elizalde in Ecuador. The procedure already back then was a surgical, technical success but unfortunately the hand was lost to severe immunological complications and rejection due to the lack of effective immunosuppressive drugs and protocols at that time [4]. Failure of this first transplant and the substantial immunological challenges preventing skin to be transplanted successfully in an allogeneic setting lead to the belief held for many years that transplantation of grafts including a skin component could not be realized at all. However, the introduction of calcineurin inhibitors (cyclosporine A in the 1980s and tacrolimus in the 1990s) and the purine analog mycophenolate mofetil (MMF) into the transplant arena enabled reproducible improvements in long-term graft survival in small and large animal models of VCA including skin [5]. Lee et al. during the same time provided data indicating that in the context of combined or "composite" tissue transplantation, the skin would not be rejected as rapidly and stringently as when skin or other tissue components are transplanted individually [6]. These findings fueled a renewed interest in VCA and the first human hand transplantation in this so called "modern" era of immunosuppression was performed in September 1998 in Lyon, France by a team led by Jean-Michel Dubernard [7]. Shortly thereafter, groups from Louisville, KY, Innsbruck, Austria and again Lyon, France followed and successfully performed several other cases of single as well as bilateral hand and forearm transplants and thereby led the groundwork for multiple teams all over the globe to initiate programs for upper extremity transplantation [8]. Since then, close to 85 upper extremity and 23 face transplantations have been performed with highly encouraging outcomes with regard to graft survival and graft function.

2 Functional and Immunological Outcomes

Functional results after VCA are dependent on the pace and degree of peripheral nerve regeneration, cortical reintegration of the graft, and intensive and continuous rehabilitation including physiotherapy and occupational therapy [9]. In those recipients compliant with immunosuppressive medication and rehabilitation, early and intermediate functional outcomes are highly encouraging, superior to those obtained with prosthesis, and in quite a few cases comparable to what can be achieved after replantation [10]. Extrinsic muscles allow for motor recovery during the early postoperative phase. Return of intrinsic muscle function has been observed in patients receiving a distal or wrist level hand transplantation. In addition to gross and fine motor function, all patients thus far regained protective sensation in their transplants. Discriminative sensation returned in the majority of recipients and their transplanted extremities were fully incorporated into the patient's body image. The functional outcomes after transplantation at more proximal levels though were less consistent and required prolonged rehabilitation [11]. However, as can be concluded from the world experience even though recovery was slow in those recipients it continued to show improvements even several years post transplant.

Despite the fact that surgical procedures and functional outcomes are largely successful, the need for long-term and high-dose multidrug immunosuppressive treatment to enable allograft survival still remains a pace-limiting obstacle toward broader and widespread application and for those procedures [10]. Conventional immunosuppressive strategies applied to VCA today are largely extrapolated from regimens used in solid organ transplantation. The overall level of immunosuppressive medication required to ensure graft survival is comparable or even slightly higher than it is for, for example, kidney transplantation [12]. According to the International Registry for Hand and Composite Tissue Transplantation the majority of hand and face transplant patients received either polyclonal (anti-thymocyte globulins, ATG) or monoclonal (alemtuzumab, basiliximab) antibody preparations as an induction agent followed by a high-dose triple drug combination for maintenance therapy including tacrolimus, MMF and steroids [2, 10]. The tacrolimus trough levels were adjusted to 10–15 ng/ml during the first 1–3 months and 5–10 ng/ml thereafter by most centers. With regard to steroid management, prednisone doses were rapidly tapered in the early post-transplant period and then maintained on lowered doses (5–15 mg/day) for 6–12 months in the majority of the patients performed to date. Of the 33 patients included in the most recent report of the international registry all recipients received tacrolimus as the baseline immunosuppressive agent, 26 received MMF, and 27 of them received steroids. During the follow-up period, eight patients were converted from tacrolimus to the mTOR inhibitor sirolimus with the rationale to minimize renal side effects, improve glycemic control, and potentially avoid chronic vascular changes (myointimal hyperproliferation) and neurotoxicity [10]. In five cases, steroids were withdrawn; two recipients received steroids and low doses of tacrolimus and everolimus; and two patients received sirolimus and MMF [10]. As of now, induction therapy followed by maintenance immunosuppression with at least a dual drug combination at optimum dose can be considered the most widely and commonly used treatment regimen for hand transplantation.

Overall such conventional regimens have proven sufficient to prevent early immunological graft loss but were not able to prevent acute rejection. 85–90 % of all VCA recipients experienced at least one acute rejection episode within the first year after transplantation regardless of their induction or maintenance immunosuppressive treatment protocol; multiple rejection episodes were observed in 56 %. This incidence is significantly higher than what is currently seen in solid organ transplantation where acute rejection rates are less than 10 % in the first year after renal transplantation [13]. However, this is probably partly due to the fact that a VCA represents a visible graft that enables immediate diagnosis of rejection based on even minor changes in appearance. Thus far, in patients compliant with immunosuppressive protocols, all episodes of acute skin rejection were reversible and no grafts in the world experience with VCA were lost due to immunological sequelae [2]. Two patients died following combined hand and face transplantation and an attempted combined upper and lower extremity transplantation. In addition to several unconfirmed cases of hand loss in China, one patient in the US lost a hand allograft as a consequence of arterial intimal hyperplasia and the first hand transplant recipient from France developed progressive acute rejection following noncompliance with immunosuppression [14].

Chronic rejection remains the leading cause for long-term graft loss in solid organ transplantation and is frequently seen after 5 years post transplant [15, 16]. Based on the world experience with hand and face transplantation this seems to be different for VCA where chronic rejection has yet to be distinctly defined and the histopathological features to be described. According to the international registry (www.handregistry.com) 14 patients received a VCA with follow-up for over 5 years and several of them are now even beyond 10 years post transplant without any objective measurable vascular changes such as myointimal hyperproliferation or other indirect signs of chronic rejection. The only clinical evidence for chronic rejection was most recently reported by Kaufman et al. who have shown vasculopathy in six out of six hand transplant recipients in their program [17]. Aggressive and severe intima hyperproliferation was observed early post transplant in two of six of the recipients in their patient series. Of concern, standard monitoring techniques such as protocol skin biopsies or angiography were inadequate to detect early potentially reversible stages of allograft vasculopathy in four out of the six recipients [17]. However, if this exceedingly lower incidence of chronic rejection in VCA as compared to solid organ transplantation is due to potential alterations in antigenicity known from combined organ transplants or when multiple tissue components are transplanted simultaneously needs to be determined [6, 18, 19].

Nevertheless, with thoughtful patient selection, detailed preoperative screening and planning, meticulous surgical technique, and diligent immunological follow-up care, excellent short- and long-term overall results can be achieved in VCA.

3 Mechanisms and Appearance of Skin Rejection

Observations made in the first decade of human upper extremity and face transplantation point towards the skin as the sentinel target for an alloimmune response and rejection. Acute rejection in VCA appears as a maculopapular erythematous rash, which can be patchy and limited to a small, focal, circumscript area of the graft or can spread over large parts of the entire transplant [20, 21]. Clinical macroscopic manifestations thereby can range from mild pink discoloration or erythema to lichenoid papules, edema, and onychomadesis. For histopathological characterization of skin rejection, a specialized Banff classification system has been established [21]. The main histological feature of acute rejection is a mononuclear, lymphocytic cellular infiltrate. It first appears in the perivascular space of the dermis during mild rejection stages and then spreads to the interface between dermis and epidermis and/or adnexal structures. A cellular infiltrate within the epidermis is typical for a moderate grade of rejection with the immunologic response reaching the outermost layer. If rejection is not successfully treated at that stage, necrosis of single keratinocytes can be observed, resulting in focal dermal–epidermal separation and significant graft damage [20, 21]. If rejection progresses further, necrosis and loss of the epidermis, as the ultimate stage of skin rejection, are considered irreversible. Immunohistochemically, the infiltrate in acute skin rejection is comprised predominantly by CD3+ T-cells spreading with progression of rejection from the perivascular space towards the dermis and then the epidermis. Among the CD3+ cells, CD8+ cells are more prominent than CD4+ cells. Depending on the grade of rejection, 10–50 % of infiltrating leukocytes stain positive for CD68. A total of 0.5–5 % of cells are positive for CD20 [22]. However, very limited information is available on the involvement of components other than the skin in this acute rejection process. Biopsy samples from bone, vessels, nerves, or muscles have not been routinely obtained after clinical VCA. The available histological findings in VCA patients are in line with results from experimental studies indicating that the skin is highly immunogenic and hence the primary/sentinel target for rejection [23]. This is further substantiated by the fact that immunological tolerance can be achieved towards all components of a VCA experimentally except the skin. However, it was also shown that skin alterations in a VCA are not exclusively limited to alloimmune-mediated injury. The clinical and histopathological features of immune-related and non-rejection processes are potentially overlapping or may coincide with acute rejection. The underlying mechanisms are largely unknown and represent a current major clinical challenge in differentiating between acute rejection and other forms of skin inflammation.

The skin of a VCA is traditionally known to be its most antigenic component and clinical practice paradigms have therefore advocated the use of high-dose multidrug immunosuppression in VCA recipients. The underlying mechanisms driving the dominant immune response towards the skin and in particular the epidermis when compared to other tissues of a VCA or solid organs remains poorly understood. Animal studies have implicated skin as being highly immunogenic, and this finding has also been noted clinically in hand transplant recipients where the epidermis gets rejected and is lost (in experimental models), while tissues other than the skin remain intact and largely unaffected [10]. The skin is an immunological organ with certain functional properties and characteristics that might contribute to the strong immune response: Skin contains a large number of antigen-presenting cells (APC) such as Langerhans cells and dermal dendritic cells; it has an extracellular matrix with densely packed glycoproteins capable of inducing cell adhesion, activation and proliferation. In addition, keratinocytes are able to express Major Histocompatibility Complex (MHC) class II molecules upon stimulation and to secrete a battery of chemokines and cytokines further attracting lymphocytes to infiltrate the epidermis.

The understanding and clinical relevance of antibody-mediated rejection (AMR) in VCA is currently not well defined. The assessment of C4d complement depositions in protocol skin biopsies has been performed routinely by some but not all hand transplant centers in an attempt to monitor for AMR. Thereby, deposits of C4d were found in approximately 50 % of all skin biopsy samples investigated and no correlation with graft function or cellular rejection could be established [24, 25].

However, donor specific antibodies (DSA) have been found in the serum of some hand transplant recipients but did not necessarily correlate with C4d deposition in corresponding skin biopsies. A recent study using a rat osteomyocutaneous transplant model for VCA showed that these grafts are rejected in an accelerated fashion but not hyperacutely in the presence of allosensitization and preformed DSA. The rejection of a vascularized composite allograft in sensitized recipients was mainly cell mediated and differed mechanistically from that for solid organ transplants [26].

4 Protocols for Prophylaxis and Treatment of Skin Rejection

Similar to maintenance immunosuppressive regimens (outlined above), treatment of acute rejection episodes mirrors therapies and concepts currently used in the field of solid organ transplantation. According to the International Registry on Hand and Composite

Tissue Transplantation (www.handregistry.com) treatment of acute skin rejection episodes included high-dose bolused intravenous steroids in 60 % of all reported cases. In 30 % of the recipients, however, increasing oral steroids was sufficient to reverse rejection. Only in 7.5 % of patients, in which rejection episodes were steroid-resistant, treatment consisted of anti-thymocyte globulins, basiliximab, or alemtuzumab [10]. In addition to systemic treatment, topical application of immunosuppressive ointments (tacrolimus, corticosteroid, or flumix) was performed taking advantage of the unique possibility of treating skin rejection locally. As under-immunosuppression was thought to be the most important cause for rejection, maintenance immunosuppression was increased at the same time in most cases.

When a second rejection episode was encountered, steroids were given intravenously with or without topical ointment in several patients. Alternatively, ATG, basiliximab or topical drugs were only given in a few select patients. In one case of a steroid and ATG resistant rejection alemtuzumab (Campath-1H) was administered and resulted in full restoration of normal skin histology [11]. Thus far, no composite tissue allograft has been lost due to acute irreversible rejection in the world experience with reconstructive transplantation (www.handregistry.com). However, the challenge remains to find a delicate balance between applying sufficient and high enough levels of immunosuppression to prevent rejection and enable graft survival and avoiding over-immunosuppression that might bear the risk of significant associated complications.

5 Unique Biological and Immunological Features of VCA

Many of the side effects of immunosuppression are a result of the fact that systemic medications are being used to treat a localized problem, i.e., the allograft itself. Reconstructive transplantation by its nature allows for the direct application of immunosuppressive agents to its skin component and thereby to the graft itself. Currently, both corticosteroids and tacrolimus are available as topical formulations. Several groups have used these agents in the perioperative period as well as to treat acute rejection episodes. Future advances in topical and targeted treatments for other autoimmune dermatological conditions may yield treatments that can be used in VCA.

To this end the concept of therapeutically targeting, for example, adhesion molecules in inflammatory skin diseases has been successfully applied for the treatment of psoriasis [27]. In an experimental small animal study Hautz et al. demonstrated that limb allograft survival is significantly prolonged by local administration of a specific selectin blocker (Efomycine M) in combination with ALS induction and low-dose tacrolimus maintenance therapy [22].

Such a combination of lymphocyte depletion and targeting lymphocyte trafficking in the skin of a VCA seems to be an appealing approach for the treatment of both acute rejection episodes as well as to minimize/spare maintenance immunosuppression. On the downside, such topical approaches might leave rejection of other tissue components of VCA undetected and allows progression of an immune response within deeper tissues such as muscle and bone. Although an immunosuppressive agent limited to the graft would be desirable, rejection represents a systemic response and it is unlikely that topical treatment alone would be sufficient to prevent or treat rejection. Apart from topical treatment the skin component offers unique and exciting opportunities for immune monitoring such as continuous observation and adequate, targeted allograft biopsy sampling by simple visual inspection of the skin. This subsequently allows for a timely intervention, treatment, and precise adjustment of immunosuppressive medication on an individualized basis.

Furthermore, VCA contain hematolymphoid precursor- and immunocompetent elements such as bone marrow and a vascularized bone marrow niche that may either hasten the rejection processes or on the other hand can result in graft versus host disease (GvHD). These factors not only govern the immune reactivity of these allogeneic tissues, but also define potential immunomodulating strategies that are different from those currently used in solid organ transplantation [28]. The fact that bone marrow elements are co-transplanted with their syngeneic microenvironments and niches also bears significant advantages over the classical approach of bone marrow transplantation for immune modulation. Such co-transplantation in the setting of VCA allows, for example, for immediate engraftment with and without immune modulation of donor hematolymphoid cells with development of mixed- or micro-chimerism and the bone marrow cells also remain in a spatial functional relationship with the stromal cells [29].

Infectious complications play an important role in VCA and are the leading cause of immunosuppression related side effects in this novel field. In particular cytomegalovirus (CMV) infections have been frequently observed after hand and face transplantation despite antiviral prophylaxis and were complicating the postoperative course after VCA [30, 31]. Viral loads thereby were found to be particularly high as compared to those found in solid organ transplant recipients. This is thought to be due to the fact that a composite tissue allograft such as a hand or forearm from a CMV-positive donor may contain a large viral load, as the mass of endothelium is high and hematopoietic precursor cells from the bone marrow component may host latent CMV [32]. Kobayashi et al. furthermore showed that skin grafts can serve as vectors for CMV infection and that CMV seronegative burn patients that required cadaveric skin allografts were particularly susceptible to CMV transmission and infection [33]. This is of particular concern for reconstructive transplantation since VCA contain large skin and mucosa components in almost all instances [34]. In addition, high-dose multidrug immunosuppression and poor HLA match in most VCA recipients significantly impair T-cell responses and limit the interaction between donor APC and recipient CD8+ T cells that is required to control the virus [30]. This may in part explain why antiviral prophylaxis and/or treatment in the setting of VCA were insufficient and ineffective to eliminate the virus. Another key issue with regard to infection and VCA is that a close correlation between CMV infection, virus replication, and acute rejection has been found in both patients after hand and face transplantation. In some of those patients, CMV infection/disease preceded severe acute skin rejection episodes and required second line treatment with cidofovir and foscarnet [32].

6 Novel Concepts for Immune Modulation in Reconstructive Transplantation

Recently, various modifications have been applied to the immunosuppressive protocols used in VCA such as steroid sparing/avoidance attempts, conversion from tracrolimus to the mTOR inhibitor sirolimus for long-term therapy or the use of topical steroid and tacrolimus ointments to reduce the overall amount of systemic immunosuppression. Although great strides in these regimens have been made, the side effects and complications related to chronic multidrug immunosuppression after hand transplantation remain considerable [10]. Obviously there is an evident need for novel concepts of systemic immunosuppression in reconstructive transplantation. Maintaining graft survival while favoring immune regulation and thereby reducing/minimizing adverse effects and improving or optimizing functional outcomes stands to significantly impact the risk–benefit equation of such reconstructive procedures.

Two immunologic responses occur following organ or tissue transplantation: the host-versus-graft response driven by host effector cells and a graft-versus-host response caused by "passenger" leucocytes which are delivered together with the graft [35]. If these two activities are not reciprocal and balanced, one cell population will predominate over the other resulting in either graft rejection or graft versus host disease (GvHD).

One of the best chances to establish a balance between host and donor immune response selectively favoring minimization of immunosuppression or tolerance is in the first few weeks post transplantation. During this time, given that optimal protocols are applied, the high degree of donor leukocyte migration provides the conditions for reciprocal exhaustion–deletion of donor-reactive recipient lymphocytes. The concept involves a depletional induction regimen before transplantation that reduces but does not completely abrogate the anti-donor immune response. Subsequently, low-dose maintenance therapy with the goal to preserve naturally occurring mechanisms of clonal exhaustion/deletion, might lead to a state of immunomodulation or operational tolerance in the recipient. An additional augmentation with donor-derived antigen, e.g., donor bone marrow cells in many instances enables donor-antigen specific immunomodulation through a sustained interaction between the recipient and donor immune cells [36]. Such a concept stimulates intrinsic mechanisms such as clonal exhaustion and deletion and finally immune ignorance to terminate the adaptive immune response and restore the quiescent state of alloreactive recipient lymphocytes [37].

Using such an approach of pre-transplant lymphocyte depletion followed by low-dose tacrolimus monotherapy and donor bone marrow augmentation in a complete MHC-mismatched swine hind-limb transplant model we were recently able to achieve indefinite graft survival without the need for long-term systemic immunosuppressive treatment [38]. Underlying regulatory mechanisms that have been identified in this model include for example effects such as macro- and micro-chimerism, and exhaustion and deletion of the recipient's T cell clones. In addition, Mathes et al. have developed a translational protocol that combines a non-myeloablative induction approach and VCA in a canine model that has led to tolerance to all components of a VCA, including skin, without the need for long-term maintenance immunosuppressive medication [39]. Such experimental evidence helped to recently refine the treatment protocols aiming to support long-term graft survival on minimal maintenance immunosuppression in human VCA.

Based on the data obtained in our laboratory in small and large animal models we implemented such a bone marrow cell based immunomodulatory protocol for the first time for patients after upper extremity transplantation [40].

Five patients received a total of eight hand/forearm transplants [bilateral hand ($n = 2$), a bilateral hand/forearm ($n = 1$) or a unilateral ($n = 2$) hand transplant] between March 2009 and September 2010. Patient I: Is a 24-year-old Marine who lost his right, dominant hand due to a blast injury in a training exercise and received a right hand transplant at the distal forearm level. Patient II: Is a 57-year-old Air Force veteran with bilateral mid-forearm and lower limb amputations due to Streptococcus A sepsis who became the first US bilateral hand/forearm transplant recipient. Patient III: A 41-year-old National Guardsman received the first US above-elbow (right) and hand transplant (left) after loss of limbs in a farming accident. Patient IV: Is a 25-year-old female with quadruple limb amputation due to Norovirus sepsis receiving a right distal-forearm level hand transplant. Patient V: Is a 33-year-old female quadruple amputee due to meningococcal sepsis underwent bilateral distal-forearm level hand transplantation. Currently, 4/5 patients are maintained on a single immunosuppressive drug (tacrolimus) at low levels and continue to have increased motor and sensory function of their transplanted hands. Patients demonstrate sustained improvements in motor function and sensory return correlating with the time after transplantation, level of amputation and participation in hand therapy. Episodes of skin rejection were few and responsive to topical therapy alone or short courses of steroids. Side effects of immunosuppression were overall mild and transient without occurrence of any systemic infectious complications.

This study is currently ongoing but data thus far suggest that the protocol is safe, efficacious, and well tolerated, and has allowed reconstructive transplantation in upper extremity amputees with low-dose tacrolimus monotherapy while minimizing cumulative risks of immunosuppression. However, the implementation of other cell-based therapies including most recent developments such as T regulatory cells or tolerogenic dendritic cells might further enable to minimize or even completely avoid immunosuppressive medication subsequent to VCA and thus ultimately optimize outcomes [41, 42].

7 Summary and Conclusion

Composite tissue transplantation has developed from myth to clinical reality as a novel treatment option for patients with devastating tissue defects and deformities over the past decade. Despite initial skepticism, both functional and immunological results by far exceeded all initial expectations. However, the need for long-term and high-dose multidrug immunosuppression to enable allograft survival still remains a pace-limiting obstacle towards broader application. To this end, as recently shown in translational large animal models and clinical trials, the unique immunological and biological features of vascularized composite allografts might not only help to advance our basic understanding of transplant immunology but also represent a most favorable scenario for minimization of immunosuppressive medication and donor antigen-specific tolerance induction. The implementation of such strategies will ultimately favor the risk–benefit equation for these life-changing types of transplants.

References

1. Swearingen B, Ravindra K, Xu H, Wu S, Breidenbach WC, Ildstad ST (2008) Science of composite tissue allotransplantation. Transplantation 86(5):627–635
2. Schneeberger S, Landin L, Jableki J, Butler P, Hoehnke C, Brandacher G, ESOT CTA Working Group (2011) Achievements and challenges in composite tissue allotransplantation. Transpl Int 24:760–769
3. Black KS, Hewitt CW, Fraser LA, Osborne JG, Achauer BM, Martin DC (1982) Cosmas and Damian in the laboratory. N Engl J Med 306:368–369
4. Gilbert R (1964) Transplant is successful with a cadaver forearm. Med Trib Med News 5:20–22
5. Benhaim P, Anthony JP, Lin LY, McCalmont TH, Mathes SJ (1993) A long-term study of allogeneic rat hindlimb transplants immunosuppressed with RS-61443. Transplantation 56:911–917
6. Lee WP, Yaremchuk MJ, Pan YC, Randolph MA, Tan CM, Weiland AJ (1991) Relative antigenicity of components of a vascularized limb allograft. Plast Reconstr Surg 87:401–411
7. Dubernard JM, Owen E, Herzberg G, Lanzetta M, Martin X, Kapila H (1999) Human hand allograft: report on first 6 months. Lancet 353:1315–1320
8. Foroohar A, Elliott RM, Kim TW, Breidenbach W, Shaked A, Levin LS (2011) The history and evolution of hand transplantation. Hand Clin 27:405–409
9. Ninkovic M, Weissenbacher A, Gabl M, Pierer G, Pratschke J, Margreiter R (2011) Functional outcome after hand and forearm transplantation: what can be achieved? Hand Clin 27:455–465
10. Petruzzo P, Lanzetta M, Dubernard JM, Landin L, Cavadas P, Margreiter R (2010) The international registry on hand and composite tissue transplantation. Transplantation 90:1590–1594
11. Schneeberger S, Ninkovic M, Gabl M, Ninkovic M, Hussl H, Rieger M (2007) First forearm transplantation: outcome at 3 years. Am J Transplant 7:1753–1762
12. Ravindra KV, Buell JF, Kaufman CL, Blair B, Marvin M, Nagubandi R (2008) Hand transplantation in the United States: experience with 3 patients. Surgery 144:638–643
13. Kaufman DB, Leventhal JR, Axelrod D, Gallon LG, Parker MA, Stuart FP (2005) Alemtuzumab induction and prednisone-free maintenance immunotherapy in kidney transplantation: comparison with basiliximab induction—long-term results. Am J Transplant 5:2539–2548
14. Kanitakis J, Jullien D, Petruzzo P, Hakim N, Claudy A, Revillard JP (2003) Clinicopathologic features of graft rejection of the first human hand allograft. Transplantation 76:688–693
15. Balk AHMM, Weimar W (1992) Chronic heart graft rejection in the clinical setting. In: Paul LC, Lolez K (eds) Organ transplantation: long-term results. Marcel Dekker, New York, pp 187–195
16. Wahlers T, Haverich A, Schäfers HJ, Hirt SW, Fieguth HG, Jurmann M (1993) Chronic rejection following lung transplantation. Incidence, time pattern and consequences. Eur J Cardiothorac Surg 7:319–323
17. Kaufman CL, Ouseph R, Blair B, Kutz JE, Tsai TM, Scheker LR (2012) Graft vasculopathy in clinical hand transplantation. Am J Transplant 12:1004–1016
18. Sarris GE, Smith JA, Shumway NE, Stinson EB, Oyer PE, Robbins RC (1994) Long-term results of combined heart-lung transplantation: the Stanford experience. J Heart Lung Transplant 13:940–949
19. Murase N, Demetris AJ, Matsuzaki T, Yagihashi A, Todo S, Fung J (1991) Long survival in rats after multivisceral versus isolated small-bowel allotransplantation under FK 506. Surgery 110:87–98
20. Schneeberger S, Gorantla VS, van Riet RP, Lanzetta M, Vereecken P, van Holder C (2008) Atypical acute rejection after hand transplantation. Am J Transplant 8:688–696
21. Cendales LC, Kanitakis J, Schneeberger S, Burns C, Ruiz P, Landin L (2008) The Banff 2007 working classification of skin-containing composite tissue allograft pathology. Am J Transplant 8:1396–1400
22. Hautz T, Zelger B, Grahammer J, Krapf C, Amberger A, Brandacher G (2010) Molecular markers and targeted therapy of skin rejection in composite tissue allotransplantation. Am J Transplant 10:1200–1209
23. Gorantla VS, Demetris AJ (2011) Acute and chronic rejection in upper extremity transplantation: what have we learned? Hand Clin 27:481–493
24. Landin L, Cavadas PC, Ibañez J, Roger I, Vera-Sempere F (2009) CD3+-mediated rejection and C4d deposition in two composite tissue (bilateral hand) allograft recipients after induction with alemtuzumab. Transplantation 87:776–781
25. Kanitakis J, McGregor B, Badet L, Petruzzo P, Morelon E, Devauchelle B (2007) Absence of c4d deposition in human composite tissue (hands and face) allograft biopsies: an immunoperoxidase study. Transplantation 84:265–267

26. Wu S, Xu H, Chen B, Wen Y, Ikusika OM, Ocker A (2011) Sensitized recipients exhibit accelerated but not hyperacute rejection of vascularized composite tissue allografts. Transplantation 92:627–633
27. Lebwohl M, Tyring SK, Hamilton TK, Toth D, Glazer S, Tawfik NH, Efalizumab Study Group (2003) A novel targeted T-cell modulator, efalizumab, for plaque psoriasis. N Engl J Med 349:2004–2013
28. Brandacher G, Gorantla VS, Lee WP (2010) Hand allotransplantation. Semin Plast Surg 24:11–17
29. Ramsamooj R, Hewitt CW (2008) In: CW Hewitt et al. (eds), Transplantation of Com posite Tissue Allografts. Springer, p 272–277
30. Schneeberger S, Lucchina S, Lanzetta M, Brandacher G, Bösmüller C, Steurer W (2005) Cytomegalovirus-related complications in human hand transplantation. Transplantation 80:441–447
31. Gordon CR, Abouhassan W, Avery RK (2011) What is the true significance of donor-related cytomegalovirus transmission in the setting of facial composite tissue allotransplantation? Transplant Proc 43:3516–3520
32. Bonatti H, Brandacher G, Margreiter R, Schneeberger S (2009) Infectious complications in three double hand recipients: experience from a single center. Transplant Proc 41:517–520
33. Kobayashi H, Kobayashi M, McCauley RL, Herndon DN, Pollard RB, Suzuki F (1999) Cadaveric skin allograft-associated cytomegalovirus transmission in a mouse model of thermal injury. Clin Immunol 92:181–187
34. Gordon CR, Zor F, Siemionow M (2011) Skin area quantification in preparation for concomitant upper extremity and face transplantation: a cadaver study and literature review. Transplantation 91:1050–1056
35. Starzl TE, Zinkernagel RM (2001) Transplantation tolerance from a historical perspective. Nat Rev Immunol 1:233–239
36. Gorantla VS, Brandacher G, Schneeberger S, Zheng XX, Donnenberg AD, Losee JE, Lee WP (2011) Favoring the risk-benefit balance for upper extremity transplantation—the Pittsburgh Protocol. Hand Clin 27(4):511–520
37. Starzl TE (2007) Acquired immunologic tolerance: with particular reference to transplantation. Immunol Res 38(1–3):6–41
38. Hettiaratchy S, Melendy E, Randolph MA, Coburn RC, Neville DM Jr, Sachs DH, Huang CA, Lee WP (2004) Tolerance to composite tissue allografts across a major histocompatibility barrier in miniature swine. Transplantation 77(4):514–521
39. Mathes DW, Hwang B, Graves SS, Edwards J, Chang J, Storer BE, Butts-Miwongtum T, Sale GE, Nash RA, Storb R (2011) Tolerance to vascularized composite allografts in canine mixed hematopoietic chimeras. Transplantation 92(12):1301–1308
40. Brandacher G, Gorantla VS, Schneeberger S, Shores JT, Imbriglia J, Azari K, Fletcher D, Zeevi A, Demetris A, Starzl TE, Losee JE, Lee WPA (2011) Hand/forearm transplantation using a novel cell-based immunomodulatory protocol—experience with five patients. Am J Transplant 11:190
41. Li XC, Turka LA (2010) An update on regulatory T cells in transplant tolerance and rejection. Nat Rev Nephrol 6(10):577–583
42. Matta BM, Castellaneta A, Thomson AW (2010) Tolerogenic plasmacytoid DC. Eur J Immunol 40(10):2667–2676

Chapter 6

Transplantation of the Sensitized Patient: Histocompatibility Testing

Robert A. Montgomery, Mary S. Leffell, and Andrea A. Zachary

Abstract

A component necessary for successful transplantation of the sensitized patient is timely and high quality support from the histocompatibility laboratory that helps guide selection of the best route to transplantation and the clinical care of the patient. Responsibilities of the laboratory include risk assessment, HLA typing, and accurate antibody characterization.

Key words Antibody monitoring, CDC crossmatch, Desensitization, Flow cytometric crossmatch, Kidney paired donation, Risk assessment, Sensitized patients, Solid phase immunoassays, Virtual crossmatch

1 Introduction

Desensitization, kidney paired donation (KPD) including domino and chain transplants, and KPD combined with desensitization have resulted in the successful transplantation of hundreds of patients disadvantaged by sensitization to HLA antigens and/or by their ABO type. These patients may have had prolonged waiting times, with its associated morbidities, or may have never been transplanted. We review here the role of the histocompatibility laboratory in support of transplantation of the sensitized patient.

2 Identifying the Most Likely Route to Transplantation

For centers with both desensitization and KPD programs, it is useful to know which route is most likely to result in transplantation. The breadth and strength of HLA antibodies are the factors with the greatest impact on the route to transplantation [1], as broadly sensitized patients, particularly those with homozygosity at any HLA locus or rare phenotypes, will have greater difficulty in finding a compatible KPD donor than those less broadly sensitized.

Andrea A. Zachary and Mary S. Leffell (eds.), *Transplantation Immunology: Methods and Protocols, Second Edition*, Methods in Molecular Biology, vol. 1034, DOI 10.1007/978-1-62703-493-7_6, © Springer Science+Business Media, LLC 2013

For patients with living potential donors, the degree of incompatibility is best assessed by a crossmatch that measures not only the strength of the donor-specific antibodies (DSA) but also the extent of antigen expression, which can vary among individuals. The titer of antibody to a potential donor determines how difficult it will be to achieve successful desensitization. It has been shown that high dose IVIg is more successful in reducing antibodies of lower titer [2–4]. Plasmapheresis and low dose IVIg or CMVIg (PP/IVIg) can overcome higher levels of donor-specific antibody (DSA) but very high DSA levels will require extensive treatment [5, 6]. Further, the elimination of DSA by this protocol is influenced by DSA specificity with 75 % of class I antibodies, 53 % of antibodies specific for DRB1 and DQB antigens, and only 10 % of antibodies to DR51, DR52, and DR53 eliminated [7]. The threshold of DSA that is acceptable for desensitization must be determined individually by each program. For patients awaiting deceased donor transplantation, the high dose IVIg protocol can be applied preemptively while the PP/IVIg protocol can be implemented immediately following transplantation for lower levels of incompatibility. Information useful to the physician includes test outcome, the strength of a positive crossmatch and the extent of contribution of different HLA antibodies, specificity of DSA present in crossmatch negative cases, the presence of factors such as autoantibodies that may influence test results, and the identity of repeated mismatches.

When the available donors have an unacceptable level of incompatibility, the likelihood of finding a compatible unrelated donor can be determined by identifying the specificity and strength of all of a patient's HLA antibodies. The antibodies that have an unacceptable strength can be identified through a series of crossmatches with donors mismatched for only a single antigen, as is done in Eurotransplant. However, this requires access to cells from an extremely large panel of HLA typed individuals and in the USA, solid phase immunoassays are most often used to characterize HLA antibodies. The data generated from these assays can then be entered into a program maintained by the United Network for Organ Sharing, the CPRA (calculated panel reactive antibody) calculator that generates the frequency of US donors with unacceptable antigens. This program is available at: http://optn.transplant.hrsa.gov/resources/professionalResources.asp?index=78.

Although SPIs are only semiquantitative, accurate and thorough interpretation of these assays permits establishing a correlation with crossmatch results that, in turn, permits highly reliable predictions of crossmatch outcome [8–10]. The high sensitivity of bead based SPIs provides an opportunity to detect very low levels of antibody, not possible previously with cell based assays [11]. This increased sensitivity also makes SPIs susceptible to variability in environmental conditions and to interference by factors present in the serum such as high levels of IgM, the presence of immune complexes, nonspecific binding of immunoglobulins to the solid matrix, and the presence of antibodies specific for the solid matrix [12, 13]. Therefore, obtaining accurate results depends on precision in test performance and on implementation of procedures to reduce or eliminate interference. Such procedures include hypotonic dialysis, dilution, and addition of EDTA [13–16].

There are some patients for whom the strength of antibody to available living donors precludes desensitization and the breadth of antibody predicts an unacceptably low probability of finding a compatible donor. When such a patient has antibodies that vary in strength, it may be possible to find a donor to whom the patient has antibodies that can be reduced effectively by desensitization. We have performed 91 such transplants using KPD combined with desensitization and found no difference in outcomes when compared to KPD in which the donors were completely compatible and no desensitization was necessary. Of course other factors, such as medical urgency, ABO types of the patient and original donor, HLA homozygosity in the donor, and number of potential donors associated with a patient, will also influence choice of transplant route and a Bayes' calculation can be applied to the collective data to calculate the probability of achieving transplantation by any particular route [17]. The probability of finding a match in a KPD can be predicted based upon verified mathematical simulations once the donor/recipient phenotypes have been established [18]. However, even if desensitization appears to be a logical choice, it is worthwhile to enter a patient into a paired donation registry as there is always the possibility of finding a compatible donor or a donor to which the patient has lower strength DSA.

3 Prior to Transplantation: Patient Evaluation

3.1 Desensitization

The laboratory's role prior to transplantation varies according to the desensitization protocol. For the protocol that employs monthly doses of high dose IVIg, testing for changes in antibody strength should occur at a sufficient time after dosing to avoid the interference in SPI known to occur when blood levels of IVIg are high. If the treatment protocol includes other agents that interfere with crossmatch tests, such as rituximab, monitoring should be based on SPIs. The PP/IVIg protocol implies a commitment to proceed with transplantation in the living donor situation since aborting treatment frequently results in substantial increases in DSA strength [19]. Monitoring prior to the start of PP/IVIg treatment should identify the trend of DSA strength as fewer treatments are required when DSA strength is static or declining compared to when it is increasing. Monitoring once treatment is initiated is to evaluate the decrease in DSA seen in serum after the initial treatment, the amount of rebound seen in the next pretreatment serum, and the level of DSA in serum obtained immediately prior to each subsequent treatment. The effectiveness of treatment in reducing DSA may dictate reducing or increasing the number of pre-transplant treatments. The response to treatment of the majority of patients is a steady decline in DSA strength. However, some antibodies are more refractory, necessitating additional treatments or immunosuppressive agents. In either protocol, a threshold should be established below which it is considered safe to transplant [20]. Reinsmoen et al have determined, for the high dose IVIg protocol, the strength of DSA associated with a reduced probability of antibody mediated rejection after transplantation thus increasing the likelihood of success [21]. In the PP/IVIg protocol the goal of pre-transplant treatment is to reduce the antibody strength below a positive cytotoxic crossmatch. Before discontinuing post-transplant PP/IVIg, it is desirable to reduce DSA to the level of a negative flow cytometric crossmatch. However, this must be weighed against the risks associated with prolonged plasmapheresis treatment.

For either protocol, it is worthwhile to identify other factors that are associated with risk of antibody mediated rejection and that may influence the specific treatment protocol. Such factors may include mismatches shared with a previous transplant [22, 23], the immunologic response to previous mismatches, and the number and specificity of mismatches in the potential donor [24, 25]. It is important to be able to identify all antibody specificities including those to DQA, DPA, and to epitopes that consist of portions of the α and β chains of DQ and DP molecules [27, 28]. Implicit in this is the requirement for typing for all the relevant HLA antigens. It is often useful to determine the paternal antigens to which a parous female has been exposed as a potential for identifying sensitization in the absence of current antibody production. However, exposure to an antigen does not guarantee that sensitization has occurred and it may not be possible to determine the total antigen exposure via pregnancy or transfusion. We have shown that cryptic sensitization can be recognized by quantifying HLA specific B cells and further that nonspecific activation of memory B cells resulting from the inflammatory response to surgery can be obviated by treatment with rituximab [29–31].

Importantly, there must be a system that assures acquisition and delivery of pretreatment and posttreatment blood specimens to the laboratory. Timeliness in testing and communicating results to the clinical team is essential. Equally important is that the clinical team inform the laboratory of any change in treatment that can affect test outcomes or of any inflammatory event such as infection or allergic reaction that may cause a rebound in DSA [32].

3.2 Kidney Paired Donation

As with desensitization, complete and accurate typing and antibody characterization is essential. Crossmatch tests provide the most accurate assessment of the compatibility of a potential donor.

However, the availability of donors for testing can pose logistical problems and represent additional cost when several donors must be tested. These problems can be overcome when the laboratory can perform virtual crossmatches with a high degree of correct prediction. The accuracy of prediction depends on the ability of the laboratory to correlate crossmatch results with those of SPIs which, in turn, is affected by differences in the sensitivity of different lots of SPI test kits, day to day variability in test sensitivity, differences among specificities in the amount and condition of antigen, and the collective strength of multiple DSAs.

4 Testing After Transplantation

The guidelines for post-transplant monitoring are the same for all sensitized patients whether transplanted by KPD or after desensitization. Sensitized patients are known to be at higher risk for the development of DSA if it is not present prior to transplantation, for an anamnestic response of historic antibody, and for increases in the breadth and strength of existing DSA [33]. An unfortunate circumstance in the USA is that post-transplant antibody testing is not reimburseable. It is an understatement to say that this is penny wise and pound foolish as the cost of antibody testing compared to the cost of a graft failed to AMR is incalculable. For the patient sensitized to donor HLA antigen, the transplantation surgery is a pro-inflammatory event that can generate an anamnestic response resulting in the reappearance of historic antibody and increase the strength and breadth of existing antibodies [30, 32]. The immediate post transplant period is critical and antibodies should be monitored frequently during the first 2 weeks after transplantation [33]. The high sensitivity of these assays, particularly the multiplexed bead assays, provides the earliest evidence of a brewing AMR. This is demonstrated in Fig. 1 that shows an increase in DSA strength well before an increase in serum creatinine is observed. We will often reinstitute empiric PP/IVIg therapy based on subclinical rises in DSA.

An important issue is recognizing when an increase in the test value represents a real increase in antibody strength. On one hand, overestimating an increase can result in expensive and unnecessary treatment but on the other, failing to recognize a real increase may result in preventable injury to the graft. Substantial increases in test values are a clear indication of antibody increases but smaller increases, such as 1000 MFI in a Luminex® bead assay can be due to day to day variability. There are several measures that can be taken to better assess such test results. Plotting the positive control value for each run against the values of beads bearing target antigens as shown in Fig. 2 or using the ratio of the test bead to the positive control bead provides an indication of the extent to which

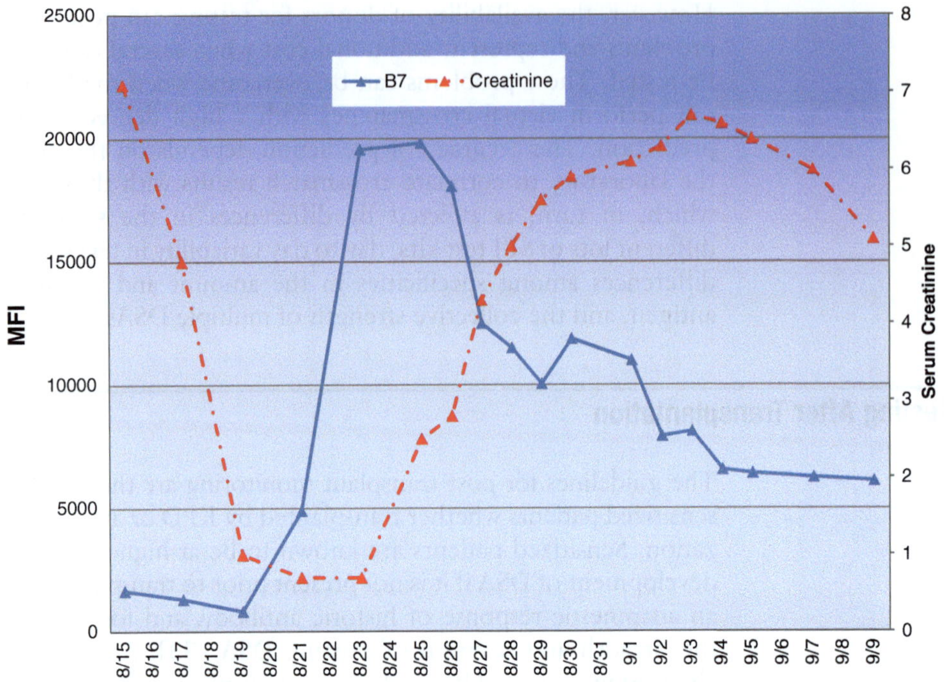

Fig. 1 An increase in donor-specific antibody is seen several days before serum creatinine increases

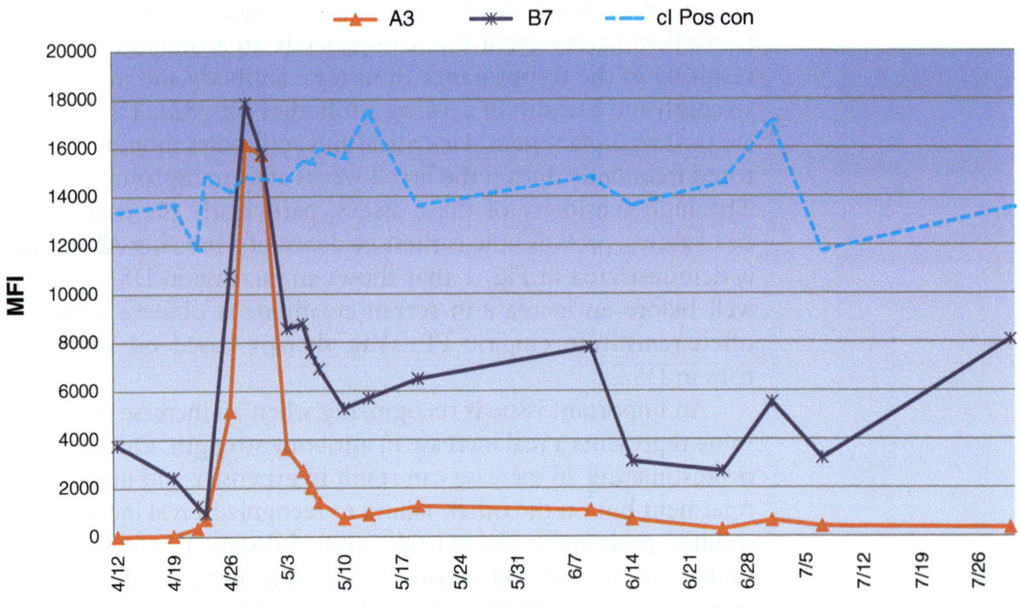

Fig. 2 A dramatic increase in the A3 and B7 DSAs was seen between 4/19 and 5/3. Treatment with PP/IVIg reduced antibody levels. Beginning on 5/17 through the remainder of the testing period, the changes in the apparent strength of B7 antibody parallel changes in the strength of the positive control (Pos con) and the course of the B7 antibody probably reflects day to day variability in test sensitivity and little if any real change in DSA strength

changes in test values are the result of day to day variability in test sensitivity. Variability in test sensitivity usually results in a change in the values of all beads—those bearing donor antigens as well as those bearing third party antigen. However, a change in the order of the beads, when listed in descending order of reaction strength, suggests a real change in antibody strength. Different reagent lots may differ in sensitivity and if a lot change occurs while a patient is being monitored, a serum, tested on the previous lot should be tested on the new lot as a reference. We have found it useful to obtain an additional serum specimen when an antibody increase is suspected as an upward trend in test values strongly suggests a real increase in antibody strength.

Increases in DSA strength may persist even in the face of aggressive treatment. It is useful to know when such an increase has crossed the threshold of crossmatch positivity. This may not always be clear from the SPIs. While we have shown better correlations between phenotype panel reactivity and crossmatch strength, not all specificities can be readily assessed in broadly reactive sera. Single antigen panels provide the opportunity to follow each antibody specificity. However, when there are multiple DSAs, the collective strength of the antibodies cannot be determined from the sum of the values of the different test beads. In such cases, it can be useful to perform a donor crossmatch, which is facilitated by freezing donor cells in advance. This may be particularly important in the KPD situation involving multiple transplant centers when it may be logistically difficult to obtain additional donor blood.

Post-transplant monitoring requires timely, ongoing communication within the entire transplant team. The laboratory must be made aware of changes in treatment and patient status and the physicians and coordinators must be provided with test results and the need for any additional blood specimens, expediently. MFI values are not an adequate indicator of antibody strength since the correlation with antibody strength varies among different beads, among different kits both within and between manufacturers, among different lots, and as noted above, can vary from day to day [16, 20, 34]. Therefore, the laboratory must make an assessment of the actual change in DSA strength.

Although antibody monitoring is most critical in the early post-transplant period, sensitized patients are always at risk for changes in DSA status. Long-term monitoring can provide an early indication of such changes. Further, it is worthwhile to test a specimen after events that are known to be pro-inflammatory such as infection and trauma.

4.1 Non-HLA Antibodies

Significant improvement in the detection and characterization of HLA antibodies has improved our understanding of the role of other antibodies. Antibodies to both autologous and allogeneic targets can effect damage to the graft [25–38]. Many laboratories have begun to explore and identify non-HLA antibodies and study their role in the transplantation of various organs. Such investigation can only enhance the success of transplantation.

5 Summary

We have provided here a brief overview of the role and responsibility of the histocompatibility laboratory in supporting the transplantation of the sensitized patient. There are many moving parts that must be considered in the effective management of immunologically and medically complex patients, many of whom have been waiting years for this opportunity to live a normal life. It requires a dedicated team of practitioners from many specialties including immunogenetics, transplant surgery, nephrology, pathology, transfusion medicine, pharmacy, administration, transplant coordination, nursing, and finance to provide optimal care for this disadvantaged group of patients. Communication and knowledge are essential to every component of the multidisciplinary team.

References

1. Montgomery RA, Lonze BE, Jackson AM (2011) Using donor exchange paradigms with desensitization to enhance transplant rates among highly sensitized patients. Curr Opin Organ Transplant 16:439–443
2. Vo AA, Lukovsky M, Toyoda M, Wang J, Reinsmoen NL, Lai CH et al (2008) Rituximab and intravenous immune globulin for desensitization during renal transplantation. N Engl J Med 359:242–251
3. Lai CH, Cao K, Ong G, Naim M, Wang Q, Mirocha J et al (2011) Antibody testing strategies for deceased donor kidney transplantation after immunomodulatory therapy. Transplantation 92:48–53
4. Alachkar N, Lonze BE, Zachary AA, Holechek MJ, Schillinger K, Cameron AM et al (2012) Infusion of high-dose intravenous immunoglobulin fails to lower the strength of human leukocyte antigen antibodies in highly sensitized patients. Transplantation 94:165–171
5. Montgomery RA, Zachary AA (2004) Transplanting patients with a positive donor-specific crossmatch: a single center's perspective. Pediatr Transplant 8:535–542
6. Zachary AA, Montgomery RA, Ratner LE, Samaniego-Picota M, Haas M, Kopchaliiska D et al (2003) Specific and durable elimination of antibody to donor HLA antigens in renal-transplant patients. Transplantation 76:1519–1525
7. Zachary AA, Montgomery RA, Leffell MS (2005) Factors associated with and predictive of persistence of donor-specific antibody after treatment with plasmapheresis and intravenous immunoglobulin. Hum Immunol 66:364–370
8. Zachary AA, Sholander JT, Houp JA, Leffell MS (2009) Using real data for a virtual crossmatch. Hum Immunol 70:574–579
9. Ferrari P, Fidler S, Holdsworth R, Woodroffe C, Tassone G, Watson N, Cantwell L, Bennett G, Thornton A, Christiansen FT, D'Orsogna L (2012) High transplant rates of highly sensitized recipients with virtual crossmatching in kidney paired donation. Transplantation 94:744–749
10. Ellis TM, Schiller JJ, Roza AM, Cronin DC, Shames BD, Johnson CP (2012) Diagnostic accuracy of solid phase HLA antibody assays for prediction of crossmatch strength. Hum Immunol 73:706–710
11. Tait BD (2009) Solid phase assays for HLA antibody detection in clinical transplantation. Curr Opin Immunol 21:573–577
12. Waterboer T, Sehr P, Pawlita M (2006) Suppression of non-specific binding in serological Luminex assays. J Immunol Methods 309:200–204
13. Zachary AA, Lucas DP, Detrick B, Leffell MS (2009) Naturally occurring interference in Luminex® assays for HLA-specific antibodies: characteristics and resolution. Hum Immunol 70:496–501

14. Schnaidt M, Weinstock C, Jurisic M, Schmid-Horch B, Ender A, Wernet D (2011) HLA antibody specification using single-antigen beads—technical solution for the prozone effect. Transplantation 92:510–515
15. Butch AW (2000) Dilution protocols for detection of hook effects/prozone phenomenon. Clin Chem 46:1719
16. Zachary AA, Vega RM, Lucas DP, Leffell MS (2012) HLA antibody detection and characterization by solid phase immunoassays: methods and pitfalls. Methods Mol Biol 882:289–308
17. Jackson AM, Leffell MS, Montgomery RA, Zachary AA (2012) A GPS for finding the route to transplantation of the sensitized patient. Curr Opin Organ Transplant 17:433–439
18. Montgomery RA (2010) Renal transplantation across HLA and ABO antibody barriers: integrating paired donation into desensitization protocols. Am J Transplant 10:449–457
19. Zachary AA, Montgomery RA, Jordan SC, Reinsmoen NL, Claas FHJ, Reed EF (2007) 14th International HLA and immunogenetics workshop: report on understanding antibodies in transplantation. Tissue Antigens 69(S1):160–173
20. Zachary A, Reinsmoen NL (2011) Quantifying HLA-specific antibodies in patients undergoing desensitization. Curr Opin Organ Transplant 16:410–415
21. Reinsmoen NL, Lai CH, Vo A, Cao K, Ong G, Naim M et al (2008) Acceptable donor-specific antibody levels allowing for successful deceased and living donor kidney transplantation after desensitization therapy. Transplantation 86:820–825
22. Cecka JM, Terasaki PI (1994) Repeating HLA antigen mismatches in renal transplants—a second class mistake? Transplantation 57:515–519
23. Opelz G (1995) Repeated HLA mismatches increase the failure rate of second kidney transplants. Collaborative Transplant Study. Transplant Proc 27:658–659
24. Claas FHJ, Dankers MK, Oudshoorn M, van Rood JJ, Mulder A, Roelen D et al (2005) Differential immunogenicity of HLA mismatches in clinical transplantation. Transpl Immunol 14:187–191
25. Wissing KM, Fomegné G, Broeders N, Ghisdal L, Hoang AD, Mikhalski D et al (2008) HLA mismatches remain risk factors for acute kidney allograft rejection in patients receiving quadruple immunosuppression with anti-interleukin-2 receptor antibodies. Transplantation 85:411–416
26. Duquesnoy RJ (2011) Humoral alloimmunity in transplantation: relevance of HLA epitope antigenicity and immunogenicity. Front Immunol 2:106
27. Tambur AR, Leventhal JR, Friedewald JJ, Ramon DS (2010) The complexity of human leukocyte antigen (HLA)-DQ antibodies and its effect on virtual crossmatching. Transplantation 90:1117–1124
28. Deng CT, El-Awar N, Ozawa M, Cai J, Lachmann N, Terasaki PI (2008) Human leukocyte antigen class II DQ alpha and beta epitopes identified from sera of kidney allograft recipients. Transplantation 86:452–459
29. Zachary AA, Kopchaliiska D, Montgomery RA, Leffell MS (2007) HLA-specific B cells: I. A method for their detection, quantification, and isolation using HLA tetramers. Transplantation 83:982–988
30. Zachary AA, Kopchaliiska D, Montgomery RA, Melancon JK, Leffell MS (2007) HLA-specific B cells: II. Application to transplantation. Transplantation 83:989–994
31. Zachary AA, Lucas DP, Montgomery RA, Leffell MS (2013) Rituximab prevents an anamnestic response in patients with cryptic sensitization to HLA. Transplantation 95(5):701–704
32. Locke JE, Zachary AA, Warren DS, Segev DL, Houp JA, Montgomery RA, Leffell MS (2009) Proinflammatory events are associated with significant increases in breadth and strength of HLA-specific antibody. Am J Transplant 9:2136–2139
33. Mohamed MA, Muth B, Vidyasagar V, Foley D, Fernandez L, Hofmann RM et al (2011) Post-transplant DSA monitoring may predict antibody-mediated rejection in sensitized kidney transplant recipients. Clin Transpl 2011:389–394
34. Leffell MS, Zachary AA (2010) Antiallograft antibodies: relevance, detection, and monitoring. Curr Opin Organ Transplant 15:2–7
35. Dragun D, Philippe A, Catar R (2012) Role of non-HLA antibodies in organ transplantation. Curr Opin Organ Transplant 17:440–445
36. Jackson AM, Lucas DP, Melancon JK, Desai NM (2011) Clinical relevance and IgG subclass determination of non-HLA antibodies identified using endothelial cell precursors isolated from donor blood. Transplantation 92:54–60
37. Li L, Sigdel T, Vitalone M, Lee SH, Sarwal M (2010) Differential immunogenicity and clinical relevance of kidney compartment specific antigens after renal transplantation. J Proteome Res 9:6715–6721
38. Zhang Q, Reed EF (2010) Non-MHC antigenic targets of the humoral response in transplantation. Curr Opin Immunol 22:682–688

Chapter 7

Thoracic Organ Transplantation: Laboratory Methods

Jignesh K. Patel and Jon A. Kobashigawa

Abstract

Although great progress has been achieved in thoracic organ transplantation through the development of effective immunosuppression, there is still significant risk of rejection during the early post-transplant period, creating a need for routine monitoring for both acute antibody and cellular mediated rejection. The currently available multiplexed, microbead assays utilizing solubilized HLA antigens afford the capability of sensitive detection and identification of HLA and non-HLA specific antibodies. These assays are being used to assess the relative strength of donor specific antibodies; to permit performance of virtual crossmatches which can reduce the waiting time to transplantation; to monitor antibody levels during desensitization; and for heart transplants to monitor antibodies post-transplant. For cell mediated immune responses, the recent development of gene expression profiling has allowed noninvasive monitoring of heart transplant recipients yielding predictive values for acute cellular rejection. T cell immune monitoring in heart and lung transplant recipients has allowed individual tailoring of immunosuppression, particularly to minimize risk of infection. While the current antibody and cellular laboratory techniques have enhanced the ability to manage thoracic organ transplant recipients, future developments from improved understanding of microchimerism and graft tolerance may allow more refined allograft monitoring techniques.

Key words Laboratory techniques, Circulating antibodies, Virtual crossmatch, Calculated panel reactive antibodies, Complement fixing antibodies, Allomap, Immune monitoring, Biomarkers

1 Introduction

Thoracic organ transplantation has become an established and acceptable therapeutic option for select patients with end-stage heart and lung disease. In the early years of thoracic transplantation, allograft rejection had been the main challenge limiting survival, a phenomenon well described in early animal experiments by Medawar et al. [1]. Acceptable survival rates only evolved with the introduction of effective immunosuppressive agents, particularly the calcineurin inhibitors, cyclosporine [3], and later tacrolimus [4]. Rejection rates sharply declined as did infection rates as host responses to bacterial and fungal infection were relatively preserved with the new immunosuppressive regimens. The improvements in

Andrea A. Zachary and Mary S. Leffell (eds.), *Transplantation Immunology: Methods and Protocols, Second Edition*, Methods in Molecular Biology, vol. 1034, DOI 10.1007/978-1-62703-493-7_7, © Springer Science+Business Media, LLC 2013

morbidity and mortality led to a remarkable expansion in solid organ transplantation. In cardiac transplantation by the late 1990s more than 2,800 transplants were being performed annually, with actuarial survival rates at 1 year and 5 years of 85 % and 75 % respectively [5]. Currently, around 3,700 heart transplants are being performed globally with a half-life of 11 years, the number being limited only by the limited supply of organ donors [6]. Although rejection rates continue to decline, the risk of rejection remains significant particularly in the early period following transplantation, necessitating routine surveillance for both acute cellular and antibody-mediated rejection (AMR). AMR is associated with worse survival and predisposes patients to vasculopathy [7]. Patients awaiting thoracic organ transplantation may manifest circulating antibodies against HLA (human leukocyte antigens). This process by which antibodies are formed is called sensitization. Sensitization occurs from exposure to blood transfusions, pregnancy, previous organ transplant, or the placement of a ventricular assist device. Identification of sensitized patients is a major concern because such patients are at increased risk of hyperacute rejection. Sensitization is associated with decreased survival, increased risk of rejection and the development of cardiac allograft vasculopathy in heart transplant recipients [7, 8]. The development of laboratory techniques has significantly contributed to the identification and management of sensitized patients at high risk of rejection.

2 Antibody Screening and Characterization

Antibody screening is routinely performed on patients waiting for solid organ transplants and measures circulating anti-HLA antibodies. The calculated panel reactive antibody (CPRA) score is given as a percentage and is a representation of the portion of the population that the anti-HLA antibody in the recipient's blood reacts with. The presence of HLA antibody after heart transplant has been shown to correlate with outcomes [9]. In a retrospective review of over 8,000 heart transplant recipients in the UNOS database, PRA was 0 % in just under 75 % of patients and just over 9 % of patients were at least moderately sensitized (PRA>10 %). Increasing PRA was correlated with both allograft rejection and adverse survival at 5 years.

Techniques for measuring HLA antibodies have evolved significantly over the last 20 years [10, 11]. Traditionally, complement-dependent cytotoxicity (CDC) assays have been performed assessing the ability of recipient serum to lyse T or B cells obtained from a panel of volunteers representative of the population. The addition of anti-human globulin (AHG) increased the sensitivity of CDC assays and allowed for detection of cytotoxic-negative, adsorption-positive HLA alloantibodies. However, because both IgG and IgM can bind complement, neither the CDC nor the AHG-CDC tests are able to distinguish between the immunoglobulin classes. The CDC also cannot distinguish between major histocompatibility (MHC) Class I and Class II antibodies or between HLA and non-HLA antibodies. Another problem with the CDC assay is that large cell panels are needed to provide coverage for detecting the most common HLA antigens, and rare or unusual antigens may be omitted [12].

More recent techniques use flow cytometry or enzyme-linked immunosorbent assay (ELISA) [11] and generally provide more reproducible results. The multiplex bead assay performed on the Luminex® platform allows for simultaneous detection of multiple antibodies, as up to 100 color-coded antigen-coated microspheres can be detected in a single well [13]. The FlowPRA® test consists of a pool of microparticle beads coated with full HLA Class I or Class II phenotype derived from purified HLA-bearing cell lines [14]. Due to variability in results between techniques, many laboratories will utilize multiple confirmatory tests.

While these assays are useful screening tools for determination of the presence of HLA antibodies further tests are required to determine specificity and quantification of alloantibodies. The importance of the strength of circulating antibody is increasingly recognized as an important factor determining the risk of a cytotoxic response. Tests based on flow cytometry to determine specificity use a panel of HLA Class I and II beads. Due to the polymorphic nature of HLA proteins, multiplex systems have been developed containing HLA Class I and II proteins from platelets, or antigens from transformed lines that are representative of all major HLA antigens. However, for determination of multiple antibody specificities and quantification of antibodies, single-antigen bead assays are now commonly deployed [15].

The ability to detect and quantify the strength of specific antibodies has allowed estimation of which recipient circulation antibodies are present at a strength that may prove to be cytotoxic for a potential donor organ. Laboratories will typically perform validation studies to determine the relationship between antibody levels determined by bead assay and flow crossmatch. For this purpose, the strength of antibody binding on beads as represented by Mean Fluoresence Intensity (MFI), Standardized Fluorescence Intensity (SFI) or Molecular Equivalent of Standardized Fluorescence (MESF) is compared to the degree of the flow crossmatch reported as median channel shift (MCS). In one study [16] pre- and post-transplant sera from 16 renal transplant patients with donor specific antibody (DSA) were tested. Strength of DSA was determined by single antigen Luminex bead assay and results expressed as standard fluorescence intensity (SFI). T-cell flow crossmatch results were expressed as mean channel shifts (MCS). AMR was determined by

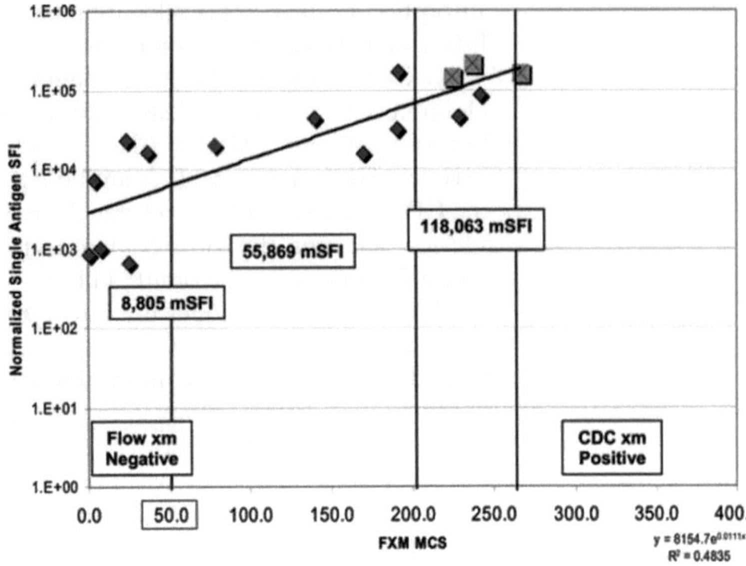

Fig. 1 Donor T-cell flow cytometric crossmatch (FXM) results expressed as MCS vs. corresponding SFI value for the highest DSA single antigen bead. (*Crossed Box operator*, patients who experienced AMR; *diamond operator*, patients with no AMR.) Reproduced from ref. 16 with permission from Wolters Kluwer Health

biopsy and C4d deposition. The results showed that patients with DSA more than 10^5 MFI and FCM more than 200 MCS were at higher risk for AMR (Fig. 1).

3 Virtual Crossmatch

Sensitized patients awaiting cardiac transplantation in the past have required the performance of a prospective crossmatch to ensure graft–host compatibility. A prospective crossmatch avoids the use of donor hearts at risk of exposure to circulating cytotoxic antibodies. This however can be logistically challenging as recipient blood has to be provided close to the site of the donor in order for the test to be performed in a timely manner. The test also requires local expertise. Recipient blood from sensitized patients has to be therefore sent out to several locations where donors could potentially become available. Recipient serum samples also need to be kept updated as clinical conditions change for the recipient who may be challenged with further potentially sensitizing events such as blood transfusions or ventricular assist device placement while awaiting transplantation. This need for a prospective crossmatch significantly limits the geographical catchment area from which sensitized patients may qualify for organ donors and therefore substantially increases the waiting time to transplant.

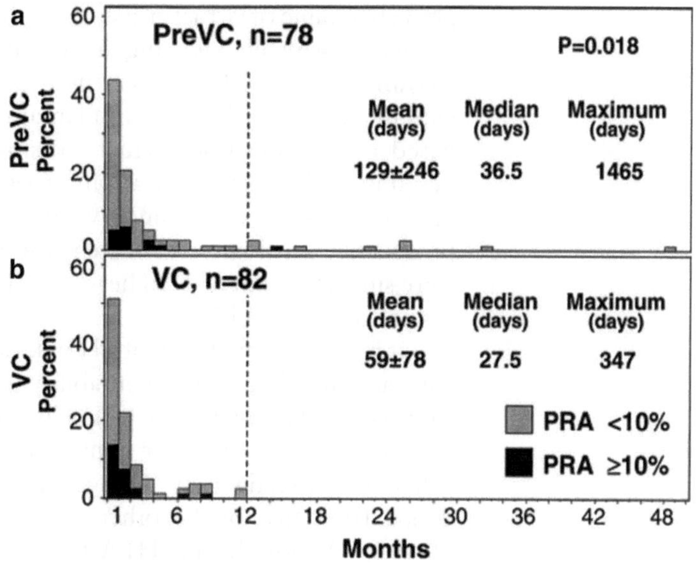

Fig. 2 Waiting time for patients before (**a**) and after (**b**) VC. No patients waited longer than a year after VC. (*PRA* panel reactive antibody, *preVC* prospective crossmatch, *VC* virtual crossmatch.) Reproduced from ref. 18 with permission from Elsevier

Fortunately, the ability now to perform high resolution alloantibody screening with solid phase assays has significantly streamlined appropriate donor selection by the use of a process termed "virtual crossmatching" [17]. In a virtual crossmatch, the recipient antibody profile is determined at the time of listing and cytotoxic antibodies to HLA antigens identified. Cytotoxicity is presumed from the strength of the antibody present [16]. These antigens are then documented as unacceptable on the transplant list. This strategy obviates the need to send out recipient blood and therefore substantially increases the geographical region from which a donor may be accepted. This approach also substantially decreases the waiting time to transplant [18] (Fig. 7.2). The virtual crossmatch also helps identify patients who are potentially at elevated risk of rejection in whom immunosuppression may need to be augmented after transplantation. The use of the virtual crossmatch has now been validated in several studies. Zangwell showed that the use of the virtual crossmatch in pediatric heart transplant recipients was associated with a significantly decreased waiting time to transplant and improved survival compared to patients listed with a prospective crossmatch [19]. In another study the accuracy of virtual crossmatch was compared to prospective AHG-CDC crossmatch [17]. Based on analysis of 257 T-cell AHG-CDC crossmatch tests, the positive predictive value of virtual crossmatch (the likelihood of an incompatible virtual crossmatch resulting in an incompatible T-cell CDC-AHG crossmatch) was 79 %, and the negative predictive value of virtual crossmatch (the likelihood of a compatible virtual crossmatch resulting in a compatible T-cell CDC-AHG crossmatch) was 92 %. When used in a cohort of 28 sensitized patients awaiting heart transplantation, 14 received allografts based on a compatible virtual crossmatch alone from donors in geographically distant locations. Compared with the other 14 sensitized patients who underwent transplant after a compatible prospective serologic crossmatch, the rejection rates and survival were similar. About 65 % of heart transplant centers now utilize the virtual crossmatch [2].

It is however unlikely that all classes and types of HLA antibodies have an equal impact on their ability to mount allograft rejection. The role of HLA-Cw and HLA-DP mismatches, for example, in allograft survival and their consideration in virtual crossmatch is still under investigation. The expression of HLA-Cw on cells is about 10 % that of the other Class I HLA alleles, HLA-A and HLA-B. Although anti-HLA-Cw antibodies in sera of highly sensitized patients are present, the probability of the single HLA-Cw mismatch in heart recipients is very low. Similarly, DP-reactive antibodies have been associated with positive B-cell crossmatch in renal transplant recipients who were zero HLA antigen mismatched (i.e., matched for A, B, and DR) [20]. Anti-HLA-DP antibodies were more common in patients with a history of rejection, and therefore these antibodies may have a greater impact in retransplantation evaluations. The impact and relevance of HLA-C and DP antibodies remains an area of active research.

4 CPRA

The degree of sensitization will determine the likelihood of a patient receiving a compatible donor. The probability of a sensitized patient receiving a compatible graft can be determined based on the frequency of HLA antigens in the population to which the patient has cytotoxic antibodies and is expressed as a ***calculated*** panel reactive antibody (CPRA). The CPRA value represents the percentage of donors in a given population to which a transplant candidate will have cytotoxic anti-HLA antibodies. Thus, the higher the CPRA, the harder it is to find a suitable donor. In the USA, the CPRA can be determined by entering HLA antigens to which the putative recipient has antibodies determined to be potentially at cytotoxic levels by bead assay into the CPRA calculator available online at the Organ Procurement and Transplantation Network website from the US Department of Health and Human Services [62]. The current CPRA data is based upon HLA frequencies derived from the HLA phenotypes of deceased kidney donors recovered over a 2 year period in 2003–2004. Ethnic frequencies were derived from more recent data in 2006–2007.

5 CPRA, Desensitization, and Monitoring

Around 10 % of patients awaiting transplantation are sensitized. A portion of these patients are highly sensitized and may require supplemental therapy to reduce circulating antibody burden to allow a sufficient reduction in their CPRA to increase their chances of obtaining a suitable organ. A number of desensitization strategies have been shown to be effective, including a combination of plasmapheresis, intravenous immune globulin, rituximab [21], and bortezomib [22]. Typically for these patients, HLA antibody type and strength is determined by bead assay prior to initiation of treatment and repeated 2 weeks after completion of treatment to assess response.

A consensus conference took place April 2008 [2] to assess the current status of sensitization in the pre-heart transplant patient, the use and efficacy of desensitization therapies, and the outcome of desensitized patients after heart transplantation. 23 of 51 centers participating in the conference reported on the type of assays routinely used for detecting circulating antibodies and determine risk of rejection. 78 % used Luminex® single antigen assay, 65 % flow cytometry, 61 % CDC, 4 % enzyme-linked immunoassay, and 91 % of centers performed testing for antibody specificities. A consensus statement for recommended interval for antibody screening and identification was published (Table 1).

6 Non-HLA Antibodies

Antibody responses to nonhuman leukocyte antigens (Non-HLA) have been reported in solid organ transplantation and may occur as alloantibodies or autoantibodies. In thoracic organ transplantation, they have been implicated in acute and chronic allograft rejection. The antigens detected include major histocompatibility class I chain-related gene A (MICA) [23, 24], angiotensin II type 1 receptor (AT_IR) [25], endothelin-1 type A receptor (ETAR) [26] endothelial cell antigens [27], vimentin [28], K-alpha-1-Tubulin (KA1T) [29], collagen-V [30], and non-HLA IgM antibodies. In cardiac transplantation, anti-MICA and anti-endothelial antibodies have been associated with increased antibody mediated rejection [31] and development of cardiac allograft vasculopathy [23]. Vimentin is an intermediate filament cytoskeletal protein found in mesenchymal cells. Approximately 30 % of heart transplant and kidney transplant recipients make de novo antivimentin antibodies after transplantation. Anti-vimentin antibodies are made significantly earlier than anti-HLA, and are likely produced as a result of antigens exposed on the surface of damaged or activated cells. Production of anti-vimentin antibodies may only reflect tissue damage, but experimental studies [32] have suggested that they

Table 1
Pre-transplant sensitization2

Consensus statements for pre-transplant sensitization [2]
The recommended frequency for antibody screening and identification is as follows:
If no evidence of sensitization, a frequency of every 6 months is advised
In patients with detectable circulating antibodies, a frequency of every 3 months
In LVAD recipients, the optimal frequency is once per month
With "interceding events" (such as blood transfusions) we recommend a PRA screen at 1–2 weeks after the event
After desensitization therapy, PRAs should be checked 1–2 weeks after therapy
In all others (pediatric, retransplant, parous women), a frequency of every 3 months is advised
Testing methodology:
Identify circulating antibodies with a solid-phase assay such as flow cytometry
Delineation of complement fixation capability of detected antibodies should be reported
Anti-HLA Class I and II specificities must be defined (any HLA antibody directed against HLA-A, -B, -Cw, -DR, and -DQ)
Quantitate circulating antibodies to assess for unacceptable antigens and to obtain the calculated PRA
In the absence of international standards, each center must develop thresholds for definitions of unacceptable antigens
Consider the use of the virtual crossmatch (utilizing the unacceptable antigens) to increase the donor pool for any one sensitized individual

Reproduced from ref. [2] with permission from Elsevier

actively participate in rejection, by activating vimentin-positive neutrophils or platelets.

The detection of these antibodies in the setting of acute and chronic rejection however at this time remains for investigational use and none of the assays used to detect these antibodies have been routinely used for clinical evaluation. The clinical significance and role of these antibodies in mediating thoracic allograft injury currently remains chiefly undetermined.

7 Complement Fixing Antibodies

Most of the solid-phase assays do not however discriminate between complement-activating and non-complement-activating antibodies, and the role of non-complement-activating antibodies in clinical transplantation is controversial. A novel C1q assay developed to detect the subset of immunoglobulin G (IgG) antibodies capable of fixing complement may allow further expansion of the donor pool by allowing exclusion of only complement fixing antibodies in the virtual crossmatch [33]. In this study the identification of complement fixing antibody in a standard virtual crossmatch was associated with a higher incidence of AMR compared to a virtual crossmatch with no complement fixing antibodies. It also appears that the ability of antibody to bind complement is independent of the strength of antibody and C1q fixation is independent of MFI values [34]. The assay also appears to be much more sensitive than the standard CDC at detecting complement fixing antibodies.

8 Post-transplant Monitoring

Post-transplant DSA monitoring is important for sensitized patients. It should be performed daily for the first week after heart transplantation to identify a possible amnestic antibody response that could lead to a delayed hyperacute rejection. This can be performed with use of donor cells in the form of a donor-specific cytotoxic crossmatch. If significant donor-specific antibody is identified, then appropriate therapy can be initiated [2]. For heart transplantation, guidelines have been recently established for further DSA monitoring [35]. Use of solid-phase assay and/or cell-based assays to assess for DSA (and quantification if antibody present) is suggested at 2 weeks and 1, 3, 6, 12 months, and then annually after transplant and when AMR is clinically suspected. However, strategies for management of post-transplant DSA particularly in the absence of clinical rejection remain controversial and an area of active research.

As the transplanted heart is denervated, symptoms resulting from graft rejection may be insidious and may not present until late in the course of a rejection episode. Surveillance percutaneous endomyocardial biopsies are therefore traditionally performed at standard intervals from the time of transplantation. Typically, a cardiac biopsy schedule would consist of performing the procedure weekly during the first month, every 2 weeks for another month and monthly until 6 months and then every 3 months until the end of the first postoperative year. This schedule reflects the general risk of allograft rejection which is highest in the first 3–6 months post-transplant. After the first year additional protocol biopsies are likely not to be of clinical significance given the very low rates of rejection observed in this period [36]. Additional biopsies however, are usually performed 7–10 days after treatment of rejection in order to confirm the resolution or when there is clinical suspicion of acute rejection. Periodic transbronchial biopsy for surveillance in asymptomatic, clinically and physiologically stable lung transplant recipients is controversial, and the practice varies among centers [37]. Transbronchial lung biopsy is safe and effective for the diagnosis of clinically suspected acute rejection and infection. When performed for a clinical indication, the sensitivity for detecting acute rejection and CMV infection is relatively high. However, the sensitivity of transbronchial biopsy for the diagnosis of bronchiolitis obliterans, the histologic counterpart of chronic allograft rejection, has been inconsistent, and a negative transbronchial biopsy does not exclude obliterative bronchiolitis.

9 AlloMap

Although the endomyocardial biopsy has served as an important tool for monitoring allograft rejection in the management of heart transplant recipients, the procedure has significant limitations. Its invasive nature may provoke anxiety and discomfort and the procedure remains particularly challenging in the pediatric population, often necessitating the use of general anesthesia. Although the procedure is safe especially in experienced hands with a complication rate well below 0.5 %, there is a finite risk of injury which may include tricuspid valve trauma and cardiac perforation. Biopsy utilizes significant resources including physician time and is associated with substantial costs. It also remains an imperfect tool for the diagnosis of rejection. The inflammatory infiltrates are often patchy and so biopsy may miss these focal sites of rejection. The pathologic finding of rejection is a relatively late phenomenon and diagnosis is only made once myocardial damage has already taken place.

A simpler noninvasive approach has long been sought in the hope of finding a marker that would reliably predict allograft rejection. Ideally, this test would be less resource-intensive and allow early detection for the onset of rejection before any significant myocardial necrosis has occurred. To date, only one noninvasive test for the detection of cardiac allograft rejection has reached routine clinical use and has been approved by the Food and Drug Administration in the USA. This technique, known as AlloMap® involves screening for genetic markers to determine a gene expression profile that may be representative of the process of acute cellular rejection. Microarray technology was utilized to screen for a number of candidate genes that were expressed in cardiac allograft cellular rejection as determined by routine endomyocardial biopsy. The selected genes were then examined in peripheral leucocytes using polymerase chain reaction from blood samples obtained at the time of endomyocardial biopsy [38]. The technique was shown to have a high negative predictive value for the diagnosis of acute cellular rejection. Furthermore, a low expression score was associated with a low future risk of rejection, suggesting that the test may be useful in identifying low risk patients who may safely avoid the need for surveillance biopsy. In one study [39], over 600 patients between 6 months and 5 years post-transplant were randomized to either routine surveillance endomyocardial biopsy or gene expression profiling. All patients were low risk with no prior evidence of rejection, and the study was powered to demonstrate non-inferiority between gene expression and biopsy. The study concluded that a strategy of monitoring for rejection that involved gene-expression profiling, as compared with routine biopsies, was not associated with an increased risk of serious adverse outcomes and resulted in the performance of significantly fewer biopsies. The study however included a majority of low-risk patients who had been more than a year post transplant. Many centers typically do not perform routine surveillance endomyocardial biopsies after the first year in such patients as the risk of allograft rejection is very low. Gene expression profiling is also limited as it is only validated for acute cellular rejection and is not applicable for the monitoring of AMR which is seen in up to 15 % of patients. It has yet to be validated in patients in the early transplant phase and in patients who are being weaned off corticosteroids. The AlloMap® test has not been validated in lung transplant recipients.

10 Immune Monitoring (Cylex®)

In stable post-transplant patients, there has been a need to reliably monitor the overall state of immunosuppression to minimize chronic exposure to immunosuppressive agents that are associated with increased morbidity, including infection, malignancy and renal insufficiency. However, the ability to minimize exposure to immunosuppressive agents needs at the same time to be balanced with the need to minimize the risk of allograft rejection. Another peripheral whole blood assay that assesses the net state of immunosuppression in transplant recipients is also now clinically available. In a meta-analysis of 504 solid organ transplant recipients (heart, kidney, kidney–pancreas, liver and small bowel) from ten U.S. centers, the Cylex ImmuKnow® assay was performed at various times post-transplant and compared with clinical course (stable, rejection, infection) [40]. In this analysis, 39 biopsy-proven cellular rejections and 66 diagnosed infections occurred. Odds ratios of infection or rejection were calculated based on measured immune response values. A recipient with an immune response value of 25 ng/ml adenosine triphosphate (ATP) was 12 times (95 % confidence of 4–36) more likely to develop an infection than a recipient with a stronger immune response. Similarly, a recipient with an immune response of 700 ng/ml ATP was 30 times (95 % confidence of 8–112) more likely to develop a cellular rejection than a recipient with a lower immune response value. The intersection of odds ratio curves for infection and rejection in the moderate immune response zone was 280 ng/ml ATP. This intersection of risk curves provides an immunological target of immune function for solid organ recipients. These data suggest that the Cylex® assay has a high negative predictive value and provides a target immunological response zone for minimizing risk and managing patients to stability. However, in a recently reported retrospective analysis of 111 cardiac transplant recipients mostly more than a year from transplant, this assay showed wide variability. No correlation was observed between the baseline Cylex® response and subsequent risk of either infection or rejection within 6 months, although the number of rejection episodes (3) and infection episodes (8) were low in the study. Lower white blood cell count and African American ethnicity were correlated with a lower Cylex® response. In a larger study of almost 300 heart transplant recipients who had 864 Cylex® assays performed, a low score was predictive of infectious risk, although in this study, due to the low number of rejection episodes, the association between a high score and rejection risk was inconclusive [41]. Cylex® scores however have not been useful in predicting acute rejection or infections in the pediatric heart transplant population [42]. Lower Cylex® scores have also been associated with infection in lung transplant recipients [43] and low values in patients colonized with fungus may identify patients at risk of developing fungal disease [44]. The assay shows some promise in monitoring the immune status in cardiac transplant recipients with post-transplant lymphoproliferative disorder in whom minimization of immunosuppression is the predominant treatment strategy [45]. Cylex® has not been utilized in patients being routinely weaned off immunosuppressive agents and its clinical utility in this regard remains unclear.

11 Other Potential Biomarkers

B-type natriuretic peptide (BNP) is well established as a neurohormonal marker that correlates with cardiac filling pressures and outcomes in patients with congestive heart failure. There is some evidence to suggest that BNP may be a useful marker to monitor in heart transplant recipients. Elevation in BNP levels have been shown to correlate with and precede histologic rejection [46], although the marker appears to be less useful for this in the first 2 months after transplantation [47]. Due to significant cross-sectional variability in BNP values, changes in levels within individuals may offer an approach to detecting allograft rejection [48]. The assay may be particularly useful at reducing the number of biopsies required in pediatric patients [49, 50]. Peripheral gene expression signatures of elevated BNP concentrations in clinically quiescent heart transplant recipients suggest that an elevated BNP concentration is associated with molecular patterns that point to ongoing active cardiac structural remodeling, vascular injury, inflammation, and alloimmune processes [51]. These findings allude to the notion that BNP elevation is not merely a hemodynamic marker but should be considered reflective of integrated processes that determine the balance between active cardiac allograft injury and repair.

C-reactive protein (CRP) is an inflammatory marker that has been studied in cardiac transplant recipients. As an acute-phase reactant, its levels are frequently associated with infection although a few studies suggest that it may be a potential marker in the assessment of acute rejection [52, 53]. CRP may however be a better biomarker for the development of cardiac allograft vasculopathy. In one study [54], early raised CRP concentrations (determined within 3 months of transplantation) were associated with development, increased severity, and enhanced rate of progression of coronary artery disease, and with heightened frequency of ischemic events and graft failure. Other studies also suggest a correlation between elevated CRP and development of allograft vasculopathy [55, 56].

Microchimerism is the presence of two genetically distinct and separately derived populations of cells, one population being at a low concentration, in the same individual or an organ. It is detected in a majority of solid-transplant recipients and its presence has been associated with the development of allograft rejection in heart transplant recipients [57]. In heart transplants, up to 10 % of myocardium may represent cells of donor origin [58]. Recent molecular techniques allow circulating molecular microchimerism detection from peripheral blood in transplant recipients [59]. The clinical utility of detecting microchimerism in peripheral blood in heart transplant recipients remains to be determined and remains an area of active research.

Another area of active research is the detection of circulating regulatory T cells (T-reg). These migrate into allografts and induce tolerance of the graft. Immunosuppressive T-reg are found among CD4+CD25++ T cells and specifically express transcription factor FOXP3. Numbers of circulating immunosuppressive T-reg are reduced in transplant recipients. Recruitment of T-reg into the cardiac allograft during transcoronary passage may induce graft tolerance during subclinical inflammation [60]. Patients with allograft rejection may demonstrate an increase in T-regs [61].

12 Conclusions

The advent of effective immunosuppressive therapy has substantially improved outcomes following thoracic organ transplantation. However, the risk of rejection, particularly in sensitized patients, and post-transplant complications, remain significant factors that limit long-term survival and contribute to significant morbidity. Fortunately advances in laboratory techniques now allow both identification and strength of circulating antibodies and studies suggest that antibody-strength is an important marker for risk of rejection. These techniques have now allowed the use of the virtual crossmatch which has significantly reduced the waiting time to transplant and expanded the donor pool. Antibody monitoring has also allowed the assessment of efficacy of desensitization regimens. For heart transplantation, invasive surveillance endomyocardial biopsies have been routinely performed for monitoring of allograft rejection. The recent development of gene expression profiling (AlloMap®) has allowed noninvasive monitoring with low scores showing a high negative predictive value for acute cellular rejection. T cell immune monitoring (Cylex®) in heart and lung transplant recipients has allowed individual tailoring of immunosuppression, particularly to minimize risk of infection. Future developments such as C1q testing to assess the ability of antibodies to activate complement may allow further refinement of the virtual crossmatch by allowing identification of truly cytotoxic antibodies. The development of these laboratory techniques have significantly enhanced our ability to manage thoracic organ transplant recipients and further improved our understanding of transplant immunology. Future developments with improved understanding of microchimerism and graft tolerance may allow more refined allograft monitoring techniques.

References

1. Billingham RE, Brent L, Medawar PB (1953) Actively acquired tolerance of foreign cells. Nature 172(4379):603–606
2. Kobashigawa J, Mehra M, West L, Kerman R, George J, Rose M et al (2009) Report from a consensus conference on the sensitized patient awaiting heart transplantation. J Heart Lung Transplant 28(3):213–225. doi:S1053-2498(08)01785-3 [pii] 10.1016/j.healun.2008.12.017
3. Oyer PE, Stinson EB, Jamieson SW (1983) Cyclosporine in cardiac transplantation: a 21/2 year follow-up. Transplant Proc 15(Suppl 1): 2546
4. Armitage JM, Kormos RL, Griffith BP, Hardesty RL, Fricker FJ, Stuart RS et al (1991) A clinical trial of FK 506 as primary and rescue immunosuppression in cardiac transplantation. Transplant Proc 23(1 Pt 2):1149–1152
5. Cheung A, Menkis AH (1998) Cyclosporine heart transplantation. Transplant Proc 30(5): 1881–1884
6. Stehlik J, Edwards LB, Kucheryavaya AY, Benden C, Christie JD, Dobbels F et al (2011) The Registry of the International Society for Heart and Lung Transplantation: twenty-eighth Adult Heart Transplant Report—2011. J Heart Lung Transplant 30(10):1078–1094. doi:S1053-2498(11)01086-2 [pii] 10.1016/j.healun.2011.08.003
7. Michaels PJ, Espejo ML, Kobashigawa J, Alejos JC, Burch C, Takemoto S et al (2003) Humoral rejection in cardiac transplantation: risk factors, hemodynamic consequences and relationship to transplant coronary artery disease. J Heart Lung Transplant 22(1):58–69
8. Itescu S, Tung TC, Burke EM, Weinberg AD, Mancini D, Michler RE et al (1998) An immunological algorithm to predict risk of high-grade rejection in cardiac transplant recipients. Lancet 352(9124):263–270
9. Nwakanma LU, Williams JA, Weiss ES, Russell SD, Baumgartner WA, Conte JV (2007) Influence of pretransplant panel-reactive antibody on outcomes in 8,160 heart transplant recipients in recent era. Ann Thorac Surg 84(5):1556–1562. doi:S0003-4975(07)01217-9 [pii] 10.1016/j.athoracsur.2007.05.095; discussion 1562–1553
10. Tinckam KJ, Chandraker A (2006) Mechanisms and role of HLA and non-HLA alloantibodies. Clin J Am Soc Nephrol 1(3):404–414. doi:CJN.00270106 [pii] 10.2215/CJN.00270106
11. Schlaf G, Pollok-Kopp B, Manzke T, Schurat O, Altermann W (2010) Novel solid phase-based ELISA assays contribute to an improved detection of anti-HLA antibodies and to an increased reliability of pre- and post-transplant crossmatching. NDT Plus 3(6):527–538

12. Altermann WW, Seliger B, Sel S, Wendt D, Schlaf G (2006) Comparison of the established standard complement-dependent cytotoxicity and flow cytometric crossmatch assays with a novel ELISA-based HLA crossmatch procedure. Histol Histopathol 21(10): 1115–1124
13. Smith JD, Hamour IM, Banner NR, Rose ML (2007) C4d fixing, luminex binding antibodies—a new tool for prediction of graft failure after heart transplantation. Am J Transplant 7(12):2809–2815. doi:AJT1991 [pii] 10.1111/j.1600-6143.2007.01991.x
14. Won DI, Jung HD, Jung OJ, Huh S, Suh JS (2007) Flow cytometry PRA using lymphocyte pools from random donors. Cytometry B Clin Cytom 72(4):256–264. doi:10.1002/cyto.b.20175
15. El-Awar N, Lee J, Terasaki PI (2005) HLA antibody identification with single antigen beads compared to conventional methods. Hum Immunol 66(9):989–997. doi:S0198-8859(05)00138-2 [pii] 10.1016/j.humimm.2005.07.005
16. Reinsmoen NL, Lai CH, Vo A, Cao K, Ong G, Naim M et al (2008) Acceptable donor-specific antibody levels allowing for successful deceased and living donor kidney transplantation after desensitization therapy. Transplantation 86(6):820–825. doi:10.1097/TP.0b013e3181856f98 00007890-200809270-00012 [pii]
17. Stehlik J, Islam N, Hurst D, Kfoury AG, Movsesian MA, Fuller A et al (2009) Utility of virtual crossmatch in sensitized patients awaiting heart transplantation. J Heart Lung Transplant 28(11):1129–1134
18. Yanagida R, Czer LS, Reinsmoen NL, Cao K, Rafiei M, De Robertis MA et al (2011) Impact of virtual cross match on waiting times for heart transplantation. Ann Thorac Surg 92(6): 2104–2110. doi:S0003-4975(11)01910-2 [pii] 10.1016/j.athoracsur.2011.07.082; discussion 2111
19. Zangwill S, Ellis T, Stendahl G, Zahn A, Berger S, Tweddell J (2007) Practical application of the virtual crossmatch. Pediatr Transplant 11(6):650–654. doi:PTR746 [pii] 10.1111/j.1399-3046.2007.00746.x
20. Vaidya S, Hilson B, Sheldon S, Cano P, Fernandez-Vina M (2007) DP reactive antibody in a zero mismatch renal transplant pair. Hum Immunol 68(12):947–949. doi:S0198-8859(07)00465-X [pii] 10.1016/j.humimm.2007.10.013
21. Kobashigawa JA, Patel JK, Kittleson MM, Kawano MA, Kiyosaki KK, Davis SN et al (2010) The long-term outcome of treated sensitized patients who undergo heart transplantation. Clin Transplant 25(1):E61–E67. doi:10.1111/j.1399-0012.2010.01334.x
22. Patel J, Everly M, Chang D, Kittleson M, Reed E, Kobashigawa J (2011) Reduction of alloantibodies via proteosome inhibition in cardiac transplantation. J Heart Lung Transplant 30(12):1320–1326. doi:S1053-2498(11)01110-7 [pii] 10.1016/j.healun.2011.08.009
23. Kauke T, Kaczmarek I, Dick A, Schmoeckel M, Deutsch MA, Beiras-Fernandez A et al (2009) Anti-MICA antibodies are related to adverse outcome in heart transplant recipients. J Heart Lung Transplant 28(4):305–311. doi:S1053-2498(09)00024-2 [pii] 10.1016/j.healun.2009.01.003
24. Angaswamy N, Saini D, Ramachandran S, Nath DS, Phelan D, Hachem R et al (2010) Development of antibodies to human leukocyte antigen precedes development of antibodies to major histocompatibility class I-related chain A and are significantly associated with development of chronic rejection after human lung transplantation. Hum Immunol 71(6):560–565. doi:S0198-8859(10)00064-9 [pii] 10.1016/j.humimm.2010.02.021
25. Reinsmoen NL, Lai C-H, Mirocha J, Cao K, Ong GD, Naim M et al (2013) Increased negative impact of anti-angiotensin type-1 receptor antibodies together with de novo donor HLA specific antibodies on graft outcome in heart transplant recipients. J Heart Lung Transplant 32(4S):S113
26. Hiemann NE, Meyer R, Wellnhofer E, Schoenemann C, Heidecke H, Lachmann N, Hetzer R et al. (2012) Dragun Non-HLA antibodies targeting vascular receptors enhance alloimmune response and microvasculopathy after heart transplantation. Transplantation. Nov 15;94(9):919–24
27. Faulk WP, Rose M, Meroni PL, Del Papa N, Torry RJ, Labarrere CA et al (1999) Antibodies to endothelial cells identify myocardial damage and predict development of coronary artery disease in patients with transplanted hearts. Hum Immunol 60(9):826–832
28. Jurcevic S, Ainsworth ME, Pomerance A, Smith JD, Robinson DR, Dunn MJ et al (2001) Antivimentin antibodies are an independent predictor of transplant-associated coronary artery disease after cardiac transplantation. Transplantation 71(7):886–892
29. Goers TA, Ramachandran S, Aloush A, Trulock E, Patterson GA, Mohanakumar T (2008) De novo production of K-alpha1 tubulin-specific antibodies: role in chronic lung allograft rejection. J Immunol 180(7):4487–4494. doi:180/7/4487 [pii]
30. Iwata T, Philipovskiy A, Fisher AJ, Presson RG Jr, Chiyo M, Lee J et al (2008) Anti-type V collagen humoral immunity in lung transplant primary graft dysfunction. J Immunol 181(8):5738–5747. doi:181/8/5738 [pii]

31. Zhang Q, Cecka JM, Gjertson DW, Ge P, Rose ML, Patel JK, Ardehali A et al (2011) HLA and MICA: targets of antibody-mediated rejection in heart transplantation. Transplantation 91(10):1153–1158. doi: 10.1097/TP.0b013e3182157d60 00007890-201105270-00015 [pii]
32. Mahesh B, Leong HS, McCormack A, Sarathchandra P, Holder A, Rose ML (2007) Autoantibodies to vimentin cause accelerated rejection of cardiac allografts. Am J Pathol 170(4):1415–1427. doi:S0002-9440(10) 61355-7 [pii] 10.2353/ajpath.2007.060728
33. Chin C, Chen G, Sequeria F, Berry G, Siehr S, Bernstein D et al (2010) Clinical usefulness of a novel C1q assay to detect immunoglobulin G antibodies capable of fixing complement in sensitized pediatric heart transplant patients. J Heart Lung Transplant 30(2):158–163. doi:S1053-2498(10)00508-5 [pii] 10.1016/j.healun.2010.08.020
34. Chen G, Sequeira F, Tyan DB (2011) Novel C1q assay reveals a clinically relevant subset of human leukocyte antigen antibodies independent of immunoglobulin G strength on single antigen beads. Hum Immunol 72(10):849–858. doi:S0198-8859(11)00171-6 [pii] 10.1016/j.humimm.2011.07.001
35. Kobashigawa J, Crespo-Leiro MG, Ensminger SM, Reichenspurner H, Angelini A, Berry G et al (2011) Report from a consensus conference on antibody-mediated rejection in heart transplantation. J Heart Lung Transplant 30(3):252–269. doi:S1053-2498(10)00731-X [pii] 10.1016/j.healun.2010.11.003
36. Mehra MR, Parameshwar J (2010) Gene expression profiling and cardiac allograft rejection monitoring: is IMAGE just a mirage? J Heart Lung Transplant 29(6):599–602
37. McWilliams TJ, Williams TJ, Whitford HM, Snell GI (2008) Surveillance bronchoscopy in lung transplant recipients: risk versus benefit. J Heart Lung Transplant 27(11):1203–1209. doi:S1053-2498(08)00581-0 [pii] 10.1016/j.healun.2008.08.004
38. Deng MC, Eisen HJ, Mehra MR, Billingham M, Marboe CC, Berry G et al (2006) Noninvasive discrimination of rejection in cardiac allograft recipients using gene expression profiling. Am J Transplant 6(1):150–160
39. Pham MX, Teuteberg JJ, Kfoury AG, Starling RC, Deng MC, Cappola TP et al (2010) Gene-expression profiling for rejection surveillance after cardiac transplantation. N Engl J Med 362(20):1890–1900
40. Kowalski RJ, Post DR, Mannon RB, Sebastian A, Wright HI, Sigle G et al (2006) Assessing relative risks of infection and rejection: a meta-analysis using an immune function assay. Transplantation 82(5):663–668. doi:10.1097/01.tp.0000234837.02126.70 00007890-200609150-00011 [pii]
41. Kobashigawa JA, Kiyosaki KK, Patel JK, Kittleson MM, Kubak BM, Davis SN et al (2010) Benefit of immune monitoring in heart transplant patients using ATP production in activated lymphocytes. J Heart Lung Transplant 29(5):504–508. doi:S1053-2498(09)01536-8 [pii] 10.1016/j.healun.2009.12.015
42. Rossano JW, Denfield SW, Kim JJ, Price JF, Jefferies JL, Decker JA et al (2009) Assessment of the Cylex ImmuKnow cell function assay in pediatric heart transplant patients. J Heart Lung Transplant 28(1):26–31. doi:S1053-2498(08)00734-1 [pii] 10.1016/j.healun.2008.10.001
43. Bhorade SM, Janata K, Vigneswaran WT, Alex CG, Garrity ER (2008) Cylex ImmuKnow assay levels are lower in lung transplant recipients with infection. J Heart Lung Transplant 27(9):990–994. doi:S1053-2498(08)00477-4 [pii] 10.1016/j.healun.2008.06.005
44. Husain S, Raza K, Pilewski JM, Zaldonis D, Crespo M, Toyoda Y et al (2009) Experience with immune monitoring in lung transplant recipients: correlation of low immune function with infection. Transplantation 87(12):1852–1857. doi:10.1097/TP.0b013e3181a75ad2 00007890-200906270-00015 [pii]
45. Gautam A, Morrissey PE, Brem AS, Fischer SA, Gohh RY, Yango AF et al (2006) Use of an immune function assay to monitor immunosuppression for treatment of post-transplant lymphoproliferative disorder. Pediatr Transplant 10(5):613–616. doi:PTR510 [pii] 10.1111/j.1399-3046.2006.00510.x
46. Masters RG, Davies RA, Veinot JP, Hendry PJ, Smith SJ, de Bold AJ (1999) Discoordinate modulation of natriuretic peptides during acute cardiac allograft rejection in humans. Circulation 100(3):287–291
47. O'Neill JO, McRae AT 3rd, Troughton RW, Ng K, Taylor DO, Yamani MH et al (2005) Brain natriuretic peptide levels do not correlate with acute cellular rejection in De Novo orthotopic heart transplant recipients. J Heart Lung Transplant 24(4):416–420. doi:S105324980400035X [pii] 10.1016/j.healun.2003.12.006
48. Kittleson MM, Skojec DV, Wittstein IS, Champion HC, Judge DP, Barouch LA et al (2009) The change in B-type natriuretic peptide levels over time predicts significant rejection in cardiac transplant recipients. J Heart Lung Transplant 28(7):704–709. doi:S1053-2498(09)00241-1 [pii] 10.1016/j.healun.2009.04.019

49. Claudius I, Lan YT, Chang RK, Wetzel GT, Alejos J (2003) Usefulness of B-type natriuretic peptide as a noninvasive screening tool for cardiac allograft pathology in pediatric heart transplant recipients. Am J Cardiol 92(11):1368–1370.doi:S0002914903012049 [pii]
50. Rossano JW, Denfield SW, Kim JJ, Price JF, Jefferies JL, Decker JA et al (2008) B-type natriuretic peptide is a sensitive screening test for acute rejection in pediatric heart transplant patients. J Heart Lung Transplant 27(6):649–654. doi:S1053-2498(08)00248-9 [pii] 10.1016/j.healun.2008.03.008
51. Mehra MR, Uber PA, Walther D, Vesely M, Wohlgemuth JG, Prentice J et al (2006) Gene expression profiles and B-type natriuretic peptide elevation in heart transplantation: more than a hemodynamic marker. Circulation 114(1 Suppl): I21–I26. doi:114/1_suppl/I-21 [pii] 10.1161/CIRCULATIONAHA.105.000513
52. Martinez-Dolz L, Almenar L, Reganon E, Vila V, Sanchez-Soriano R, Martinez-Sales V et al (2009) What is the best biomarker for diagnosis of rejection in heart transplantation? Clin Transplant 23(5):672–680. doi:CTR1074 [pii] 10.1111/j.1399-0012.2009.01074.x
53. Balduini A, Campana C, Ceresa M, Arbustini E, Bosoni T, Serio A et al (2003) Utility of biochemical markers in the follow-up of heart transplant recipients. Transplant Proc 35(8):3075–3078. doi:S0041134503011394 [pii]
54. Labarrere CA, Lee JB, Nelson DR, Al-Hassani M, Miller SJ, Pitts DE (2002) C-reactive protein, arterial endothelial activation, and development of transplant coronary artery disease: a prospective study. Lancet 360(9344):1462–1467. doi:S0140-6736(02)11473-5 [pii] 10.1016/S0140-6736(02)11473-5
55. Raichlin ER, McConnell JP, Lerman A, Kremers WK, Edwards BS, Kushwaha SS et al (2007) Systemic inflammation and metabolic syndrome in cardiac allograft vasculopathy. J Heart Lung Transplant 26(8):826–833. doi:S1053-2498(07)00400-7 [pii] 10.1016/j.healun.2007.05.008
56. Hognestad A, Endresen K, Wergeland R, Stokke O, Geiran O, Holm T et al (2003) Plasma C-reactive protein as a marker of cardiac allograft vasculopathy in heart transplant recipients. J Am Coll Cardiol 42(3):477–482. doi:S0735109703006454 [pii]
57. Sahota A, Gao S, Hayes J, Jindal RM (2000) Microchimerism and rejection: a meta-analysis. Clin Transplant 14(4 Pt 1):345–350
58. Quaini F, Urbanek K, Beltrami AP, Finato N, Beltrami CA, Nadal-Ginard B et al (2002) Chimerism of the transplanted heart. N Engl J Med 346(1):5–15. doi:10.1056/NEJMoa012081346/1/5 [pii]
59. Pujal JM, Gallardo D (2008) PCR-based methodology for molecular microchimerism detection and quantification. Exp Biol Med (Maywood) 233(9):1161–1170. doi:0802-RM-35 [pii] 10.3181/0802-RM-35
60. Schmidt-Lucke C, Aicher A, Romagnani P, Gareis B, Romagnani S, Zeiher AM et al (2007) Specific recruitment of CD4+CD25++ regulatory T cells into the allograft in heart transplant recipients. Am J Physiol Heart Circ Physiol 292(5):H2425–H2431. doi:01197.2006 [pii] 10.1152/ajpheart.01197.2006
61. Chen M, Mohtize M, Mattei MF, Villemot JP, Kohler C, Faure GC et al (2010) Reduced levels of both circulating CD4+ CD25+ CD127(low/neg) and CD4+ CD8(neg) invariant natural killer regulatory T cells in stable heart transplant recipients. Clin Exp Immunol 163(1):104–112. doi:10.1111/j.1365-2249.2010.04281.x
62. http://optn.transplant.hrsa.gov/resources/allocationcalculators.asp?index=78 Accessed on 1st May 2013

Part II

Methods Chapters

Chapter 8

HLA Typing by Sequence-Specific Primers

Mike Bunce and Ben Passey

Abstract

HLA typing by sequence-specific primers (PCR-SSP) is a commonly used technique in HLA typing in which multiple pairs of *cis*-located allele-specific primers are used to determine the alleles present in a given DNA sample. Although the technique is around two decades old, it still offers a relatively straight forward way of typing and has the benefit of using commonly available laboratory equipment. Here we describe the background of the PCR-SSP, how to design and validate reactions, and common problems that arise.

Key words Polymerase chain reaction, HLA genotyping, Sequence-specific primers, PCR-SSP, Amplification refractory mutation system, ARMS

1 Introduction

PCR primers that are not matched at the 3′ end with target DNA are generally not extended because Taq polymerase lacks 3′ to 5′ exonuclease proofreading ability [1]. This feature of the enzyme was first exploited in 1988 when PCR based methods to detect *cis-located* DNA polymorphisms performed by utilizing the 3′ primer mismatch methods were described by Wu et al. [2] and Newton et al. [3], the latter of which coined the term amplification refractory mutation system (ARMS). The ARMS method was applied to histocompatibility testing, originally by Fugger et al. [4], and then in its present form by Olerup and Zetterquist [5] who renamed the method PCR-SSP (PCR by sequence-specific primers). PCR-SSP methods and designs were soon published by others to cover all HLA loci [6, 7]. PCR-SSP proved useful in HLA typing as it utilized commonly available laboratory equipment and was a simpler, quicker and less ambiguous method of genotyping than the prevailing methods at the time.

PCR-SSP has certain common features whether the user is developing their own system or utilizing commercial kits. All reactions in a given set utilize the same PCR parameters and conditions,

Andrea A. Zachary and Mary S. Leffell (eds.), *Transplantation Immunology: Methods and Protocols, Second Edition*, Methods in Molecular Biology, vol. 1034, DOI 10.1007/978-1-62703-493-7_8, © Springer Science+Business Media, LLC 2013

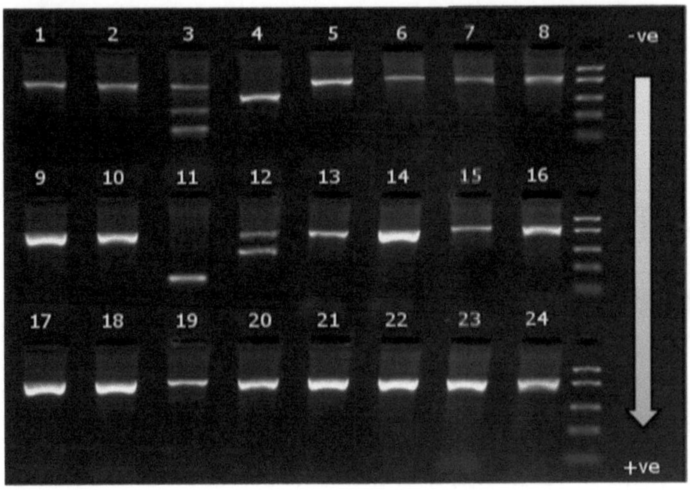

Fig. 1 An example of a 24 reaction HLA-A typing plate. The *arrow* indicates the direction of migration during electrophoresis. In this example the positive reactions are 3, 4, 11, and 12, which indicate the presence of A*02 and A*24 which can be deduced from the interpretation Table 1

and all PCR reactions are multiplexed to include primers for the amplification of a housekeeping gene that indicates successful PCR (whether the PCR for the alleles is positive or negative). Generally, post-PCR processing requires agarose gel electrophoresis to identify positive and negative amplifications, but increasingly methods for non-gel based detection are being utilized.

PCR-SSP can be applied to HLA typing as a high resolution method where the primers in a single PCR-SSP reaction identify a single allele. Alternatively, PCR-SSP can be applied to HLA genotyping in a group-specific or low-resolution approach where, for example, to genotype for HLA-A a set of primers would be designed to amplify groups of alleles based on the first two digits of the allele name. A reaction would be developed for HLA-A*01 alleles and another for A*02 alleles, and so on until all allelic groups are identified. The drawback of the approach is that HLA is highly polymorphic and therefore in most cases it is no longer possible to design a single PCR-SSP reaction for most allelic groups. To design a typing system to amplify all HLA alleles in an unambiguous approach requires that each allelic group is amplified in at least two reactions where the priming positions are different. An example of a 24 reaction HLA typing plate is shown in Fig. 1 and its interpretation is illustrated in Table 1.

To achieve consistent high quality PCR-SSP typing it is important to design and test all the PCR primers in a consistent manner, suitable for the PCR buffer being used and the PCR parameters and protocols being used (*see* **Note 1**). PCR primer design methods are suggested in Subheading 4, but these should be tailored to suit the

Table 1
HLA-A PCR-SSP example interpretation table

Reaction Number	1	2	3	4	5	6	7	8
BP sizes	660	125, 225	215, 420	580, 630	175	210	540, 570	540
Common	A*01	A*01, 11, 36, 80	A*02	A*02, 03, 11, 24, 68, 69	A*03, 30, 34, 80	A*03	A*11, 66	A*23, 30, 32
Rare		A*03, 26, 31, 74		A*01, 25, 26, 29, 31, 32, 33, B*46	A*01, 11, 24, 31, 32	A*02, 24, 32, 68	A*01, 03, 25, 26, 68	A*02, 24, 29, 31
Reaction Number	**9**	**10**	**11**	**12**	**13**	**14**	**15**	**16**
BP sizes	140	160, 190, 695	215	495, 500	135	140	190	425, 430
Common	A*23	A*30	A*24	A*24	A*36	A*25	A*25, 26, 43, 66	A*26, 43
Rare	A*24, 29, 31, 32, 33		A*33	A*02, 32, 68		A*24, 32, 68	A*02, 31	A*02, 25
Reaction Number	**17**	**18**	**19**	**20**	**21**	**22**	**23**	**24**
BP sizes	130	190	125	205	175	195	130	185, 190, 205, 235, 240
Common	A*29	A*31	A*32, 74	A*33	A*34	A*68	A*33, 34, 66, 68, 69	A*43, 80
Rare		A*29		A*02, 24, 31, 68	A*03, 25, 26, 31	A*02, 11, 25, 26	A*02, 03, 11, 26	A*01, 02, 11, 26, 30, 31, 34

stringency of the overall PCR system being used. The PCR buffer utilized is of upmost importance to the efficiency and accuracy of the PCR-SSP system being implemented; different combinations and concentrations of PCR buffer ingredients(*see* **Note 2**), in particular dNTPs and free magnesium (*see* **Note 3**), are of critical importance to achieve reliable and accurate amplification.

Individual-specific primer pairs (primer mixes) should be empirically tested (*see* **Note 4**) with appropriate DNA sample to ensure that the reaction is appropriately positive with homozygous and heterozygous reference DNA samples. A good range of negative sample should be tested, and particular attention should be made to testing the primer mixes with samples most likely to give false positives (*see* **Note 4**). Once a reaction is working the primer mix can be stored frozen until ready to use whilst all the required primer mixes for a given set of reactions is developed and ready to be used as a full SSP genotyping set.

2 Materials

It is important to prepare all solutions using molecular grade water that is certified endonuclease free. Similarly, all plastic ware should also be certified.

1 M Tris–HCl, pH 9. Add 121.1 g tris base {$NH_2C(CH_2OH)_3$} to a suitable sterile 1 l container and dissolve in 800 ml molecular grade water. Adjust to pH 9 using concentrated hydrochloric acid. Adjust the final volume to 1 l with molecular grade water. Mix well and sterile filter or autoclave if required.

1 M Potassium Chloride Solution. Add 74.55 g potassium chloride {KCl} to a suitable sterile 1 l container. Add molecular grade water to a final volume of 1 l. Mix well and sterile filter or autoclave if required.

0.1 M Ammonium Sulfate Solution. Add 13.214 g ammonium sulfate {$(NH_4)_2SO_4$} to a suitable sterile 1 l container. Add molecular grade water to a final volume of 1 l. Mix well and sterile filter or autoclave if required.

1 M Magnesium Chloride Solution. Add 203.3 g magnesium chloride hexahydrate {$MgCl_2\ 6H_2O$} to a suitable sterile 1 l container. Add molecular grade water to a final volume of 1 l. Mix well and sterile filter or autoclave if required. Magnesium chloride solution can deteriorate once made; therefore, it is suggested that once a new stock is made it is frozen in suitably sized aliquots.

2× TBE Buffer (0.18 M Tris–Borate, 4 mM EDTA). Add 216 g tris base {$NH_2C(CH_2OH)_3$} and 110 g boric acid {H_3BO_3} to a suitable, sterile 10 l container and dissolve with 9 l distilled water. Add 8 ml 0.5 M EDTA pH 8.3 {$C_{10}H_{16}N_2O_8$}. Add distilled water to a final volume of 10 l. Mix well.

Table 2
Potassium chloride 10× PCR buffer

Solution	Volume to add for 10× (ml)	10× buffer concentration	Working PCR concentration
1 M KCl	50	500 mM	50 mM
1 M Tris–HCl pH 9.0	10	100 mM	10 mM
1 M $MgCl_2$	20	20 mM	2 mM
100 mM dNTPs	2	2 mM	200 μM
Tween 20	1	1 %	0.1 %
Molecular grade sterile water	37		
Total	100		

0.5× TBE Buffer. Add 250 ml 2× TBE buffer and 750 ml distilled water to a suitable, sterile 1 l container and mix well.

1 % Agarose Gel. Add 10 g molecular biology grade agarose to a 2 l pyrex beaker with 400 ml 0.5× TBE buffer. Microwave for 3 min at full power (750 W), remove the beaker and swirl to help dissolve the agarose. Repeat until the agarose is fully dissolved, taking care not to allow the agarose to get too hot and bubble over. Add 0.5× TBE to a final volume of 1 l before adding 10 μl 10 mg/ml ethidium bromide (*see* **Note 5**). Mix well and store at 50 °C until required (use within 24 h).

100 mM dNTP Mix. 100 mM stock of dNTPs means that the final concentration of each dNTP (dATP, dCTP, dGTP, and dTTP) is 100 mM. Store at −20 °C.

Taq Polymerase. Usually suspended in a 50 % glycerol buffer at 5 U/μl and stored at −20 °C until required.

10× PCR Buffer. PCR buffers utilized in PCR-SSP are usually either potassium chloride or ammonium sulfate based. Commercial PCR buffers are normally very good but you may wish to make your own. In general, it is best to make a 10× concentration PCR buffer to be used at 1× in the final PCR. Make up stock solutions of $MgCl_2$, tris and potassium chloride or ammonium sulfate as appropriate from Tables 2 and 3. Combine Tris-HCl and the potassium chloride or ammonium sulfate with the water and $MgCl_2$, add the dNTPs and filter if required (using 0.22 μm filter) before adding the Tween 20. Aliquot into appropriate volumes and store at below −20 °C.

Primers. If primers are lyophilized they should be resuspended in TE buffer (10 mM Tris pH 8.0, 1 mM EDTA) to a stock concentration of 200 μM. Before resuspending the primers briefly

Table 3
Ammonium sulfate 10× PCR buffer

Solution	Volume to add for 10× (ml)	10× buffer concentration	Working PCR concentration
0.1 M Ammonium sulfate	20	200 mM	20 mM
1 M Tris–HCl pH 9.0	50	500 mM	50 mM
1 M $MgCl_2$	20	20 mM	2 mM
100 mM dNTPs	2	2 mM	200 μM
Tween 20	1	1 %	0.1 %
Molecular grade sterile water	27		
Total	100		

centrifuge them to ensure that all material is deposited in the bottom of the tube, and mix well once resuspended. Ideally they should be aliquoted before freezing to avoid repeated freezing–thawing, which can damage the primers. Primers are generally used a 50–100 pmol in the final reaction (*see* Subheading 3 for more details).

3 Methods

3.1 Reaction Components

PCR-SSP reactions are usually set to a volume between 10 and 25 μl. Generally the primer mixes are prepared at 10× concentration and stored as frozen aliquots until required. They should not be repeatedly freeze-thawed as this can damage the oligonucleotides. Alternatively, primer mixes can be dispensed directly into the PCR plate and either stored frozen under a layer of mineral oil, or dried down (*see* **Note 6**). A dye such as cresol red may be added to the 10× primer mix to aid accurate pipetting. 10× PCR buffers can be pre-prepared and frozen as aliquots. Again, it is important not to repeatedly freeze-thaw these buffers as it may damage the buffer components. Taq polymerase should be stored in a buffer containing 50 % glycerol and be kept in the freezer until required.

3.2 Template DNA Requirements

Template DNA is typically extracted from EDTA or citrate anticoagulated whole blood. Heparinized samples can be problematic as heparin is a known inhibitor of PCR—such samples should be avoided if possible. If heparinized samples must be used, then it is recommended that the extracted DNA is treated with heparinase II before PCR. There are several DNA extraction methods, and a variety of commercial products available—choose a method that will give sufficient yield of DNA to run the PCR-SSP assays you are planning. As a guide, PCR-SSP should be capable of amplifying from between 1 and 10 ng/μl genomic DNA (concentration in final reaction), with an $OD_{260/280}$ of between 1.6 and 2. Samples that fall outside these parameters may still be viable and should be tested empirically.

A note on the use of storage buffers containing EDTA. Excessive amounts of EDTA will chelate free magnesium ions in the PCR mix, and can therefore inhibit the reaction. Many DNA extraction methods recommend resuspending in TE buffer. If TE is used then the EDTA concentration in the buffer should not exceed 1 mM (some alternative recipes include up to 10 mM EDTA), alternatively the DNA can be resuspended in molecular grade water.

3.3 PCR-SSP Setup

A typical PCR-SSP reaction will consist of the following:

1 μl 10× primer mix (containing both allele-specific and control primers)

1 μl 10× PCR buffer

0.1 μl Taq polymerase (5 U/μl)

1 μl template DNA (10–100 ng/μl)

6.9 μl molecular grade water

1. Dispense the various 10× primer mixes into known positions in the PCR plate either at the time of testing, or pre-aliquoted as noted above. Prepare a working reaction mix as a bulk stock, containing PCR buffer, polymerase, DNA and water. The working reaction mix is then dispensed directly onto the pre-aliquoted primers in the PCR plate (taking care to avoid carry-over from one well to another).
2. Cover the PCR reactions with a layer of mineral oil, or seal with a PCR film to avoid evaporation. Depending on the model of thermal cycler a foam or metal PCR mat may be required to ensure that even pressure is applied to the PCR plate during the reaction. The thermal cycler should have heating and cooling ramp rates of at least 1 °C/s, and be equipped with a heated lid.

Normally a single PCR program is set in place for PCR-SSP, and the reactions are optimized to work with these parameters. Touchdown PCR is often used, in which the annealing temperatures of the first few cycles are higher in order to discourage none-specific binding of primers (and therefore false positive reactions). In later cycles the annealing temperature is reduced to encourage more binding and increase PCR yield. A typical PCR-SSP protocol may consist of 96 °C for 60 s; 5 cycles of: 96 °C for 25 s, 70 °C for 45 s, 72 °C for 25 s; 21 cycles of: 96 °C for 25 s, 65 °C for 50 s, 72 °C for 30 s; 4 cycles of: 96 °C for 20 s, 55 °C for 60 s, 72 °C for 90 s; 20 °C for 30 s to cool.

3.4 Electrophoresis

There are a variety of different gel tanks available on the market. Ideally the one selected should have enough wells to accommodate all of the PCRs, and have 9 mm well spacing to be compatible with most multi-channel pipettes.

Prepare 1 % agarose gels and run with 0.5× TBE buffer for around 20 min at 200 V. Gel loading buffer with dye is recommended to aid loading and visualize migration across the gel. A DNA size marker should also be run in each row of the gel to aid sizing of the bands. These parameters may need to be altered if there is insufficient separation of bands upon visualization. Gels should be illuminated at 312 nm wavelength (UV) and photographed before interpretation.

3.5 Interpretation of Results

Examine the gel image examined for the presence of a control band in each well, and whether an allele-specific band is present. If there is an allele-specific band present but no control band then it is likely that the control reaction has been out competed. For this reason it is recommended that the control primers should always be used at a lower concentration, in order to increase the chance of them being out-competed by the allele-specific primers and not the other way around. If the control band is absent but there is an allele-specific band present, then the result is still viable. If there is no control or allele-specific band then the reaction has failed.

The pattern of positive reactions should be compared to the expected reactivity of each reaction in order to determine which alleles are present in the sample tested.

4 Notes

1. Primer design

   Primer Melting Temperature (Tm) by definition is the temperature at which one half of the DNA duplex will dissociate to become single stranded. Most PCR-SSP protocols have a PCR protocol with annealing at 65 °C. Primers with melting temperatures in the range of 60–65 °C generally produce the best results in PCR-SSP protocols. Primers with melting temperatures above 65 °C have a tendency for secondary annealing and false positives, whilst shorter primers may give weak or unreliable amplification. Aiming for a 65 °C primer length will generate PCR primers of between 18 and 25 bp.

   The Tm of a primer is affected by base composition and sequence of bases, length of the primer and salt concentration of the PCR buffer. In general, using the buffer compositions given in the methods section a simple calculation of G/C = 4 °C and A/T = 2 °C suffices for the majority of primers. Excellent free online tools for primer Tm calculation and general primer design can be found on the Internet, for example the Netprimer tool available at www.premierbiosoft.com is very useful.

The design of the primer is critical to its performance, and in particular an understanding of mismatch tolerance is important. In PCR-SSP the type and the position of mismatches within the first five or six bases from the 3′ end is critical. It should be noted that although SSP relies on non-extension of a 3′ mismatch it is sometimes possible to get extension of the primer even when the primer is exactly matched at the terminal 3′ end. Primers detecting T/C or G/A polymorphisms are at the most risk of extension and hence false positive amplification. However, it is unavoidable in designing PCR-SSP for HLA to not include T/C and G/A mismatches, thus it can be a useful strategy to include deliberate mismatches within the first six bases from the 3′ end to improve specificity of a primer. The closer to the 3′ end the deliberate mismatch is placed the stronger the destabilizing effect. In addition the selection of a T/G, T/A, or C/G or C/A deliberate mismatch will generate stronger destabilizing effects than T/C or G/A deliberate mismatches.

In general the specificity of a primer should be calculated from the matches and mismatches within the first six 3′ bases of the primer; this is termed the significant length of a primer and should be tested empirically to evaluate the efficacy of the design.

The use of the GC clamp rule can influence the choice of exactly where to place the deliberate mismatches. The presence of G or C bases within the last five bases from the 3′ end of primers can help improve specific binding at the 3′ end due to the stronger bonding of these bases. More than 3G's or C's should be avoided in the last five bases at the 3′ end of the primer.

Several general approaches to PCR primer design hold true for PCR-SSP design. It is advisable to keep the GC content (the number of G's and C's in the primer as a percentage of the total bases) of the primer in the region of 40–60 %. Excessive runs of greater than five of an individual base should generally be avoided as they can misprime. Long runs of consecutive di-nucleotide repeats should similarly be avoided because they can also misprime.

During primer design every effort should be made to avoid significant secondary structures affecting primers. Presence of the primer secondary structures produced by self-primer or cross-primer interactions can lead to poor product yield and/or primer-dimer artifact. Primers should be designed to minimize the risk of the following secondary structure problems.

3′ Hairpins: A hairpin is formed when a primer folds on itself and creates a stable bond. Each primer designed should be tested with an appropriate algorithm to assess the potential for hairpins. Internal and 5′ hairpins with a ΔG of −3 kcal/mol are generally tolerated, whereas 3′ end hairpins where the terminal base is matched should be avoided when the ΔG is lower than −1.8 kcal/mol. The ΔG value represents the energy required to break the secondary structure. Larger negative values for ΔG indicates stable, undesirable hairpins.

Dimers: Primer self-dimers are formed by interactions between identical primers (where the primer is complementary to itself) whereas cross-dimers are formed by interaction between sense and antisense primers, where they are complementary. The more likely a primer dimer is to form, the less primer will be available to hybridize to the template DNA, and therefore the PCR yield will be lower. Internal dimers with a ΔG of −8 kcal/mol are acceptable, but 3′ end dimer with a ΔG of −4 kcal/mol or lower can be problematic.

Investigation of secondary structures should be performed to investigate the interactions between allele primers, control primers and between allele and control primers.

2. Reaction design

   Allele-specific amplicon size. PCR-SSP is best suited to allelic amplicons of between 150 and 700 bp. If using potassium chloride buffer it is best to select priming position to generate amplicons of no greater than 300 bp.

   Control amplicon size: it is preferable to design primers to generate a PCR product 200 bp larger than the largest allele amplification in your system in order to allow greatest separation between allele and control in gel electrophoresis. It is recommended that in general the control amplicon primers should be at a lower concentration and less effective in PCR than the allele primers so that the allele amplification is not out-competed by the control primers.

   Ammonium sulfate based PCR buffers are useful for GC rich targets and PCR amplicons greater than 700 bp. PCR-SSP reactions spanning HLA class I introns are generally best designed in ammonium sulfate based buffer as potassium chloride buffers can fail to amplify across introns 2 and 3 in particular. KCl buffers are a better choice if the PCR mixture is to be used in a dried pellet approach as KCl gives added stability in this regard.

3. dNTPs and $MgCl_2$

   Concentration of dNTPs can be increased to generate stronger amplification and $MgCl_2$ can be increased for stronger amplification, but both approaches can induce false positives so titration should be done with care. In addition, dNTPs are chelated by $MgCl_2$ so that an increase in dNTPs creates a lower availability of $MgCl_2$ so conversely if you raise dNTPs too far you can get false negative reactions or reaction failure due to low $MgCl_2$. It is often best to raise or lower dNTPs and $MgCl_2$ together to achieve stronger reactions.

4. Primer Mix Testing
   The specificity of the primers designed should be tested empirically with samples selected to test for unwanted 3′ mismatch extension that can cause false positives. For example if the forward primer matches HLA-A*01 & A*03 and the reverse primer detects HLA-A*03 & A*11, the combined specificity should detect A*03 only. Testing with DNA samples positive for HLA-A*01 or A*11 will test the propensity for the forward or reverse primers respectively to false prime.

   False positive reactions during testing can be alleviated by using lower concentrations of primer or redesigns of the primer to incorporate more mismatches in the significant length. Lowering the Tm of the primer by redesigning to a shorter length by removing 5′ bases can help. Finally, reducing magnesium chloride concentration or raising PCR annealing temperature can help reduce false positives. It should be noted that raising the PCR annealing temperature will affect all PCR-SSP reactions within the system designed.

   False negative or weak allele PCR can be alleviated by increasing the concentration of primers, increasing the magnesium chloride concentration, or increasing dNTP concentration. If the control amplification remains stronger than the allele amplification in a given SSP reaction the control primer concentration should be reduced to avoid PCR competition.

   Final concentration in PCR mix is normally in the range 1.5–3 mM, with 2 mM being the most commonly used. The $MgCl_2$ to dNTP ratio is critical (as discussed above); generally if you increase $MgCl_2$ concentrations it is best to also increase dNTP concentration as well otherwise some PCR-SSP reactions may fail.

5. Ethidium Bromide and alternatives
   Ethidium bromide is a carcinogen and mutagen and care should be taken whilst handling. Relatively nontoxic substitutes are not available, such as GelRed, which work reasonably well. If you are using ethidium bromide already for SSP work you should validate the use of GelRed as there are subtle differences in sensitivity between different DNA stains that can cause smearing or lack of differentiation in gels. This problem can be frequently alleviated by reducing the amount of PCR product loaded.

6. Drying PCR reactions prior to use.
   For most storage requirements freezing 10 μl SSP reactions in PCR plates or strips works well. The dried down option is utilized mainly by commercial companies, but can be copied in the laboratory. To make your own dried-down PCR plates pre-seed the PCR vessels with 10 μl of primer mix and leave to evaporate for approximately 3 days at 28 °C, then seal the

plates with adhesive plate sealer or strip cap and store in the fridge until required.

Following is a brief troubleshooting guide to common problems experienced with PCR-SSP.

No amplification in any reaction

- Insufficient quantity of template DNA, or too much template DNA.
- PCR inhibitors present (e.g., heparin, EDTA).
- Poor quality DNA sample—check $OD_{260/280}$ is between 1.6 and 2.
- Missing reagents—ensure that PCR buffer, polymerase, primers, and template DNA were added correctly.
- Defective reagents—if problem persists try remaking the PCR ingredients.
- Thermal cycler problems—ensure that the thermal cycler is functioning and the heated lid is operational, and the correct PCR protocol is selected.
- Electrophoresis problems—ensure that adequate volumes of amplicon are added to the gel, electrophoresis is occurring correctly and ethidium bromide is present in the gel.
- Evaporation of reagents—ensure that the plate is sealed correctly (or adequate mineral oil is used).

Random PCR failure

- Electrophoresis problems—inadequate reagent loaded, gels not being run for the correct amount of time (i.e., bands not separated, or gel run too far), wells in gel not formed correctly.
- Thermal cycler problems—insufficiently tightened lid, thermal cycler out of calibration, wrong PCR protocol selected.
- Evaporation of reagents—ensure that the plate is sealed correctly (or adequate mineral oil is used).
- Missing reagents—ensure that PCR buffer, polymerase, primers, and template DNA were added correctly.
- Defective reagents—if problem persists try remaking the PCR ingredients.
- Insufficient quantity of template DNA, or too much template DNA.
- PCR inhibitors present (e.g., heparin, EDTA).
- Poor quality DNA sample—check $OD_{260/280}$ is between 1.6 and 2.

Weak amplification

- Primers incorrectly designed—refer to primer design recommendations.
- Insufficient quantity of template DNA, or too much template DNA.
- Electrophoresis problems—inadequate reagent loaded
- Thermal cycler problems—insufficiently tightened lid, thermal cycler out of calibration, wrong PCR protocol selected.

Nonspecific amplification

- Primers not specific—redesign primers following the recommendations in the methods section.
- Insufficient quantity of template DNA, or too much template DNA.
- Reactions loaded onto the gel in the incorrect order.
- New allele identified.

Amplification pattern not interpretable

- Primers not specific—redesign primers following the recommendations in the methods section.
- Reactions loaded onto the gel in the incorrect order.
- New allele identified.

Electrophoresis problems

- Insufficient separation, or running too far.

References

1. Tindall KR, Kunkel TA (1988) Fidelity of DNA synthesis by the *Thermus aquaticus* DNA polymerase. Biochemistry 27:6008–6013
2. Wu DY, Ugozzoli L, Pal BK, Wallace RB (1989) Allele-specific enzymatic amplification of beta-globin genomic DNA for diagnosis of sickle cell anaemia. Proc Natl Acad Sci USA 86:2757–2760
3. Newton CR, Graham A, Heptinstall LE, Powell SJ, Summers C et al (1989) Analysis of any point mutation in DNA. The amplification refractory mutation system (ARMS). Nucleic Acid Res 17:2503–2516
4. Fugger L, Morling N, Ryder LP, Odum N, Svejgaard A (1990) Technical aspects of typing for HLA-DP alleles using allele-specific DNA in vitro amplification and sequence-specific oligonucleotide probes. Detection of single base mismatches. J Immunol Methods 129:175–185
5. Olerup O, Zetterquist H (1992) HLA-DR typing by PCR amplification with sequence-specific primers (PCR-SSP) in 2 hours: an alternative to serological DR typing in clinical practice including donor-recipient matching in cadaveric transplantation. Tissue Antigens 39:225–235
6. Browning MJ, Krausa P, Rowan A, Bicknell DC, Bodmer JG et al (1993) Tissue typing the HLA-A locus from genomic DNA by sequence-specific PCR: comparison of HLA genotype and surface expression on colorectal tumour cell lines. Proc Natl Acad Sci USA 90: 2842–2845
7. Bunce M, O'Neill CM, Barnardo MC, Krausa P, Browning MJ et al (1995) Phototyping: comprehensive DNA typing for HLA-A, B, C, DRB1, DRB3, DRB4, DRB5 and DQB1 by PCR with 144 primer mixes utilising sequence-specific primers (PCR-SSP). Tissue Antigens 46

Chapter 9

Human Leukocyte Antigen (HLA) Typing by DNA Sequencing

Ana Lazaro, Bin Tu, Ruyan Yang, Yi Xiao, Kanthi Kariyawasam, Jennifer Ng, and Carolyn Katovich Hurley

Abstract

DNA sequencing is a powerful technique for identifying allelic variation within the human leukocyte antigen (HLA) genes. Sequencing is usually focused on the most polymorphic exons of the class I (HLA-A, -B, -C) and class II (HLA-DR, -DQ, and -DP) genes. These exons encode the antigen recognition site, the region of the HLA molecule that binds peptides and interacts with the T cell receptor for antigen and natural killer cell immunoglobulin-like receptors (KIR). Sanger sequencing of amplified DNA from each HLA gene from a preparation containing one or two alleles yields a sequence that is used to identify the alleles by comparison with a reference database.

Key words Human leukocyte antigens, DNA sequencing, Alleles

1 Introduction

The human leukocyte antigen (HLA) genes are encoded by 12 loci including three class I loci (HLA-A, -B, -C) and nine class II loci (HLA-DRA, -DRB1, -DRB3, -DRB4, -DRB5, -DQA1, -DQB1, -DPA1, -DPB1). These genes likely arose from gene duplications and crossing over since they share extensive sequence homology. Each gene is divided into 5–8 exons that encode the signal peptide, two or three extracellular domains, transmembrane region, and cytoplasmic tail. The coding sequence of each gene is approximately 1,100 base pairs in length for a class I gene and about 800 base pairs in length for a class II gene; if introns are included, an HLA gene is about 3,000 base pairs in length for a class I gene and about 5,000–10,000 bases in length for a class II gene. While most

---

Ana Lazaro and Bin Tu have contributed equally to first authorship.

Andrea A. Zachary and Mary S. Leffell (eds.), *Transplantation Immunology: Methods and Protocols, Second Edition*, Methods in Molecular Biology, vol. 1034, DOI 10.1007/978-1-62703-493-7_9, © Springer Science+Business Media, LLC 2013

HLA genes are present in a diploid state, individuals vary in the number of DRB genes carried from two to four. Usually two DRB1 loci are present, one on each copy of chromosome six; the additional loci can be one or two of the following loci, DRB3, DRB4, or DRB5 [1].

The HLA loci are polymorphic; DRA has only seven alleles while HLA-B has over 2,200. Alleles at a locus may differ by synonymous substitutions that do not alter the protein sequence or by nonsynonymous substitutions that alter the protein sequence. Some alleles are not expressed as full length proteins. For example, the 2,271 HLA-B alleles known at the time this chapter was written encode 1,737 different proteins and there are 73 non-expressed alleles. The nomenclature used to designate HLA alleles and a description of the DNA sequence variation are described on two reference Web sites: http://hla.alleles.org/ and http://www.ebi.ac.uk/imgt/hla/ [2].

The protein structures formed by the assembly of a HLA class I polypeptide with beta-2 microglobulin and by the assembly of HLA class II alpha and beta polypeptides are very similar. The amino-terminal regions of the HLA polypeptides form an antigen recognition site (ARS), binding antigenic peptides within the cell for transport to the cell surface and interacting with antigen-receptors on T lymphocytes to trigger an adaptive immune response. The remainder of the HLA protein forms a scaffold for the ARS. The majority of the genetic variation within an HLA allele alters the sequence of the ARS, giving that region different specificities for antigenic peptide binding and T cell antigen receptor interaction. Natural killer (NK) cell immunoglobulin-like receptors also interact with the ARS to influence NK cell killing. Many DNA sequencing strategies focus solely on the exons that encode the ARS.

1.1 Overview of Methods

This protocol describes the amplification and sequencing of HLA genes from genomic DNA. The polymerase chain reaction (PCR) is used to obtain an amplicon covering the exons encoding the antigen recognition site of each gene. These are exons 2 and 3 for class I and exon 2 for class II genes. The nucleotide sequences of the exons carried by each amplicon are determined using Sanger sequencing [3]. Figure 1 shows the annealing sites of locus-specific PCR amplification and sequencing primers in an HLA-A locus allele, A*01:01:01:01.

For the HLA loci, we present two different strategies to obtain HLA assignments (Fig. 2). In one strategy, both alleles of the locus are amplified together by PCR and sequenced concurrently. The allele assignments are made by comparison to a HLA reference database. If alternative genotypes are obtained (i.e., the result is ambiguous) and this level of resolution does not meet the testing requirements, the alleles can be separated from one another for sequencing by performing a group-specific PCR amplification or

```
gDNA                 -291       -281       -271       -261       -251       -241       -231       -221       -211       -201
 A*01:01:01:01  CAGGAGCAGA GGGGTCAGGG CGAAGTCCCA GGGCCCCAGG CGTGGCTCTC AGGGTCTCAG GCCCCGAAGG CGGTGTATGG ATTGGGGAGT CCCAGCCTTG

gDNA                 -191       -181       -171       -161       -151       -141       -131       -121       -111       -101
A*01:01:01:01   GGGATTCCCC AACTCCGCAG TTTCTTTTCT CCCTCTCCCA ACCTACGTAG GGTCCTTCAT CCTGGATACT CACGACGCGG ACCCAGTTCT CACTCCCATT

gDNA                  -91        -81        -71        -61        -51        -41        -31        -21        -11         -1
A*01:01:01:01   GGGTGTCGGG TTTCCAGAGA AGCCAATCAG TGTCGTCGCG GTCGCTGTTC TAAAGTCCGC ACGCACCCAC CGGGACTCAG ATTCTCCCCA GACGCCGAGG

gDNA                   10         20         30         40         50         60         70         80         90        100
A*01:01:01:01   |ATGGCCGTCA TGGCGCCCCG AACCCTCCTC CTGCTACTCT CGGGGGCCCT GGCCCTGACC CAGACCTGGG CGG|GTGAGTG CGGGGTCGGG AGGGAAACCG

gDNA                  110        120        130        140        150        160        170        180        190        200
A*01:01:01:01   CCTCTGCGGG GAGAAGCAAG GGGCCCTCCT GGCGGGGGCG CAGGACCGGG GGAGCCGCGC CGGGAGGAGG GTCGGGCAGG TCTCAGCCAC TGCTCGCCCC

gDNA                  210        220        230        240        250        260        270        280        290        300
A*01:01:01:01   CAG|GCTCCCA CTCCATGAGG TATTTCTTCA CATCCGTGTC CCGGCCCGGC CGCGGGGAGC CCCGCTTCAT CGCCGTGGGC TACGTGGACG ACACGCAGTT

gDNA                  310        320        330        340        350        360        370        380        390        400
A*01:01:01:01   CGTGCGGTTC GACAGCGACG CCGCGAGCCA GAAGATGGAG CCGCGGGCGC CGTGGATAGA GCAGGAGGGG CCGGAGTATT GGGACCAGGA GACACGGAAT

gDNA                  410        420        430        440        450        460        470        480        490        500
A*01:01:01:01   ATGAAGGCCC ACTCACAGAC TGACCGAGCG AACCTGGGGA CCCTGCGCGG CTACTACAAC CAGAGCGAGG ACG|GTGAGTG ACCCCGGCCC GGGGCGCAGG

gDNA                  510        520        530        540        550        560        570        580        590        600
A*01:01:01:01   TCACGACCCC TCATCCCCCA CGGACGGGCC AGGTCGCCCA CAGTCTCCGG GTCCGAGATC CACCCCGAAG CCGCGGGACT CCGAGACCCT TGTCCCGGGA

gDNA                  610        620        630        640        650        660        670        680        690        700
A*01:01:01:01   GAGGCCCAGG CGCCTTTACC CGGTTTCATT TTCAGTTTAG GCCAAAAATC CCCCCGGGTT GGTCGGGGCG GGGCGGGGCT CGGGGGACTG GGCTGACCGC

gDNA                  710        720        730        740        750        760        770        780        790        800
A*01:01:01:01   GGGGTCGGGG CCAG|GTTCTC ACACCATCCA GATAATGTAT GGCTGCGACG TGGGGCCGGA CGGGCGCTTC CTCCGCGGGT ACCGGCAGGA CGCCTACGAC

gDNA                  810        820        830        840        850        860        870        880        890        900
A*01:01:01:01   GGCAAGGATT ACATCGCCCT GAACGAGGAC CTGCGCTCTT GGACCGCGGC GGACATGGCA GCTCAGATCA CCAAGCGCAA GTGGGAGGCG GTCCATGCGG

gDNA                  910        920        930        940        950        960        970        980        990       1000
A*01:01:01:01   CGGAGCAGCG GAGAGTCTAC CTGGAGGGCC GGTGCGTGGA CGGGCTCCGC AGATACCTGG AGAACGGGAA GGAGACGCTG CAGCGCACGG |GTACCAGGGG

gDNA                 1010       1020       1030       1040       1050       1060       1070       1080       1090       1100
A*01:01:01:01   CCACGGGGCG CCTCCCTGAT CGCCTATAGA TCTCCCGGGC TGGCCTCCCA CAAGGAGGGG AGACAATTGG GACCAACACT AGAATATCAC CCTCCCTCTG

gDNA                 1110       1120       1130       1140       1150       1160       1170       1180       1190       1200
A*01:01:01:01   GTCCTGAGGG AGAGGAATCC TCCTGGGTTT CCAGATCCTG TACCAGAGAG TGACTCTGAG GTTCCGCCCT GCTCTCTGAC ACAATTAAGG GATAAAATCT
```

Fig. 1 The genomic sequence of HLA-A*01:01:01:01 showing the position of exons 1 (nucleotides 1–73), 2 (nucleotides 204–473), and 3 (nucleotides 715–990) *vertical lines* mark their 5′ and 3′ boundaries). The annealing sites for locus-specific amplification primers, 5A2 and 3A2 (Table 2), are shown in with a *double underline*; the annealing sites for sequencing primers which flank exon 2 and flank exon 3 are *underlined* (Table 3)

by using an allele specific sequencing primer. The secondary testing allows the laboratory to determine the phase of two or more polymorphisms (i.e., which alternative nucleotides are found within the same allele). This additional information allows the laboratory to distinguish among alternative genotypes. A protocol for separating alleles by bacterial cloning and sequencing is also provided. In a second strategy, group-specific PCR amplification primers are used in the first step. If low resolution types are available, the specific primer sets can be selected. If not available, all the primer sets are used. Using this strategy, the two alleles may be separated and can be sequenced separately. However, some of the time, both alleles will amplify with the same group-specific primer pair. If this is the case, alternative genotypes can be resolved as described in the first strategy.

The disadvantage of using group-specific primers when the low resolution typing assignment is not known is that the complete panel of primers must be used. If this panel is large (e.g., DRB1 requires 12 or more primer pairs), then it is labor intensive and wasteful of reagents since many amplifications will be negative.

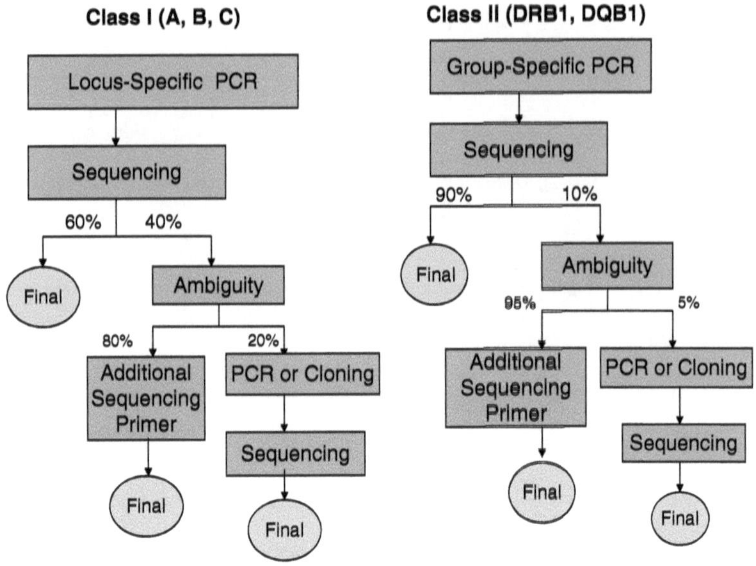

Fig. 2 Strategies to obtain HLA allele assignments. The approximate percentage of samples that must undergo further testing are indicated. The percentages will vary depending on the frequency of specific HLA alleles in the population and the characteristics of the alleles

For DRB1, because of extensive sharing of sequences with DRB3, DRB4, and DRB5 loci, a single locus specific primer pair is not possible so only a group-specific primer strategy is provided.

Sequencing exons other than those specifying the ARS. The focus is on the ARS exons; however, in some cases, alternative genotypes will differ for the presence of non-expressed alleles. In order to determine if the non-expressed allele is present, the sequence of other regions of the gene may be required. For example, HLA-C*04:01 and non-expressed HLA-C*04:09N are identical in nucleotide sequence in exons 2 and 3. Since both are frequent alleles, the laboratory may wish to distinguish between these alleles. This is accomplished by amplification and sequencing of exon 7 where the nucleotide sequence difference distinguishing these alleles is found. The position in the gene of the sequence information needed to resolve expressed from non-expressed alleles can vary; some differences are found in the 5′ or 3′ untranslated regions or in the introns. In some cases, because there is little information on the DNA sequences found in regions outside of the commonly typed exons for specific HLA alleles and reference cells are not available, the assay may lack the appropriate controls and information to interpret the results. Laboratories may use information on the predicted frequency of the non-expressed allele or the predicted haplotype carrying the non-expressed allele to determine whether further testing is required. Unfortunately, this frequency information is very limited.

Commercial sequencing reagents. Kits designed for sequencing HLA alleles are available commercially from several vendors. The advantage of these kits is that the vendor has provided the quality control and the strategy. The disadvantage is that the sequences of the oligonucleotide reagents in the kit are not provided, making trouble-shooting difficult. Furthermore, if the kit does not provide a necessary reagent to resolve an ambiguity or to isolate a novel allele, it may take some time before the vendor can provide the needed reagent. The use of in-house reagents as described here allows more flexibility and timeliness in addressing issues of resolution. The disadvantage is that use of "in-house" reagents requires more quality control within the laboratory and a more advanced level of understanding of HLA diversity. Furthermore, the HLA interpretation software used to assign alleles from the primary sequence data may not be designed to accommodate these in-house reagents so interpretation may be more cumbersome.

1.2 Use of Methods in Clinical Practice

DNA sequencing is commonly used for unrelated donor and umbilical cord blood selection in hematopoietic stem cell transplantation (HSCT) used to treat leukemia, lymphoma, or other serious diseases affecting the hematopoietic system. Sequencing may also be used to identify an HLA-matched family donor for HSCT when similar HLA alleles are segregating in the family or where parents are unavailable. Selection of a donor who is allele-matched with the patient for HLA-A,-B, -C, and -DRB1 increases survival following transplantation [4, 5]. When the best matched donor carries a different allele at one of these four loci, matching for HLA-DQB1 and HLA-DRB3, -DRB4, and -DRB5 alleles may also be considered by the transplant center. While the matching requirements for umbilical cord blood are less stringent, most transplant centers type units at higher resolution, selecting better matched units with the expectation of a better outcome [6, 7]. If the patient is to receive a mismatched transplant and the patient is sensitized to specific HLA allelic products, the transplant center may type other HLA loci if involved in the sensitization including DQA1, DPA1, and DPB1. This information will be used in donor selection in order to reduce the risk of graft failure [4, 8].

Sequencing is less commonly used in solid organ transplantation since the focus is on donor selection to avoid rejection by patients sensitized to specific HLA mismatches. However, in cases where patients are sensitized to specific HLA allelic products, sequencing may be used to guide donor selection.

2 Materials

Use molecular biology reagent grade water (e.g., catalogue number W4502, Sigma-Aldrich) unless noted. Storage conditions of commercial reagents are indicated by the vendor. If reagents are frozen, thaw completely and be sure salts are in solution before use. A brief centrifugation of reagents will ensure that small quantities are in the bottom of the tube prior to opening.

2.1 DNA Preparation

1. Whole blood drawn into a standard blood tube containing the anticoagulant acid citrate dextrose (ACD) (*see* **Note 1**). Alternatively, epithelial cells collected by swabbing the buccal surfaces of the mouth with an applicator with a sterile cotton tip (e.g., catalogue number 1495996CLC, Fisher Scientific) (*see* **Note 2**).
2. QIAamp[R] DNA Blood Mini Kit (QIAGEN, Valencia, CA, USA): The kit contains buffers AL, AW1, AW2, protease and solvent for protease, spin columns, collection tubes and instruction manual. The buffers in the kit, AW1 and AW2, are provided as concentrates. When opening a new bottle, add the appropriate amount of 96–100 % ethanol (as written on the label). To reconstitute the protease, add the supplied solvent to the protease powder and invert the bottle several times to mix. Store for 2 months at 4 °C after preparation.
3. 96–100 % ethanol.
4. Phosphate buffered saline (PBS).
5. 1.5 ml microcentrifuge tubes.
6. Pipettor (5–200 μl) and tips.
7. Heat block or water bath at 56 °C.
8. Vortex mixer.
9. Centrifuge capable of holding 1.5 ml tubes with a maximum speed of 20,000 × *g* (14,000 rpm).

2.2 Polymerase Chain Reaction Co-amplification of Both Alleles at an HLA Class I Locus

1. Genomic DNA prepared as described in Subheading 3.1 at approximate concentration of 10–30 ng/μl; 5 μl is required for each PCR amplification.
2. ABC buffer: 150 mM ammonium sulfate, 0.5 M Tris–HCl (pH 8.8), 0.5 mM EDTA, 15 mM $MgCl_2$, 0.1 % gelatin, 100 mM β-mercaptoethanol. Mix 75 ml 1 M ammonium sulfate, 250 ml 1 M Tris–HCl (pH 8.8), 0.5 ml 0.5 M EDTA, 7.5 ml 1 M $MgCl_2$, 50 ml 1 % gelatin, and add water to 500 ml. After autoclaving, add 3.45 ml 14.4 M β-mercaptoethanol, mix, and store as 1.5 ml aliquots at 4 °C.
3. 10 mM PCR nucleotide dNTP mixture (e.g., catalogue number 11581295001; Roche, Mannheim, Germany).
4. HLA locus-specific PCR primers: 20 μM of each oligonucleotide primer in water, store at −20 °C. HLA-A locus primers 5A2 and 3A2; HLA-B locus primers 5B3, 5B1, 3B1, and 3B1-AC; HLA-C locus primers 5CIn1-61 and 3BCIn3-12 (Tables 1, 2, 4, 5, 7, and 8) (*see* **Notes 3** and **4**).

Table 1
HLA-A PCR amplification primer pairs

Sense primer	Antisense primer	Amplification specificity[a]
Locus specific primer pairs		
5A2	3A2	Locus specific primer pair to obtain amplicon carrying exon 2, exon 3
AIn1-46-F	3AIn3-62-R	Locus specific primer pair to obtain amplicon carrying exon 2, exon 3; alternative to primer pair above
Group-specific primer pairs		
AIn1-A-F	3AIn3-62-R	Allele group-specific primer pair amplifying alleles with A at a polymorphic position 153 in intron 1 (e.g., A*02*01:01:01)
AIn1-G-F	3AIn3-62-R	Allele group-specific primer pair amplifying alleles with G at a polymorphic position 153 in intron 1 (e.g., A*01:01:01:01)
AIn1-T-F	3AIn3-62-R	Allele group-specific primer pair amplifying alleles with T at a polymorphic position 153 in intron 1 (e.g., A*29:01)
AIn1-226	AIn3-249	A*02 group-specific primer pair to obtain complete A*02 group allele sequences of exon 2, exon 3
5′FR-296m	AIn3-249	A*03 group-specific primer pair to obtain complete A*03 group allele sequences of exon 2, exon 3
AIn1-214	AIn3-249	A*24 group-specific primer pair to obtain complete A*24 group allele sequences of exon 2, exon 3
BW4	3A2	Allele group-specific primer pair amplifying alleles carrying TCGCGCTCC at CDS 311–319 to obtain exon 3 and partial exon 2 sequences
5A2	A-GTR	Allele group-specific primer pair amplifying alleles carrying GT at CDS 570–570

[a]CDS, coding sequence where nucleotide 1 is the first nucleotide of exon 1

5. Dimethyl sulfoxide (DMSO).
6. Reagent grade water.
7. Taq DNA polymerase (5 U/μl) (e.g., Roche).
8. DNA control (*see* **Note 5**).
9. 1.5 ml sterile disposable tubes.
10. Semi-skirted PCR tray (e.g., Fisher Scientific, Dallas, TX, USA).
11. Tray seals (e.g., One Lambda, Canoga Park, CA, USA).
12. Single channel and multichannel (8 or 12 channel) pipettors (0.5–200 μl) and tips.
13. Thermal cycler (e.g., model 2720, Applied Biosystems, Foster City, CA, USA).
14. Vortex mixer.
15. Centrifuge capable of holding plates with a maximum speed of 20,000 × *g* (14,000 rpm) (e.g., model 5804 (for plates with A-2-deep well plate rotor), Eppendorf, Hauppauge, NY, USA).

Table 2
Sequences and annealing sites of HLA-A PCR amplification primers[a]

Name	Sequence 5′–3′[b,c]	Annealing site region/3′ nucleotide[d]
5′FR-296 m	CCA GGC GTG GCT CAC AGA	Sense, 5′ noncoding, -248
AIn1-A-F	GGG GCG CAR GAC CCG GGA	Sense, intron 1, 153
AIn1-G-F	GGG CGC AGG ACC GGG GG	Sense, intron 1, 153
AIn1-T-F	GGG RCG CAG GAC CCG GGT	Sense, intron 1, 153
AIn1-46-F	CCT CTG YGG GGA GAA GCA A	Sense, intron 1, 119
5A2	CCC AGA CGC CGA GGA TGG CCG	Sense, CDS 7
AIn1-226	CTC TGT GGG GAG AAG CAA C	Sense, intron 1, 120
AIn1-214	CGC CTG GCG GGG GGG CAA	Sense, intron 1, 143
BW4	GAG AAC CTG CGG ATC GCG CTC C	Sense, exon 2, CDS 319
A-GTR	AG GTA TCT GCG GAG CCA C	Antisense, exon 3, CDS 570
3AIn3-62-R	GTC CCA ATT GTC TCC CCT CCTT	Antisense, intron 3, 1053
AIn3-249	CAG AGT CAC TCT CTG GTA CAG	Antisense, intron 3, 1138
3A2	GCA GGG CGG AAC CTC AGA GTC ACT CTC T	Antisense, intron 3, 1145

[a]Sequences of many of the reagents were based on reagents described by Cao (1999 5860 /id), Cereb (1995 186 /id), Kotsch (1997 5798 /id), SY Yang (personal communication)
[b]Sequences are divided into triplets for the ease of reading; they do not necessarily correspond to codons
[c]International Union of Biochemistry (IUB) nucleotide codes for multiple nucleotides e.g., R = AG, S = GC
[d]Nucleotide numbering of primers annealing in introns or 5′ of exon 1 is based on the numbering of the genomic sequence of A*01:01:01:01 in the IMGT/HLA database where +1 is the first nucleotide of exon 1 specifying the ATG codon of the signal peptide. CDS numbering is based on exons only where +1 is the first nucleotide of exon 1 specifying the ATG codon of the signal peptide

2.3 Allele Group-Specific Amplification of HLA Class I Loci, HLA-A and HLA-B

1. Genomic DNA prepared as described in Subheading 3.1.
2. Positive and negative control genomic DNA (*see* **Note 5**).
3. 10× buffer : 500 mM Tris–HCl, pH 8.8; 150 mM ammonium sulfate; 500 μM EDTA, 0.1 % w/v gelatin; 100 mM 14.4 M β-mercaptoethanol. For 100 ml of stock (10×) solution: 15 ml 1 M ammonium sulfate (132.1 g/l), 50 ml 1 M Tris–HCl, pH 8.8 (121.1 g/l, use HCl to adjust pH), 0.1 ml 0.5 M EDTA, pH 8.0 (186.1 g/l, use NaOH to adjust pH), 100 mg Knox gelatin, 34.8 ml water. Autoclave and store at room temperature. The working solution is 1 ml 10× PCR buffer and 7 μl β-mercaptoethanol. The working solution is made fresh just before use in the pre-PCR area. Do not autoclave after adding β-mercaptoethanol.
4. 10 mM PCR nucleotide dNTP mixture (e.g., catalogue number 11581295001; Roche, Mannheim, Germany).

5. Group-specific PCR primers: 10 μM of each oligonucleotide primer in water, store at –20° C. Three HLA-A locus primer pairs: (1) AIn1-A-F and 3AIn3-62-R; (2) AIn1-G-F and 3AIn3-62-R, and (3) AIn1-T-F and 3AIn3-62-R. Two HLA-B locus primers: (1) BIn1-TA and BIn3-R, BIn3-AC and (2) BIn1-CG and BIn3-R, BIn3-AC (Tables 1, 2, 4, and 5) (*see* **Notes 3** and **4**).
6. Dimethyl sulfoxide (DMSO).
7. 50 mM magnesium chloride.
8. Reagent grade water.
9. Platinum Taq DNA polymerase (5 U/μl) (e.g., Invitrogen, Grand Island, NY, USA).
10. Semi-skirted PCR tray (e.g., Fisher Scientific, Dallas, TX, USA).
11. Tray seals (e.g., One Lambda, Canoga Park, CA, USA).
12. Single channel and multichannel (8 or 12 channel) pipettors (0.5–200 μl) and tips.
13. Thermal cycler (e.g., model 2720, Applied Biosystems, Foster City, CA, USA).
14. Vortex mixer.
15. Centrifuge capable of holding plates with a maximum speed of 20,000×*g* (14,000 rpm) (e.g., model 5804 (for plates with A-2-deep well plate rotor), Eppendorf, Hauppauge, NY, USA).

2.4 Allele Group-Specific Polymerase Chain Reaction Amplification of HLA-DRB Loci with Intron Primers

1. Genomic DNA prepared as described in Subheading 3.1 at approximate concentration of 100 ng/μl.
2. Positive and negative control genomic DNA (*see* **Note 5**).
3. PCR primers as described in the publication from Kotsch et al. [9] at a concentration of 5 pmol/μl (*see* **Note 3**). In addition to the published primer sequences, the primer pair, CGG CGT CTC TGT CAG TRT CTT CCC (intron 1, 118–138) and I2RB28, is used to amplify DRB5.
4. 5× PCR buffer : 75 mM $(NH_4)_2$ SO_4, 12.5 mM $MgCl_2$, 300 mM Tris–HCl, pH 9.0. Make the buffer by mixing 37.5 ml 1 M ammonium sulfate, 150 ml 1 M Tris–HCl (pH 9.0), 6.25 ml 1 M $MgCl_2$, water to 500 ml. Store at –20 °C.
5. Dimethyl sulfoxide (DMSO).
6. 1.25 mM dNTP: Make solution by adding 12.5 μl of each 100 mM nucleotide stock (e.g., Invitrogen, Grand Island, NY, USA; catalogue number 10297-018) to 950 μl of water.
7. Taq DNA polymerase (5 U/μl) (e.g., Invitrogen, Grand Island, NY, USA).
8. Semi-skirted PCR tray (e.g., Fisher Scientific, Dallas, TX, USA).
9. Tray seals (e.g., One Lambda, Canoga Park, CA, USA).

10. Single channel and multichannel (8 or 12 channel) pipettors (0.5–200 μl) and tips.
11. Thermal cycler (e.g., model 2720, Applied Biosystems, Foster City, CA, USA).
12. Vortex mixer.
13. Centrifuge capable of holding plates with a maximum speed of 20,000×*g* (14,000 rpm) (e.g., model 5804 (for plates with A-2-deep well plate rotor), Eppendorf, Hauppauge, NY, USA).

2.5 Polymerase Chain Reaction Amplification of DQB1

1. Genomic DNA prepared as described in Subheading 3.1 at concentration of at least 20 ng/μl.
2. Positive and negative control genomic DNA (*see* **Note 5**).
3. PCR primers: 20 pmol/μl, oligonucleotide sequences described by Dunn et al. [10] (*see* **Notes 3** and **4**).
4. Gold Taq Polymerase (5 U/μl) (cat # 1435094, Roche, Mannheim, Germany).
5. 10× PCR Gold Buffer (cat # 1435094, Roche).
6. 5 M betaine (e.g., catalogue number B0300-5VL, Sigma-Aldrich, St. Louis, MO, USA).
7. 10 mM PCR nucleotide dNTP mixture (e.g., catalogue number 11581295001; Roche).
8. 1.5 mM $MgCl_2$.
9. Reagent grade water.
10. Semi-skirted PCR tray (e.g., Fisher Scientific, Dallas, TX, USA).
11. Tray seals (e.g., One Lambda, Canoga Park, CA, USA).
12. Single channel and multichannel (8 or 12 channel) pipettors (0.5–200 μl) and tips.
13. Thermal cycler (e.g., model 2720, Applied Biosystems, Foster City, CA, USA).
14. Vortex mixer.
15. Centrifuge capable of holding plates with a maximum speed of 20,000×*g* (14,000 rpm) (e.g., model 5804 (for plates with A-2-deep well plate rotor), Eppendorf, Hauppauge, NY, USA).

2.6 Gel Electrophoresis

1. 100 base pair (bp) DNA ladder (e.g., TrackIt™100 bp DNA ladder, Invitrogen, Grand Island, NY, USA) (*see* **Note 6**).
2. Agarose (e.g., UltraPure™Agarose, Invitrogen, Grand Island, NY, USA).
3. 10× TBE buffer (e.g., UltraPure™ 10× TBE buffer, Invitrogen) diluted with deionized water at an operational resistivity of 18.2 MΩ/cm at 25 °C to 1×.

4. GelRed™ nucleic acid gel stain 10,000× (Biotium, Inc., Hayward, CA, USA).
5. 5× sucrose cresol (0.04 % cresol red in 30 % sucrose) gel loading solution.
6. Microwave oven to melt the agarose.
7. Flat bed slab gel unit (e.g., tray 11.9 cm (length) × 11.5 cm (width)) and power supply (e.g., RunOne™ Electrophoresis Unit, Embi Tec, San Diego, CA, USA).
8. UV transilluminator.
9. Gel photography system.

2.7 Purification of PCR Amplicons Using AMPure

1. Agencourt AMPure kit (Beckman Coulter, Beverly, MA, USA).
2. 70 % ethanol in water (e.g., Warner-Graham Company, Cockeysville, MD, USA).
3. Agencourt SPRIPlate 96R magnet plate (Beckman Coulter).

2.8 DNA Sequencing

1. Amplified DNA purified with AMPure from Subheading 3.7 at concentration of 50–100 ng/μl.
2. Big Dye Terminator Cycle Sequencing Kits with AmpliTaq DNA Polymerase, FS (catalogue number P/N4303150, Life Technologies, Austin, TX, USA).
3. Better Buffer (The Gel Company, San Francisco, CA, USA).
4. HLA locus sequencing primers: 5 pmol/μl in water. Store at −20 °C. HLA-A locus sequencing primers include 5AIn1-46, 3In2-65, 5In2-148, 3AIn3-66. HLA-B locus sequencing primers include 5Bin1-57, BEx2R, BEx3F, and 3Bin3-37. HLA-C locus sequencing primers include CEx2F, CEx2R, CEx3F, 3BCIn3-12 (Tables 3, 6, and 9). Sequencing primers for DRB1 [9] and DQB1 [10] have been described. An additional sequencing primer for DRB1 is GTG AGC GCG GCT GAG G (intron 2, 1–16, antisense) used to obtain a read of DRB1*07 (*see* **Notes 3** and **4**).
5. Agencourt CleanSEQ kit (Beckman Coulter, Beverly, MA, USA).
6. Ethanol: 73 % solution in water. Add water to 73 ml 200 proof ethanol to make 100 ml final volume.
7. Reagent grade water.
8. Semi-skirted PCR tray (Fisher Scientific, Dallas, TX, USA).
9. Tray seals (One Lambda, Canoga Park, CA, USA).
10. Agencourt SPRIPlate 96R magnet plate (Beckman Coulter).
11. Single channel and multichannel pipettors (0.5–200 μl) and tips.
12. Thermal cycler (e.g., model 2720, Applied Biosystems, Foster City, CA, USA).

Table 3
HLA-A sequencing primers[a]

Primer	Sequence 5'–3'[b,c]	Annealing site region/3' nucleotide[d]	Comments
Locus specific sequencing primers			
5AIn1-46	GAA ACS GCC TCT GYG GGG AGA AGC AA	Sense, intron 1, 119	Locus specific sequencing primer for exon 2, forward
3In2-65	TCG GAC CCG GAG ACT GTG	Antisense, intron 2, 538	Locus specific sequencing primer for exon 2, reverse
AIntlF	GCG CCK GGA SGA GGG T	Sense, intron 1, 157	Locus specific sequencing primer for exon 2, forward; alternative to 5AIn1-46
Int2R	GGA TCT CGG ACC CGG AG	Antisense, intron 2, 545	Locus specific sequencing primer for exon 2, reverse; alternative to 3In2-65
5In2-148	GTT TCA TTT TCA GTT TAG GCC A	Sense, intron 2, 622	Locus specific sequencing primer for exon 3, forward
3AIn3-66	TGT TGG TCC CAA TTG TCT CCC CTC	Antisense, intron 3, 1054	Locus specific sequencing primer for exon 3, reverse
Int2F	TTA CCC GGT TTC ATT TTC AG	Sense, intron 2, 637	Locus specific sequencing primer for exon 3, forward; alternative to 5In2-148
AInt3R	TCC TTG TGG GAG GCC AG	Antisense, intron 3, 1041	Locus specific sequencing primer for exon 3, reverse; alternative to 3AIn3-66
Secondary assay—group-specific sequencing primers			
KA1S	ATG AGG TAT TTC TTC ACA	Sense, exon 2, CDS 102	Sequencing primer for alleles carrying TTCACA at CDS 97–102 in exon 2
KA1S-M	CTC CAT GAG GTA TTT CTT	Sense, exon 2, CDS 98	Sequencing primer for alleles carrying CTT at CDS 96–98 in exon 2
A-AC	ATG AGG TAT TTC TAC ACC	Sense, exon 2, CDS 102	Sequencing primer for alleles carrying ACACC at CDS 98–102 in exon 2
RBW4T	TA GTA GCG GAG CGC GAT C	Antisense, exon 2, CDS 309	Sequencing primer for alleles carrying TCGCGCTCC at CDS 311–319 in exon 2
A-GTR	AG GTA TCT GCG GAG CCA C	Antisense, exon 3, CDS 570	Sequencing primer for alleles carrying GT at CDS 570–570 in exon 3
KA31-M1	TC CGC GGG TAC CAC CAG T	Sense, exon 3, CDS 418	Sequencing primer for alleles carrying ACCAGT at CDS 413–418 in exon 3
KA31-M2	TTC CTC CGC GGG TAC CAC	Sense, exon 3, CDS 414	Sequencing primer for alleles carrying AC at CDS 413–414 in exon 3

[a]Sequences of some of the reagents were based on reagents described by Cereb (1995 186 /id), Kotsch (1997 5798 / id). Other sequences were based on regions interrogated by oligonucleotide probes (Cao, 1999 5860 /id)
[b]Sequences are divided into triplets for the ease of reading; they do not necessarily correspond to codons
[c]International Union of Biochemistry (IUB) nucleotide codes for multiple nucleotides e.g., R = AG, S = GC
[d]Nucleotide numbering is based on genomic sequence of A*01:01:01:01 in the IMGT/HLA database where +1 is the first nucleotide of exon 1 specifying the ATG codon of the signal peptide. CDS numbering is based on exons only where +1 is the first nucleotide of exon 1 specifying the ATG codon of the signal peptide

13. Centrifuge capable of holding plates with a maximum speed of 20,000×*g* (14,000 rpm) (e.g., model 5804 (for plates), Eppendorf, Hauppauge, NY, USA).
14. 3,730×l DNA Analyzer with POP7, 1× running buffer with EDTA, and manual (Applied Biosystems, Foster City, CA).

2.9 Sequence Analysis

1. HLA analysis software: For example, Assign™ (Conexio Genomics, Applecross, Western Australia), with manual.
2. HLA nucleotide sequence database: IMGT/HLA curated coding region sequence database at http://www.ebi.ac.uk/imgt/hla/. This Web site also contains a list of alternative HLA genotypes that share identical sequences in the exons sequenced, a list of alleles identical in the commonly characterized exons, and a list of alleles with known deletions in the coding region.
3. List of primers used to resolve alternative genotypes (*see* **Note 7**).
4. Frequency data on alleles and haplotypes (e.g., http://bioinformatics.nmdp.org lists this information for populations in the USA; http://www.allelefrequencies.net lists this information for worldwide populations).

2.10 HLA Allele Isolation by Cloning

1. Purified HLA amplicon containing two alleles.
2. TOPO TA® Cloning Kit with TOP10 *E. coli* (Invitrogen, Grand Island, NY, USA).
3. Top10 One Shot Kit (Invitrogen).
4. LB agar plates containing 50 μg/ml ampicillin.
5. 40 mg/ml X-gal (5-bromo-4-chloro-3-indolyl-b-D-galactopyranoside) in dimethylformamide.
6. 100 mM isopropyl β-D-1-thiogalactopyranoside (IPTG) in water.
7. Sterile reagent grade water.
8. Sterile toothpicks.
9. Sterile bacterial cell spreader.
10. 1.5 ml sterile disposable tubes.
11. 37 °C shaking and non-shaking bacterial incubators.
12. Centrifuge capable of holding 1.5 ml tubes with a maximum speed of 20,000×*g* (14,000 rpm) (e.g., model 5424 (for tubes), Eppendorf, Hauppauge, NY, USA).
13. Heating block at 42 and 94 °C.
14. Ice.

3 Methods

3.1 DNA Preparation

1. Label the appropriate number of 1.5 ml microcentrifuge tubes and QIAamp spin columns with sample identifier. *See* **Note 8** on laboratory requirements.
2. Add 200 μl whole blood sample to the tube (*see* **Note 9**). If the sample volume is less than 200 μl, add PBS to bring sample to volume. For buccal swab samples, add 400 μl of PBS to each tube containing an applicator.
3. Pipet 20 μl protease into the blood/swab sample in the tube.
4. Add 200 μl Buffer AL to the blood sample (*see* **Note 10**). For buccal swabs, add 400 μl Buffer AL to the swab-containing tube. Immediately mix by vortexing for 15 s.
5. Incubate at 56 °C for 10 min.
6. Briefly centrifuge the microcentrifuge tube to remove condensation drops from the inside of the lid (*see* **Note 11**).
7. Add 200 μl 96–100 % ethanol to the blood sample and mix again by vortexing for 15 s. For a buccal swab sample, add 400 μl 96–100 % ethanol to the swab-containing tube. Again briefly centrifuge the microcentrifuge tube.
8. Carefully apply the lysate of the blood sample to the QIAamp spin column in a collection tube without wetting the rim of the spin column. Centrifuge at 6,000 × *g* (8,000 rpm) for 1 min. Place the QIAamp spin column into a clean 2 ml collection tube and discard the tube containing the filtrate. For buccal swab samples, the lysate must be divided into two parts and each passed through the same spin column consecutively.
9. After placing the spin column into a clean collection tube, carefully add 500 μl Buffer AW1 without wetting the rim of the spin column. Centrifuge at 6,000 × *g* (8,000 rpm) for 1 min.
10. Place the spin column into a clean 2 ml collection tube and discard tube with the filtrate. Carefully add 500 μl Buffer AW2 without wetting the rim. Centrifuge at 20,000 × *g* (14,000 rpm) for 3 min.
11. Place the QIAamp spin column in a clean 1.5 ml microcentrifuge tube and discard the tube with the filtrate. Add 200 μl water for blood samples (or 100 μl water for swab samples) and incubate at room temperature for 1–5 min.
12. Centrifuge at 6,000 × *g* (8,000 rpm) for 1 min. The isolated DNA is in the liquid fraction.
13. Discard the spin column. Make sure the sample tube is labeled correctly. Store at 4 °C for short term, or −20 to −80 °C for long term storage (*see* **Note 12**). *See* **Note 13** for a discussion of potential problems.

3.2 Polymerase Chain Reaction Co-amplification of Both Alleles at an HLA Class I Locus

1. This protocol and reagents were originally based on a protocol for probe-based typing [11, 12]. Both alleles at a class I locus (HLA-A, HLA-B, or HLA-C) are amplified simultaneously to yield amplicons carrying exons 2 and 3. The advantage of this protocol is that prior knowledge of the allele groups present is not required.
2. Prepare master PCR mix: For each sample, 32.75 μl water, 5 μl ABC Buffer, 5 μl DMSO, 0.5 μl 20 μM forward primer, 0.5 μl 20 μM reverse primer, 1 μl 10 mM dNTP. A list of primer pairs is provided in Tables 1, 2, 4, 5, 7, and 8.

Table 4
HLA-B PCR amplification primer pairs

Sense primer	Antisense primer	Amplification specificity[a]	Comments/approximate amplicon size
Locus specific amplification primers			
5B3 + 5B1	3B1 3B1-AC	Locus specific primer pair to obtain complete sequences of exon 2, exon 3	Mix primers in the following ratio: 2 parts 5B3 to 1 part 5B1 (to amplify majority of allele); 2 parts 3B1 to 1 part 3B1-AC (to amplify B*73)
BIn1b-F	BIn3-R BIn3-AC	Locus specific primer pair to obtain complete sequences of exon 2, exon 3	Add 4 parts of BIn3 to 1 part of BIn3-AC; BIN3-AC is used to amplify B*73:01 ; alternative to primer pair above
Group-specific amplification primer pairs			
BIn1-TA	BIn3-R BIn3-AC	Group-specific primer pair amplifying alleles carrying TA at a polymorphic position in intron 1 (e.g., B*07:02:01); most HLA-B alleles will amplify with either this primer or BIn1-CG	Add 4 parts of BIn3 to 1 part of BIn3-AC; BIN3-AC is used to amplify B*73:01
BIn1-CG	BIn3-R BIn3-AC	Group-specific primer pair amplifying alleles carrying AC at a polymorphic position in intron 1 (e.g., B*13:01); most HLA-B alleles will amplify with either this primer or BIn1-TA	Add 4 parts of BIn3 to 1 part of BIn3-AC; BIN3-AC is used to amplify B*73:01
GAT	3B1	Group-specific primer pair amplifying alleles carrying GAT at CDS 204–206	
GAC	3B1	Group-specific primer pair amplifying alleles carrying GAC at CDS 204–206	
AGA	3B1	Group-specific primer pair amplifying alleles carrying AGA at CDS 204–206	
GAA	3B1	Group-specific primer pair amplifying alleles carrying GAA at CDS 204–206	
BW4	3B1	Group-specific primer pair amplifying alleles carrying TCGCGCTCC at CDS 311–319	
BW6	3B1	Group-specific primer pair amplifying alleles carrying ACCTGCGCG at CDS 311–319	

(continued)

Table 4
(continued)

Sense primer	Antisense primer	Amplification specificity[a]	Comments/approximate amplicon size
5B3	RTTGG	Group-specific primer pair amplifying alleles carrying TTGG at CDS 354–357	
5B3	RCT	Group-specific primer pair amplifying alleles carrying CT at CDS 559–560	
BEx261G	3B1	Group-specific primer pair amplifying alleles carrying GAG at CDS 259–261	

[a]CDS, coding sequence where nucleotide 1 is the first nucleotide of exon 1

Table 5
Sequences and annealing sites of HLA-B PCR amplification primers[a]

Name	Sequence 5′–3′[b,c]	Annealing site region/3′ Nucleotide[d]
5B1	GCA CCC ACC CGG ACT CAG AAT CTC CT	Sense, 5′ to exon 1, -12
5B3	GGG TCC CAG TTC TAA AGT CCC CAC G	Sense, 5′ to exon 1, -37
BIn1b-F	GGG AGG AGM RAG GGG ACC GCA G	Sense, intron 1, 129
BIn1-TA	GGC GGG GGC GCA GGA CCT GA	Sense, intron 1, 149
BIn1-CG	CGG GGG CGC AGG ACC CGG	Sense, intron 1, 149
GAT	AC GCC RCG AGT CCG AGG ATT GC	Sense, exon 2, CDS 206
RTGG	C CTC CAG GTA GGC TCT CCA	Antisense , exon 3, CDS 528
RCT	GAG CCA CTC CAC GCA CAG	Antisense , exon 3, CDS 559
GAC	AC GCC GCG AGT CCG AGT AC	Sense, exon 2, CDS 206
AGA	AC GCC GCG AGT CCG AGA GA	Sense, exon 2, CDS 206
GAA	AC GCC RCG AGT CCG AGG AA	Sense, exon 2, CDS 206
BW4	GAG AAC CTG CGG ATC GCG CTC C	Sense, exon 2, CDS 319
BW6	GAG AGC CTG CGG AAC CTG CGC G	Sense, exon 2, CDS 319
3B1	CCA TCC CCG GCG ACC TAT AGG AGA TG	Antisense, intron 3, 1020
BEx261G	CCG GAG TAT TGG GAC CGG GAG	Sense, exon 2, CDS 261
3B1-AC	AGG CCA TCC CGG GCG ATC TAT	Antisense, intron 3, 1028
BIn3-R	GGA GSC CAT CCC CGS CGA CCT AT	Antisense, intron 3, 1029
BIn3-AC	GGA GGC CAT CCC GGG CGA TCT AT	Antisense, intron 3, 1029

[a]Sequences of some reagents have been described by Cereb (1997 187 /id), Cao (1999 5860 /id), Voorter (2001 134 /id)
[b]Sequences are divided into triplets for the ease of reading; they do not necessarily correspond to codons
[c]International Union of Biochemistry (IUB) nucleotide codes for multiple nucleotides e.g., K = GT
[d]Nucleotide numbering of primers annealing in introns or 5′ of exon 1 is based on the numbering of the genomic sequence of B*07:02:01 in the IMGT/HLA database where +1 is the first nucleotide of exon 1 specifying the ATG codon of the signal peptide. CDS, coding sequence where nucleotide 1 is the first nucleotide of exon 1

Table 6
HLA-B sequencing primers

Primer	Sequence 5′–3′[a, b]	Annealing site region/3′ nucleotide[a]	Comments[c, d]
Locus specific sequencing primers			
5BIn1-57	GGG AGG AGC GAG GGG ACC SCA G	Sense, intron 1, 129	Locus-specific sequencing primer for exon 2, forward
BIn1S	GCC GGG AGG AGG GTC	Sense, intron 1, 171	Locus-specific sequencing primer for exon 2, forward, alternative to 5Bin1-57
In2R	GGA TCT CGG ACC CGG AG	Antisense, intron 2, 543	Locus-specific sequencing primer for exon 2, reverse
BEx2R	CAC TCA CCG GCC TCG CTC TGG	Antisense, exon 2, CDS 329	Locus-specific sequencing primer for exon 2, reverse, alternative to In2R
BEx3F	GGK CCA GGG TCT CAC A	Sense, exon 3, CDS 352	Locus-specific sequencing primer for exon 3, forward
B5.5	GGG GGA CGG KGC TGA CCG	Sense, intron 3, 701	Locus-specific sequencing primer for exon 3, forward, alternative to Ex3F
3BIn3-37	GGA GGC CAT CCC CGG CGA CCT AT	Antisense, intron 3, 1028	Locus-specific sequencing primer for exon 3, reverse
BIn3S	AGG CTC CCC ACT G	Antisense, intron 3, 1003	Locus-specific sequencing primer for exon 3, reverse, alternative to 3Bin3-37
Secondary assays—group-specific sequencing primers			
B18In1_188	TCT CAG CCC CTC CTT GCC CCA	Sense, intron 1, 188	Sequencing primer for B*18 alleles
GAC	AC GCC GCG AGT CCG AGT AC	Sense, exon 2, CDS 206	Sequencing primer for alleles carrying GAC at CDS 204–206
GAT	AC GCC RCG AGT CCG AGG ATT GC	Sense, exon 2, CDS 206	Sequencing primer for alleles carrying GAT at CDS 204–206
GAA	AC GCC RCG AGT CCG AGG AA	Sense, exon 2, CDS 206	Sequencing primer for alleles carrying GAA at CDS 204–206
AGA	AC GCC GCG AGT CCG AGA GA	Sense, exon 2, CDS 206	Sequencing primer for alleles carrying GAA at CDS 204–206
BEx261G	CCG GAG TAT TGG GAC CGG GAG	Sense, exon 2, CDS 261	Sequencing primer for alleles carrying GAG at CDS 259–261
RBW4T	TA GTA GCG GAG CGC GAT C	Antisense, exon 2, CDS 309	Sequencing primer for alleles carrying GATCGC at CDS 309–314
RBW6	TA GTA GCC GCG CAG GTT C	Antisense , exon 2, CDS 309	Sequencing primer for alleles carrying GAACCT at CDS 309–314
BW4	GAG AAC CTG CGG ATC GCG CTC C	Sense, exon 2, CDS 319	Sequencing primer for alleles carrying TCGCGCTCC at CDS 311–319
BW6	GAG AGC CTG CGG AAC CTG CGC G	Sense, exon 2, CDS 319	Sequencing primer for alleles carrying ACCTGCGCG at CDS 311–319
RBW4C	TA GTA GCG GAG CGC GGT G	Antisense, exon 2, CDS 309	Sequencing primer for alleles carrying CACCGC at CDS 309–314
BEx2-5	CTC CTC RCC CCC AGG CTC C	Sense, exon 2, CDS 78	Sequencing primer for exon 2 of B*18 alleles because deletion removes annealing site of generic primer

(continued)

Table 6
(continued)

Primer	Sequence 5'–3'[a, b]	Annealing site region/3' nucleotide[a]	Comments[c, d]
RTTGG	CAG CCA TAC ATC GTC TGC CAA	Antisense, exon 3, CDS 354	Sequencing primer for alleles carrying TTGG at CDS 354–357
RGA	GAG CCA CTC CAC GCA CTC	Antisense, exon 3, CDS 559	Sequencing primer for alleles carrying A at CDS 559–560
RCT	GAG CCA CTC CAC GCA CAG	Antisense , exon 3, CDS 559	Sequencing primer for alleles carrying CT at CDS 559–560
RAC	GAG CCA CTC CAC GCA CGT	Antisense, exon 3, CDS 559	Sequencing primer for alleles carrying AC at CDS 559–560
RGAC	C CTC CAG GTA GGC TCT GTC	Antisense, exon 3, CDS 528	Sequencing primer for alleles carrying GAC at CDS 538–540
RCAGT	AGC GCG CTC CAG CTT GTC	Antisense, exon 3, CDS 603	Sequencing primer for alleles carrying CAAGCTGGAGCGCGCT at CDS 603–618
RGCCG	CGC GCG CTG CAG CGT CTC	Antisense, exon 3, CDS 603	Sequencing primer for alleles carrying GACGCTGCAGCGCGCG at CDS 603–618
CI322M	CAG GGT CTC ACA CTT GG	Sense, exon 3, CDS 357	Sequencing primer for alleles carrying TTGG at CDS 354–357
CI324M	GG CCA GGG TCT CAC ATC A	Sense, exon 3, CDS 355	Sequencing primer for alleles carrying TCA at CDS 353–355
RCGG	C CTC CAG GTA GGC TCT CCG	Antisense, exon 3, CDS 528	Sequencing primer for alleles carrying CGG at CDS 538–540
RCTG	C CTC CAG GTA GGC TCT CAG	Antisense, exon 3, CDS 528	Sequencing primer for alleles carrying CTG at CDS 538–540
RTGG	C CTC CAG GTA GGC TCT CCA	Antisense, exon 3, CDS 528	Sequencing primer for alleles carrying TGG at CDS 538–540

[a]Sequences are divided into triplets for the ease of reading; they do not necessarily correspond to codons
[b]International Union of Biochemistry (IUB) nucleotide codes for multiple nucleotides e.g., R = AG, S = GC
[c]Nucleotide numbering of primers annealing in introns or 5′ of exon 1 is based on the numbering of the genomic sequence of B*07:02:01 in the IMGT/HLA database where +1 is the first nucleotide of exon 1 specifying the ATG codon of the signal peptide
[d]All alleles known at time chapter was written, IMGT/HLA database 3.5.0. Because limited number of intron sequences, it is possible that some alleles will not amplify. Homozygotes need to be tested with second amplification

3. Add 0.25 μl AmpliTaq polymerase to 44.75 μl PCR master mix for each sample (*see* **Note 14**).
4. Add 5 μl of DNA (*see* **Note 15**).
5. Cover the plate tightly with a tray seal, place in thermal cycler, close and tighten lid.
6. PCR cycle parameters for HLA-A and HLA-B loci: 94 °C for 2 min, 8 cycles of 94 °C for 22 s, 65 °C for 50 s, 72 °C for 30 s; 30 cycles of 94 °C for 22 s, 62 °C for 50 s, 72 °C for 30 s; 72 °C for 5 min. PCR cycle parameters for the HLA-C locus: 94 °C

Table 7
HLA-C PCR amplification primer pairs

Sense primer	Antisense primer	Amplification specificity
Locus specific amplification primers		
5CIn1-61	3BCIn3-12	Locus specific primer pair to obtain amplicon carrying exon 2, exon 3
Group-specific amplification primers to resolve some alternative genotypes		
C07split	3BCIn3-12	Group-specific primer pair amplifying ambiguities involving, for example, C*07:01:01G+C*07:02:01G from C*07:19+C*07:27:01
5CIn1-61	RCT	Group-specific primer pair amplifying ambiguities involving alleles carrying CT at CDS[a] 559–560
CIn4-F3	C'3UTR-2912G	Amplification to isolate exon 7 to distinguish C*04:09N from other expressed alleles in C*04:01:01G

[a]CDS, coding sequence where nucleotide 1 is the first nucleotide of exon 1

Table 8
Sequences and annealing sites of HLA-C PCR amplification primers[a, b]

Name	Sequence 5'–3'[b, c]	Annealing site region/3' nucleotide[d]
5CIn1-61	AGC GAG GKG CCC GCC CGG CGA[c]	Sense, intron 1, 135
3BCIn3-12	GGA GAT GGG GAA GGC TCC CCA CT	Antisense, intron 3, 1007
C07split	GGG ACC GGG AGA CAC AGA AC	Sense, exon 2, CDS 270
RCT	GAG CCA CTC CAC GCA CAG	Antisense, exon 3, CDS 559
CIn4-F3	CAG CYR GGT CAG GGC TGA G	Sense, intron 4, 1938
C'3UTR-2912G	GAA ATC CTG CAT CTC AGT CC	Antisense, intron 4, 1938

[a]Sequences of some of the reagents were based on reagents described by Cereb (1995 186 /id)
[b]Sequences are divided into triplets for the ease of reading; these do not necessarily correspond to codons
[c]International Union of Biochemistry (IUB) nucleotide codes for multiple nucleotides e.g., R = AG, S = GC
[d]Nucleotide numbering of primers annealing in introns or 5′ of exon 1 is based on the numbering of the genomic sequence of C*01:02:01 in the IMGT/HLA database where +1 is the first nucleotide of exon 1 specifying the ATG codon of the signal peptide. CDS numbering is based on exons only where +1 is the first nucleotide of exon 1 specifying the ATG codon of the signal peptide

for 2 min, 39 cycles of 94 °C for 22 s, 59 °C for 50 s, 72 °C for 30 s; 72 °C for 10 min. A hold at 4 °C completes each cycle (*see* **Notes 8** and **16**).

7. Check for specific amplification by agarose electrophoresis (Subheading 3.6). The amplicons are approximately 900–1,100 bp in length.
8. Treat the PCR amplicons with AMPure to eliminate unincorporated primers and nucleotides (Subheading 3.7) prior to sequencing (Subheading 3.8).

Table 9
HLA-C sequencing primers

Primer	Sequence 5′–3′[a,b]	Annealing site region/3′ nucleotide[c,d]	Comments
Locus specific sequencing primers			
CEx2F	GGG TCG GGC GGG TCT CAG CC	Sense, intron 2, 188	Locus-specific sequencing primer for exon 2, forward
CEx2R	GGA GGG GTC GTG ACC TGC GC	Antisense, intron 2, 494	Locus-specific sequencing primer for exon 2, reverse
CEx3F	TGA CCR CGG GGG CG GGG CC	Sense, intron 2, 718	Locus-specific sequencing primer for exon 3, forward
3BCIn3-12	GGA GAT GGG GAA GGC TCC CCA CT	Antisense, intron 3, 1007	Locus-specific sequencing primer for exon 3, reverse
Secondary assay—group-specific sequencing primers used to resolve alternative genotypes, select primer based on ambiguous genotypes obtained			
CEx103G	GAG GTA TTT CTA CAC CG	Sense, exon 2, CDS 103	Sequencing primer for alleles carrying CG at CDS 102–103
GAC	AC GCC GCG AGT CCG AGT AC	Sense, exon 2, CDS 206	Sequencing primer for alleles carrying GAC at CDS 204–206
GAT	AC GCC RCG AGT CCG AGG ATT GC	Sense, exon 2, CDS 206	Sequencing primer for alleles carrying GAT at CDS 204–206
GAA	AC GCC RCG AGT CCG AGG AA	Sense, exon 2, CDS 206	Sequencing primer for alleles carrying GAA at CDS 204–206
AGA	AC GCC GCG AGT CCG AGA GA	Sense, exon 2, CDS 206	Sequencing primer for alleles carrying AGA at CDS 204–206
RBW4C	TA GTA GCG GAG CGC GGT G	Antisense, exon 2, CDS 309	Sequencing primer for alleles carrying CACCGC at CDS 309–314
KC39RM	GTA GTA GCC GCG CAG T	Antisense, exon 2, CDS 302	Sequencing primer for alleles carrying AC at CDS 312–312
CI324M	GG CCA GGG TCT CAC ATC A	Sense, exon 3, CDS 355	Sequencing primer for alleles carrying TCA at CDS 353–355
CI322M	CAG GGT CTC ACA CTT GG	Sense, exon 3, CDS 357	Sequencing primer for alleles carrying TTGG at CDS 354–357
RCGG	C CTC CAG GTA GGC TCT CCG	Antisense, exon 3, CDS 528	Sequencing primer for alleles carrying CGG at CDS 538–540
RCTG	C CTC CAG GTA GGC TCT CAG	Antisense, exon 3, CDS 528	Sequencing primer for alleles carrying CTG at CDS 538–540
RTGG	C CTC CAG GTA GGC TCT CCA	Antisense, exon 3, CDS 528	Sequencing primer for alleles carrying TGG at CDS 538–540
RGAC	C CTC CAG GTA GGC TCT GTC	Antisense, exon 3, CDS 528	Sequencing primer for alleles carrying GAC at CDS 538–540
CEx538T-R	CTC CAG GTA GGC TCT CA	Antisense, exon 3, CDS 538	Sequencing primer for alleles carrying TGA at CDS 539–541
RGA	GAG CCA CTC CAC GCA CTC	Antisense, exon 3, CDS 559	Sequencing primer for alleles carrying A at CDS 559–560
RCT	GAG CCA CTC CAC GCA CAG	Antisense , exon 3, CDS 559	Sequencing primer for alleles carrying CT at CDS 559–560
RAC	GAG CCA CTC CAC GCA CGT	Antisense, exon 3, CDS 559	Sequencing primer for alleles carrying AC at CDS 559–560

(continued)

Table 9
(continued)

Primer	Sequence 5′–3′[a,b]	Annealing site region/3′ nucleotide[c,d]	Comments
CEx601A-R	GCG CGC TGC AGC GTC TT	Antisense, exon 3, CDS 601	Sequencing primer for alleles carrying AAG at CDS 601–603
RCAGT	AGC GCG CTC CAG CTT GTC	Antisense, exon 3, CDS 603	Sequencing primer for alleles carrying CAAGCTGGAGCGCGCT at CDS 603–618
RGCCG	CGC GCG CTG CAG CGT CTC	Antisense, exon 3, CDS 603	Sequencing primer for alleles carrying GACGCTGCAGCGCGCG at CDS 603–618

[a]Sequences are divided into triplets for the ease of reading; they do not necessarily correspond to codons
[b]International Union of Biochemistry (IUB) nucleotide codes for multiple nucleotides e.g., R = AG, S = GC
[c]Nucleotide numbering of primers annealing in introns or 5′ of exon 1 is based on the numbering of the genomic sequence of C*01:02:01 in the IMGT/HLA database where +1 is the first nucleotide of exon 1 specifying the ATG codon of the signal peptide
[d]All alleles known at time chapter was written, IMGT/HLA database 3.5.0. Because of the limited number of intron sequences, it is possible that some alleles will not amplify. Homozygotes need to be tested with a second amplification

3.3 Allele Group-Specific Amplification of HLA Class I Loci, HLA-A and HLA-B

1. This protocol and reagents were originally described by Cereb et al. [12, 13] and a personal communication from Dr. S Y Yang (HLA-A). HLA-A and HLA-B alleles are amplified in 2–3 broad groups based on polymorphisms lying in the intron preceding exon 2. The advantages of this protocol is that the alleles may be separated and the intron primers will allow complete coding sequence analysis of exons 2 and 3 (*see* **Note 17**).
2. Prepare master mix: For each sample, 8.65 μl water, 2.5 μl 10× buffer, 0.6 μl 50 mM $MgCl_2$, 2 μl DMSO, 1 μl 10 pmol/μl sense primer, 1 μl 10 pmol/μl antisense primer, 4 μl 10 mM dNTP, 0.25 μl 5 U/ml Taq Platinum (*see* **Note 14**). For each locus, one to several amplifications are set up unless a lower resolution typing has been performed that will determine which primer pairs should be selected (*see* **Note 17**).
3. Add 5.0 μl genomic DNA (*see* **Note 15**).
4. Cover plate tightly with tray seal and place in thermal cycler.
5. PCR conditions and amplification (*see* **Note 16**):

HLA-A	HLA-B
96 °C for 5 min	96 °C for 5 min
5 cycles of 96 °C for 20 s, 58 °C for 50 s, 72 °C for 30 s	5 cycles of 96 °C for 20 s, 63 °C for 30 s, 72 °C for 60 s
30 cycles of 96 °C for 22 s, 55 °C for 50 s, 72 °C for 30 s	30 cycles of 96 °C for 22 s, 58 °C for 30 s, 72 °C for 60 s
72 °C for 10 min followed by 4 °C hold until required	72 °C for 10 min followed by 4 °C hold until required

6. Check amplification by agarose electrophoresis (*see* **Note 18**) (Subheading 3.6). The amplicons are approximately 800 bp in length.
7. Treat the PCR amplicons with AMPure to eliminate unincorporated primers and nucleotides (Subheading 3.7) prior to sequencing (Subheading 3.8).

3.4 Allele Group-Specific Polymerase Chain Reaction Amplification of HLA-DRB Loci with Intron Primers

1. This protocol, described by Kotsch et al. [9], is based on group-specific amplification of distinct DRB lineages (e.g., DRB1*01; DRB1*03, DRB1*08, DRB3, DRB4, DRB5). The PCR primers anneal in introns bracketing exon 2. The amplicons range in size from 384 base pairs to 1,018 base pairs (*see* **Note 18**). For DRB, multiple amplification reactions are set up unless a lower resolution typing has been performed that will determine which primer pairs should be selected (*see* **Note 17**).
2. Prepare reaction solution: For each primer pair, 4 μl 5× PCR buffer, 0.4 μl DMSO, 4 μl 1.25 mM dNTP, 1 μl sense primer, 1 μl antisense primer, 9.4 μl genomic DNA, 0.2 μl Taq polymerase to total volume of 20 μl (*see* **Notes 14** and **15**).
3. PCR cycle parameters: 96 °C for 5 min, 10 cycles of 96 °C for 30 s, 63 °C for 50 s; 20 cycles of 96 °C for 30 s, 60 °C for 50 s, 72 °C for 30 s; 72 °C for 5 min (*see* **Note 16**). The reaction can be stored at 4 °C.
4. Check amplification by agarose gel electrophoresis (Subheading 3.6).
5. Treat the PCR amplicons with AMPure to eliminate unincorporated primers and nucleotides (Subheading 3.7) prior to sequencing (Subheading 3.8).

3.5 Polymerase Chain Reaction Amplification of DQB1

1. This protocol and reagents were originally described by Dunn et al. [10]. For DQB1, multiple amplification reactions are set up unless a lower resolution typing has been performed that will determine which primer pairs should be selected (*see* **Note 17**).
2. Prepare PCR master mixes: For each reaction: 2.5 μl 10× PCR Gold Buffer, 2.5 μl betaine, 0.50 μl 10 mM dNTP, 1.5 μl 1.5 mM $MgCl_2$, 0.25 μl sense primer, 0.25 μl antisense primer, 3 μl genomic DNA, 0.30 μl Gold Taq polymerase, water to final volume of 25.0 μl (*see* **Notes 14** and **15**).
3. Seal the plate and place in thermal cycler.
4. Amplification conditions are as follows: 96 °C 12 min; 20 cycles of 96 °C 20 s, 65 °C 45 s, 72 °C 45 s; 15 cycles of 96 °C 20 s, 60 °C 45 s, 72 °C 45 s; 10 cycles of 96 °C 20 s, 55 °C 45 s, 72 °C 45 s; 72 °C 5 min (*see* **Note 16**). The reaction can be stored at 4 °C.

5. Check amplification by agarose gel electrophoresis as described in Subheading 3.6. The amplicons should be approximately 600 bp in size (*see* **Note 18**).
6. Treat the PCR amplicons with AMPure to eliminate unincorporated primers and nucleotides (Subheading 3.7) prior to sequencing (Subheading 3.8).

3.6 Gel Electrophoresis

1. Prepare a 1 or 2 % agarose gel in 1× TBE (*see* **Note 19**). Add 4 μl of GelRed™ to 80 ml of the gel solution prior to pouring the gel into the apparatus.
2. After the amplification cycles are complete, confirm amplification by electrophoresis. Mix 3–5 μl of each amplification reaction with 1 μl of 5× sucrose cresol solution and load the entire sample into one well of the polymerized agarose gel. Electrophorese the DNA ladder as a molecular weight marker following manufacturer's instructions for dilution. The ladder should be mixed with 5× sucrose cresol solution as described above. Electrophorese at 100 V for 10 min until the cresol red dye has reached the bottom of the gel (*see* **Note 20**).
3. Visualize the bands by placing the gel on a UV transilluminator (*see* **Note 20**). Photograph the gel. Using the molecular weight markers, determine the approximate molecular weight of the amplicons by comparison. The expected sizes of the amplicons for each locus can be determined using the information in Tables 2, 5, and 8 and in publications for DRB and DQB1 [9, 10]. The presence of additional bands indicates a potential problem (*see* **Note 20**).

3.7 Purification of PCR Amplicons Using AMPure

1. Add the AMPure solution directly to each PCR reaction in the PCR plate. The volume of AMPure to add is 1.8 times the reaction volume (*see* **Note 21**).
2. Mix thoroughly by pipeting and place the PCR plate onto a magnetic plate to separate the AMPure beads from the solution. Incubate at room temperature for approximately 5–10 min.
3. With the PCR plate on the magnet, aspirate the cleared solution with a pipet and discard.
4. Keeping the PCR plate on the magnet, dispense 200 μl of 70 % ethanol to each well. Allow to sit at least 30 s at room temperature. Aspirate the wash solution with a pipet, discard, and repeat. Be sure to remove as much ethanol as possible to shorten the drying time. Dry at room temperature for 10 min.
5. To elute the purified DNA, add 30–50 μl (*see* **Note 22**) of reagent grade water to each well and mix well by pipeting up and down. Place the plate back on the magnet.
6. Remove the eluate containing the amplified DNA to a clean 96-well plate to begin the DNA sequencing reactions (Subheading 3.8).

3.8 DNA Sequencing

1. Thaw the Terminator Ready Reaction Mix and leave it on ice (*see* **Note 23**).
2. In a plate, assemble the sequencing reactions (one for each primer) on ice adding reagents in the following order: 2 μl purified PCR product, 6 μl water, 1 μl primer, 1 μl Terminator Ready Reaction Mix, 5 μl Better Buffer to a final reaction volume of 15 μl (*see* **Note 24**).
3. Place tray seal over entire tray and quick spin the samples in the centrifuge to ensure all liquid is at the bottom of the container. Place samples in thermocycler and start the program: denature DNA at 96 °C for 2 min, 25 cycles 96 °C 10 s, 50 °C 5 s, 60 °C 4 min, finishing with a 4 °C hold (*see* **Note 16**).
4. Following amplification, use the Agencourt CleanSEQ kit to remove excess dye terminators from the sequence reaction by adding 10 μl of CleanSEQ magnetic beads solution to each well of the sequencing plate.
5. For each sequencing reaction, add 75 μl 73 % ethanol to each well and mix thoroughly.
6. Place the sequencing plate onto the magnet to separate the beads from the solution. Incubate approximately 3 min at room temperature.
7. With the sequencing plate on the magnet, aspirate the cleared solution with a pipet and discard.
8. Keeping the plate on the magnet, dispense 100 μl 73 % ethanol to each well and allow it to sit for at least 30 s at room temperature. Aspirate the solution and discard.
9. Add 30–40 μl of water to each well (*see* **Note 25**). Keeping the plate on the magnet, transfer 5 μl into 95 μl of reagent grade water pre-loaded into a 96-well plate for loading onto the sequencer. The reactions are now ready to electrophorese on the DNA analyzer.
10. Follow the instructions for operation of the DNA analyzer. The samples are electrophoresed using ABI RunModule "Rapidseq 36_POP7" with the default values. Longer electrophoresis times may be required for some sequences.
11. Sample files are analyzed as described in Subheading 3.9.

3.9 Sequence Analysis

1. Consult the software user manual on how to use the HLA sequence assignment software, Assign™ or another commercially available software product (*see* **Note 26**).
2. Import the sequencing files from the DNA sequencer software into Assign™ following instructions in the software's user's guide. For each locus sequenced, the Assign™ report will list (1) the allele combination(s) potentially carried by the sample (i.e., the genotype) and (2) the genotypes that differ by one to

a few nucleotides from the assignment(s). Sequencing may result in a single allele if a group-specific PCR primer or cloning has been used to isolate one of the two alleles in the sample (*see* **Note 27**).

3. Manually review the chromatographs associated with each locus sequenced and compare to a consensus sequence which shows all the positions of potential polymorphism. Review both strands of the sequence to ensure they are complementary. Carefully check the positions that contain double peaks where the two alleles differ in sequence to ensure correct base assignments. If clear sequences are not obtained for most positions of both strands for a specific region, repeat the sequencing reaction to obtain the missing data.
4. Review the alternative allele assignments which are mismatched to the sequence at single nucleotide positions. Look at each of these positions in the chromatograms to ensure that the software has assigned the correct nucleotide(s). Be alert for known sequence artifacts which may confuse the interpretation of the sequence (*see* **Note 28**).
5. Compare the assigned genotype(s) with any prior HLA typing data for that sample. Previous data will likely be at a lower level of resolution (*see* **Note 17**). If the sequence assignment is included within the low resolution assignment, the result is acceptable. If the alleles differ, the result is discrepant. If discrepant, review both typing results and consider retesting the sample.
6. If the assignment is homozygous, retest the sample unless the low resolution data are consistent with the sequencing assignment. Failure of one allele to amplify is more likely if the DNA was poorly amplified. Use of a different amplification primer pair should address any issues with loss of a primer annealing site. If the sample has been amplified with a group-specific primer, a single allele may be expected.
7. It is likely that more than one genotype will be perfectly matched to the sequence (*see* **Note 27**). In these cases, evaluate the genotypes to determine if further testing is required based on the following criteria:
   (a) Alternative alleles with names greater than six digits long (e.g., B*15:01:01:01 or B*15:01:01:02N): These alleles differ in sequence only outside of the coding region. If one of the alternatives is a non-expressed (or null, N) allele and this is in a potential transplant donor or patient, additional testing may be required.
   (b) Alternative alleles that are identical in sequence in exons 2 and 3 (class I) or in exon 2 (class II) as listed on the IMGT/HLA Web site (top portion of the table of ambiguous

combinations, e.g., A*01:01:01 or A*01:04N). These alleles are not usually distinguished from one another in matching. However, if one of the alternatives is a non-expressed allele and this is a potential transplant donor or patient, additional testing may be required.

(c) Alternative genotypes that are identical in exons 2 and 3 (class I) or exon 2 (class II) when sequenced as a mixture (e.g., A*31:02,*32:03 or A*31:07,*74:07). These combinations are listed in the bottom portion of the table of ambiguous assignments on the IMGT/HLA Web page. These combinations usually can be resolved by either amplification of a single allele by PCR followed by sequencing or by sequencing with a group-specific sequencing primer as described below.

8. If the resolution is not sufficient, subsequent typing steps (allele group-specific PCR or use of an allele-specific sequencing primer) will isolate one of the two alleles for additional sequence analysis. This secondary testing will eliminate some of the possible genotypes (*see* **Note 7**).
9. Review the frequencies of alleles and haplotypes in the assignment. If the allele assigned is rare or if the haplotype is unusual (e.g., an unusual HLA-B/-C or HLA-DRB1/-DQB1 combination), carefully review the results.
10. The sequence interpretation library should be updated with newer versions of the IMGT/HLA database as required (*see* **Note 29**).

3.10 HLA Allele Isolation by Cloning

1. Cloning is required only if the alleles in a heterozygote must be separated for sequencing and there are no appropriate PCR or sequencing primers available to separate the alleles.
2. Amplify the alleles at a locus and purify the PCR products using AMPure as described in Subheading 3.7.
3. Using the TOPO TA cloning kit, clone the PCR product into the pCR 2.1-TOPO vector following the manufacturer's instructions (*see* **Note 30**).
4. Add 2 μl of the TOPO cloning reaction to a vial of One Shot Chemical *E. coli* and mix gently. Incubate on ice for 5–30 min.
5. Heat-shock the cells for exactly 30 s at 42 °C. Do not shake during this incubation.
6. Add 250 μl of SOC at room temperature to the tube.
7. Incubate in a 37 °C shaker (250 rpm) for 1 h.
8. Apply 40 μl Xgal (40 mg/ml) and 40 μl 100 mM IPTG to the surface of an LB agar plate containing ampicillin and let dry.
9. To optimize distinct colonies, plate 50 and 100 μl of each transformation onto two separate agar plates. Incubate at 37 °C overnight but not longer than 18 h.

10. Pick several isolated white colonies from the agar plate using a sterile toothpick (*see* **Note 31**). Transfer each colony of bacteria into a 0.5 ml tube containing 50 μl sterile water and vortex to mix (*see* **Note 32**).
11. Place the tubes in a heating block at 94 °C for 5 min to lyse the bacteria and to inactivate nucleases. Centrifuge at 12,000 × *g* for 1 min to remove cell debris.
12. Use 2–5 μl of the supernatant in a 50 μl PCR reaction with the same primers and protocol as used in the original amplification of genomic DNA in **step 1** of this protocol. The amplification method used will depend on the primers and locus (e.g., Subheading 3.3 for a group-specific primer pair amplifying HLA-A).
13. Verify amplification on a 1 % agarose gel as described in Subheading 3.6.
14. Purify the PCR fragments using AMPure as described in Subheading 3.7 and proceed with DNA sequencing in Subheading 3.8.

4 Notes

1. Blood (8.5 ml) is collected by venipuncture into a yellow top ACD-A tube. ACD is the preferred anticoagulant. Other anticoagulants (e.g., heparin) may inhibit DNA amplification during the polymerase chain reaction. Blood can be aliquoted into 2 ml tubes and stored at −20 °C until use. Blood should be treated as a biohazard and handled with caution.
2. A buccal swab is collected by inserting a cotton-tipped applicator in the mouth and, with a firm scraping motion, twirling the applicator on the inside of one of the cheeks approximately 10–12 times, moving it around all areas on that side of the mouth. This process can be repeated for all the four quadrants of the mouth using separate applicators. After swabbing, gently wave each applicator in the air for 1 min to dry. Place the applicator in a 1.5 ml microfuge tube, snap off the stick and close the tube. Store the tube at 4 °C until the extraction is performed. Applicators containing epithelial samples can also be stored at room temperature in a sealed envelope. Cotton-tipped applicators should be quality controlled before use. Two applicators from a new batch should be tested for the ability to extract DNA from two different individuals. Results should be generated using regular sample procedures. New lots will pass quality control if 100 % of the tested applicators generate DNA that can be used for regular typing procedures. HLA assignments from the tested applicators should be consistent with previous HLA assignments of the individuals.

3. Primers can be commercially synthesized by a number of vendors. Desalted primers are diluted in reagent grade water. Aliquot diluted primers and store at −20 °C. The aliquot in current use can be stored at 4 °C. Repeated freezing and thawing of diluted oligonucleotide primers should be avoided. The rate of degradation of the oligonucleotide stocks when stored at −20 °C or at 4 °C can vary. Each time an oligonucleotide is used in an assay, its specificity should be monitored. In locus-specific amplifications, the appearance of a single amplicon at the expected size upon gel electrophoresis can be used to monitor specificity (*see* **Note 5**). For group-specific amplifications, the amplification of reference DNA monitors specificity. For sequencing primers, the quality of the sequence electropherogram can be used as a monitor of the quality of primer. Oligonucleotides can be designed in-house for use in PCR amplification or DNA sequencing when required to resolve alternative genotypes and no reagent currently exists. Comparison of allele sequences will identify the regions to target for primer annealing; software programs, sometimes provided for free by the vendor providing synthesis, will help define annealing conditions and identify secondary structure that might prevent amplification. Newly synthesized oligonucleotides should be tested for their ability to specifically anneal to and amplify alleles carrying the complementary sequence before use in clinical testing.
4. Tables 1 and 4 list alternative PCR primer pairs that can be used for locus specific amplification. These primers can be used, for example, to evaluate the possibility that one allele failed to amplify (i.e., when a homozygous assignment was obtained using the first set of primers). Tables 1, 4, and 7 also include PCR primer pairs that might be used in a secondary assay when the desired resolution is not obtained from the locus-specific amplification. For example, Table 1 lists a primer pair, AIn1-226 and AIn3-249, that can be used to specifically amplify an HLA-A*02 allele for sequencing if further resolution is required. Tables 3, 6, and 9 also include alternate sequencing primers that can be used with a locus-specific amplicon as well as sequencing primers that can be used in a secondary assay when the desired resolution is not obtained from the locus-specific sequencing primers. For example, sequencing primer KA1S can be used to obtain a sequence that will discriminate the genotype A* 02:11:01, A*33:24 from the genotype A*02:01:01:01G, A*33:03:01 by linking the polymorphic nucleotide sequence TTCACA found at coding sequence (CDS) 97–102 to a polymorphism found at CDS 290–292.

5. A control DNA that has been previously amplified successfully should be included in the assay to control for correct set-up of the PCR reaction and the quality of test DNA. A negative control with water instead of DNA will provide a control for contamination with previously amplified DNA. Locus-specific (or "generic") primers usually amplify all alleles at a locus. Group-specific primers amplify a subset of alleles at a locus. In order to ensure that amplification is specific, reference DNA containing alleles that should amplify with the primer pair and reference DNA containing alleles that should not amplify with the primer pair should be included as controls in the amplification reaction. Reference DNA carrying known alleles can be obtained from the National Marrow Donor Program Research Repository (Minneapolis, MN, USA; http://www.cibmtr.org/samples/) or the Research Cell Bank (Fred Hutchinson Cancer Research Center, Seattle, WA, USA; http://www.ihwg.org) or by subscribing to an external proficiency testing program (e.g., American Society for Histocompatibility and Immunogenetics, http://www.ashi-hla.org/lab-center/pt-program/; UCLA Immunogenetics Center International Cell/DNA Exchange, Los Angeles, CA, USA; http://www.hla.ucla.edu/cellDna.htm).
6. The DNA ladder should range in size between 100 base pairs (bp) and 2,000 bp. It is helpful to have markers every 100 bp. A high DNA mass ladder (e.g., Invitrogen, Grand Island, NY, USA) is also helpful when judging the approximate quantity of amplicon present.
7. If the desired resolution is not reached, one or more allele-specific sequencing primers or a group-specific amplification followed by sequencing will be required (*see* also **Note 4**). Tables 1–9 include additional sequencing primers and additional group-specific amplification primers that can be employed as a secondary step to reach the desired resolution. Figure 3 illustrates how an additional sequencing primer can be used to distinguish two genotypes that have identical DNA sequences in exons 2 and 3.
8. DNA amplicons generated in previous PCR reactions are a potential source of sample contamination. By separating the source of the amplicons (i.e., post-PCR activities as defined by thermal cycling and subsequent steps) from the pre-PCR activities (as defined by all steps up to and including assembly of the PCR reaction just prior to placing in the thermal cycler), the potential for contamination is greatly reduced. Ideally, the pre-PCR and post-PCR procedures should be performed in two different rooms, but, if not available, different areas of the laboratory should be set aside. If all activities are to be performed in a single room, pre-PCR activities should occur

```
cDNA                 10         20         30         40         50         60         70         80         90        100
B*07:02:01   ATGCTGGTCA TGGCGCCCCG AACCGTCCTC CTGCTGCTCT CGGCGGCCCT GGCCCTGACC GAGACCTGGG CCG|GCTCCCA CTCCATGAGG TATTTCTACA
B*07:05:01   ---------- ---------- ---------- ---------- ---------- ---------- ---------- ---|------- ---------- ----------
B*08:01:01   ---------- ---------- ---------- ---------- ---------- ---------- ---------- ---|------- ---------- ------G---
B*08:07      ********** ********** ********** ********** ********** ********** ********** ***|------- ---------- ------G---

cDNA                110        120        130        140        150        160        170        180        190        200
B*07:02:01   CCTCCGTGTC CCGGCCCGGC CGCGGGGAGC CCCGCTTCAT CTCAGTGGGC TACGTGGACG ACACCCAGTT CGTGAGGTTC GACAGCGACG CCGCGAGTCC
B*07:05:01   ---------- ---------- ---------- ---------- ---------- ---------- ---------- ---------- ---------- ----------
B*08:01:01   --G--A---- ---------- ---------- ---------- ---------- ---------- ----G----- ---------- ---------- ----------
B*08:07      --G--A---- ---------- ---------- ---------- ---------- ---------- ----G----- ---------- ---------- ----------

cDNA                210        220        230        240        250        260        270        280        290        300
B*07:02:01   GAGAGAGGAG CCGCGGGCGC CGTGGATAGA GCAGGAGGGG CCGGAGTATT GGGACCGGAA CACACAGATC TACAAGGCCC AGGCACAGAC TGACCGAGAG
B*07:05:01   ---------- ---------- ---------- ---------- ---------- ---------- ---------- ---------- ---------- ----------
B*08:01:01   ---------- ---------- ---------- ---------- ---------- ---------- ---------- -T----A--A -CA------- ----------
B*08:07      ---------- ---------- ---------- ---------- ---------- ---------- ---------- -T----A--A -CA------- ----------

cDNA                310        320        330        340        350        360        370        380        390        400
B*07:02:01   AGCCTGCGGA ACCTGCGCGG CTACTACAAC CAGAGCGAGG CCG|GGTCTCA CACCCTCCAG AGCATGTACG GCTGCGACGT GGGGCCGGAC GGGCGCCTCC
B*07:05:01   ---------- ---------- ---------- ---------- ---|------- ---------- ---------- ---------- ---------- ----------
B*08:01:01   ---------- ---------- ---------- ---------- ---|------- ---------- ---------- ---------- ---------- ----------
B*08:07      ---------- ---------- ---------- ---------- ---|------- ---------- ---------- ---------- ---------- ----------

cDNA                410        420        430        440        450        460        470        480        490        500
B*07:02:01   TCCGCGGGCA TGACCAGTAC GCCTACGACG GCAAGGATTA CATCGCCCTG AACGAGGACC TGCGCTCCTG GACCGCCGCG GACACGGCGG CTCAGATCAC
B*07:05:01   ---------- -A-------- ---------- ---------- ---------- ---------- ---------- ---------- ---------- ----------
B*08:01:01   ---------- -A-------- ---------- ---------- ---------- ---------- ---------- ------G--- -----C---- ----------
B*08:07      ---------- ---------- ---------- ---------- ---------- ---------- ---------- ------G--- -----C---- ----------

cDNA                510        520        530        540        550        560        570        580        590        600
B*07:02:01   CCAGCGCAAG TGGGAGGCGG CCCGTGAGGC GGAGCAGCGG AGAGCCTACC TGGAGGGCGA GTGCGTGGAG TGGCTCCGCA GATACCTGGA GAACGGGAAG
B*07:05:01   ---------- ---------- ---------- ---------- ---------- ---------- ---------- ---------- ---------- ----------
B*08:01:01   ---------- ---------- ------T--- -------GAC ---------- --------AC ---------- ---------- ---------- ----------
B*08:07      ---------- ---------- ------T--- -------GAC ---------- --------AC ---------- ---------- ---------- ----------

cDNA                610        620        630        640        650        660        670        680        690        700
B*07:02:01   GACAAGCTGG AGCGCGCTG|A CCCCCCAAAG ACACACGTGA CCCACCACCC CATCTCTGAC CATGAGGCCA CCCTGAGGTG CTGGGCCCTG GGTTTCTACC
B*07:05:01   ---------- ---------|- ---------- ---------- ---------- ---------- ---------- ---------- ---------- ----------
B*08:01:01   ----C----- -------G-|- ---------- ---------- ---------- ---------- ---------- ---------- ---------- --C-------
B*08:07      ----C----- -------G-|* ********** ********** ********** ********** ********** ********** ********** **********
```

Fig. 3 An example of two genotypes (B*07:02:01, *08:01:01 and B*07:05:01, *08:07) that cannot be distinguished when both alleles are sequenced concurrently. The sequences of the four alleles are coding sequences (i.e., exons only). *Vertical lines* mark the exon boundaries. A *double underline* marks the annealing site of a group-specific sequencing primer (called RAC) added to sequence one strand of the HLA-B locus amplicon. The resultant sequence is *underlined*. Note that the two B*08 alleles can be distinguished from one another at nucleotide 412 where B*08:01:01 encodes an A and B*08:07 encodes a G. Based on this information, the laboratory can distinguish between the two genotypes

inside a laminar flow hood, preferably equipped with a UV light. The walls of the hood should be wiped with a freshly made 10 % bleach solution (1 part regular bleach: 9 parts tap water) before processing samples or preparing PCR samples. Dedicated equipment (e.g., pipettors, test tube racks) and lab coats should be set aside for pre-PCR procedures.

9. Typically, 200 μl of whole blood from a healthy individual will yield 3–12 μg of DNA. The amount of DNA isolated from a buccal swab with a cotton-tipped applicator (*see* **Note 2**) will depend on the number of epithelial cells collected during the swabbing and will usually yield 1–4 μg of DNA. Because this amount is usually less than that obtained from blood, amplification and sequencing protocols may need to be adjusted.
10. Never add Buffer AL directly to the protease. To obtain complete lysis, the sample and the Buffer AL must be mixed immediately and thoroughly.

11. The speed of the quick spin should be above 1,000 rpm. Set the speed to 8,000 rpm; press the button for 5 s and release to achieve this speed.

12. DNA should be stored in a neutral to slightly basic buffered solution to prevent degradation. Tris EDTA (TE) buffer can be used for storage. TE contains EDTA which has a high affinity towards divalent ions like Ca^{2+} and Mg^{2+}. These ions are cofactors for many enzymes including nucleases that digest DNA molecules. Since repeated access to a tube of genomic DNA may introduce nucleases, TE buffer will protect DNA from degradation during long term storage. However, since EDTA can bind divalent ions, it can inhibit Taq polymerase in the PCR reaction. If DNA is stored in deionized water which is often at an acidic pH, DNA degradation can occur by acid hydrolysis.

13. Refer to the QIAamp^{R} DNA Mini Kit handbook for troubleshooting problems.

14. Avoid pipeting less than 0.5 μl of the Taq because the solution is viscous. Usually a larger volume of master mix is prepared so that pipeting volumes are optimized.

15. It is critical to have high quality DNA for the PCR reaction. To quantify the DNA and to determine its purity, read its optical density (OD) using a spectrophotometer. The NanoDrop spectrophotometer (e.g., NanoDrop ND-1000, NanoDrop Technologies, Inc. Wilmington, DE USA) uses very small quantities of the solution so it or a similar instrument is recommended. The DNA concentration at OD 260 nm should be >10 ng/μl (OD at 260 nm × dilution factor × 50 = ng/μl). The purity as measured by the ratio of the absorbance at 260 nm to the absorbance at 280 nm (measuring protein contamination) should be in the 1.65–1.9 range.

16. The thermal cycler should be calibrated at regular intervals to ensure that the temperatures required for PCR are achieved in all of the wells of the thermal cycler. This should be done at least every 6 months or more frequently depending on the usage. The Driftcon Temperature Verification System (CYCLERtest, Landgraaf, Netherlands) is one instrument that might be used if this calibration is performed in-house.

17. Often samples have already been HLA typed by a lower resolution method, for example by sequence specific priming (SSP), sequence specific oligonucleotide probe hybridization (SSOP), or by serologic typing. These methods narrow down the alleles that an individual may carry but not to allele-level resolution. The typing result may also be reported using letter codes (e.g., DRB1*04:AB, *15:BCD). The interpretation of these letter codes can be found at http://bioinformatics.nmdp.org [14]. The alleles included within a serologic assignment can be found

at http://http://www.ebi.ac.uk/imgt/hla/ under the HLA Dictionary. These low resolution assignments can be used to select a subset of group-specific primers that will amplify the alleles of interest.

18. Since not all alleles have been sequenced for intron 1 and intron 3, it is possible that sequence variation in some alleles may cause primers to fail to anneal. Failure to hybridize will cause amplification to fail. Sequences for HLA introns can be found on the IMGT/HLA Web site [2] as well as in a number of publications (for example, for class I [12, 15, 16]).

19. Do not boil the agarose too vigorously as the water in the flask will evaporate and alter the gel concentration. An alternative to GelRed™ nucleic acid gel stain is to use ethidium bromide to stain DNA. This is not recommended because ethidium bromide is a carcinogen and must be handled with care. DNA is negatively charged and will move toward the positive pole. Unincorporated primers will also stain with the nucleic acid stain. Wear gloves and UV safety glasses when photographing the agarose gel.

20. The molecular weight markers should be present as single sharp bands. The cresol red dye runs at approximately 125 base pairs. Each PCR reaction should yield a single bright band of the expected size (Tables 2, 5, 8) [9, 10]. The presence of additional bands suggests that the amplification conditions were less stringent than required and the primer annealing temperature should be raised until a single band is produced. The absence of a band may indicate that the amplification conditions are too stringent or that an allele group is not present. To reduce stringency, lower the annealing temperature until a single strong band is produced. Amplification of a locus or of one of two alleles at a locus may fail if the allele carries a nucleotide sequence variation in a primer annealing site.

21. The AMPure kit will remove unincorporated primers, dNTPs and salts following the PCR reaction. An alternative to the use of AMPure is the use of ExoSapIT. ExoSAP-IT eliminates unincorporated primers and the dNTPs following the PCR reaction but is not as efficient as AMPure. It might be used in cases where the sample volume is too small for use with AMPure. Use a 1:1 dilution of ExoSAP-IT (USB, Affymetrix, Santa Clara, CA, USA) made by adding 1 μl enzyme to 1 μl of water for each sample. Add 2 μl of diluted ExoSAP-IT to each reaction tube and centrifuge briefly to combine enzyme and PCR amplicon. Put the tubes in the thermal cycler and run the following thermal cycling profile: 37 °C for 15 min, 80 °C for 15 min, 4 °C hold. Dilute the PCR product with water at a ratio of 1 (DNA):4 (water) (v/v) or less if the PCR reaction

appears weak on the agarose gel. Mix well. Perform a sequencing reaction as described in Subheading 3.8.

22. Comparison of the intensity of staining of a reference mass ladder (*see* **Note 6**) to the staining intensity of an amplicon following gel electrophoresis can be used to estimate the amount of amplified DNA in the reaction. In turn, this information can be used to determine the amount of water used to elute purified DNA from the AMPure beads. If the concentration of DNA is low, elute with 30 µl instead of 50 µl of water.
23. The Big Dye Terminator Cycle Sequencing Kit contains a fluorescent dye and should be kept away from direct sunlight.
24. The primer in a sequencing reaction will anneal to a sequence flanking a specific exon to yield sequence data from one strand of the DNA. Through the use of a primer annealing 5′ of an exon and a second primer annealing 3′ of an exon, the sequences of both DNA strands for that exon will be obtained. The availability of data from both strands provides a more accurate sequencing result. Note that the protocol provided in this chapter for DQB1 sequencing uses only a single primer to obtain the sequence of a single DNA strand of DQB1 exon 2 [10].
25. The amount of dilution will depend on the concentration of DNA as judged by gel electrophoresis after PCR amplification.
26. Assign™ is used to obtain HLA allele assignments from the DNA sequences obtained. For laboratories designing their own oligonucleotide reagents or evaluating novel sequences, a software program like Sequencher (Gene Codes Corporation, Ann Arbor, MI, USA) with its library of full length genomic sequences and coding region sequences is used to confirm the annealing site of PCR and sequencing primers, to design new primers, and to aid in assigning alleles in unusual sequences.
27. The primarily heterozygous sequences are compared to a database of known HLA sequences to identify genotypes (combination of two alleles). At positions where the two alleles differ in the nucleotide sequence, two peaks will appear, usually with half the intensity of the neighboring peaks representing single nucleotides. Many alleles share the nucleotide sequence of exons 2 and 3 (class I) or exon 2 (class II) (e.g., A*02:01:01:01, A*02:09, and 28 other alleles have identical sequences in exons 2 and 3 and are often designated as A*02:01:01G). In addition, combinations of two alleles may also be indistinguishable from one another when sequenced as a mixture. Use of PCR primers to selectively isolate a single allele for sequencing or use of a sequencing primer to produce the sequence of a single allele will allow the localization of nucleotide polymorphisms to a single strand therefore identifying the allele present or excluding a specific allele. Sometimes, the 5′ or 3′ ends of an exon are not

covered by sequence from both strands due to the positioning of the sequencing primers. In these cases, a single clear sequence may be acceptable.

28. Single stranded DNA fragments migrate on the sequencing gel based on their size; however, in some circumstances, secondary structure may alter that migration. This leads to "sequence artifacts" where the peaks in an electropherogram may not accurately represent the DNA sequence. Comparison to reference sequences will help identify these artifacts. Novel alleles carrying new allele sequences are not unusual; it is estimated that a novel allele is found once in every 1,000 sequences in a well HLA-characterized population. Review the data for frameshifts indicating that one of the alleles has an insertion or deletion of nucleotides. A frameshift will result in a region of sequence where almost all peaks are double nucleotide calls. The presence of a frameshift may require isolation of single alleles for sequencing. The allele library used by the software for interpretation may or may not contain alleles with insertions or deletions.
29. The HLA allele database, IMGT/HLA, is updated quarterly with new, modified, or deleted alleles. Updates to the HLA library used in interpretation of results by the Assign™ software should be validated by interpreting the sequence data from a small panel of cells carrying known HLA alleles.
30. The amplified DNA should be obtained by PCR just prior to cloning.
31. The efficiency at which inserts are obtained should be at least 70–80 %. The white colonies contain inserted DNA (e.g., one allele of HLA-C); the blue colonies do not contain an insert.
32. Several independent clones should be sequenced from each isolated allele. Since each bacterium incorporates one DNA fragment from the PCR amplicon, it is possible that PCR amplification artifacts due to mis-incorporation of nucleotides will be found within the sequence. Usually selection of at least eight colonies should be sufficient to obtain both alleles and to achieve a consensus sequence for each allele.

References

1. Posch PE, Hurley CK (2011) Histocompatibility: HLA and other systems. In: Porwit A, McCullough J, Erber WN (eds) Blood and bone marrow pathology, 2nd edn. Elsevier, Edinburgh, pp 641–676
2. Robinson J, Waller MJ, Fail SC, McWilliam H, Lopez R, Parham P et al (2009) The IMGT/HLA database. Nucleic Acids Res 37(Database issue):D1013–D1017
3. Sanger F, Nicklen S, Coulson A (1977) DNA sequencing with chain terminating inhibitors. Proc Natl Acad Sci USA 74:5463–5467
4. Bray RA, Hurley CK, Kamani NR, Woolfrey A, Muller C, Spellman S et al (2008) National marrow donor program HLA matching guidelines for unrelated adult donor hematopoietic cell transplants. Biol Blood Marrow Transplant 14(9 Suppl):45–53

5. Lee SJ, Klein J, Haagenson M, Baxter-Lowe LA, Confer DL, Eapen M et al (2007) High-resolution donor-recipient HLA matching contributes to the success of unrelated donor marrow transplantation. Blood 110(13):4576–4583
6. Barker JN, Scaradavou A, Stevens CE (2010) Combined effect of total nucleated cell dose and HLA match on transplantation outcome in 1061 cord blood recipients with hematologic malignancies. Blood 115(9):1843–1849
7. Kamani N, Spellman S, Hurley CK, Barker JN, Smith FO, Oudshoorn M et al (2008) State of the art review: HLA matching and outcome of unrelated donor umbilical cord blood transplants. Biol Blood Marrow Transplant 14(1):1–6
8. Spellman S, Bray R, Rosen-Bronson S, Haagenson M, Klein J, Flesch S et al (2010) The detection of donor-directed, HLA-specific alloantibodies in recipients of unrelated hematopoietic cell transplantation is predictive of graft failure. Blood 115(13):2704–2708
9. Kotsch K, Wehling J, Blasczyk R (1999) Sequencing of HLA class II genes based on the conserved diversity of the non-coding regions: sequencing based typing of HLA-DRB genes. Tissue Antigens 53:486–497
10. Dunn PP, Day S, Williams S, Bendukidze N (2005) HLA-DQB1 sequencing-based typing using newly identified conserved nucleotide sequences in introns 1 and 2. Tissue Antigens 66(2):99–106
11. Cao K, Chopek M, Fernandez-Vina MA (1999) High and intermediate resolution DNA typing systems for Class I HLA-A, -B, -C genes by hybridization with sequence specific oligonucleotide probes (SSOP). Rev Immunogenet 1:177–208
12. Cereb N, Maye P, Lee S, Kong Y, Yang SY (1995) Locus-specific amplification of HLA class I genes from genomic DNA: locus-specific sequences in the first and third introns of HLA-A, -B, and -C alleles. Tissue Antigens 45(1):1–11
13. Cereb N, Yang SY (1997) Dimorphic primers derived from intron 1 for use in the molecular typing of HLA-B alleles. Tissue Antigens 50(1):74–76
14. Bochtler W, Maiers M, Oudshoorn M, Marsh SG, Raffoux C, Mueller C et al (2007) World Marrow Donor Association guidelines for use of HLA nomenclature and its validation in the data exchange among hematopoietic stem cell donor registries and cord blood banks. Bone Marrow Transplant 39(12):737–741
15. Summers CW, Hampson VJ, Taylor GM (1993) HLA class I non-coding nucleotide sequences, 1992. Eur J Immunogenet 20(3):201–240
16. Blasczyk R, Kotsch K, Wehling J (1998) The nature of polymorphism of the HLA-DRB intron sequences is lineage specific. Tissue Antigens 52:19–26

Chapter 10

Next-Generation HLA Sequencing Using the 454 GS FLX System

Elizabeth A. Trachtenberg and Cherie L. Holcomb

Abstract

Next-generation sequencing (NGS) of HLA class I and II loci (HLA-A, HLA-B, HLA-C, DRB1, DRB3, DRB4, DRB5, DQA1, DQB1, DPB1) is described here in detail using the 454 Life Sciences GS FLX System and Titanium chemistry. An overview of the protocol with our experience on sequence performance efficiencies, read depth and ambiguity analyses using the GS FLX System are also presented. A total of 14 HLA primer pairs with multiplex identifiers (MIDs) are used in clonal, amplicon-based pyrosequencing of up to 44 samples per plate using the GS FLX. Genotype assignment and ambiguity reduction analysis is performed using Conexio Assign ATF 454 software. Clonal NGS gives a significant reduction in genotyping ambiguity during analysis of the highly complex HLA system.

Key words HLA class I and II sequencing, Clonal pyrosequencing, Next-generation sequencing (NGS), 454 Life Sciences GS FLX Titanium Chemistry, 454 Life Sciences GS FLX 454 System, HLA genotype ambiguity reduction

1 Introduction

High resolution HLA class I and II genotyping continues to be a challenge because of the extreme level of polymorphism in these loci. Allelic ambiguities, the biggest problem in high resolution HLA typing, stem from incomplete genomic coverage and inability to set phase, and are time consuming to resolve. Next-generation, clonal sequencing significantly resolves phase ambiguities and provides higher resolution HLA genotypes. This chapter describes next-generation HLA sequencing using the 454 Life Sciences GS FLX System (GS FLX) and Titanium chemistry, detailing test procedures, and listing manufacturer and laboratory provided materials and reagents needed for the testing. Further information for the protocols may be found by visiting the Web sites of the manufacturers of the instruments, reagents, and robotics.

Elizabeth A. Trachtenberg and Cherie L. Holcomb have contributed equally to this manuscript.

Andrea A. Zachary and Mary S. Leffell (eds.), *Transplantation Immunology: Methods and Protocols, Second Edition*, Methods in Molecular Biology, vol. 1034, DOI 10.1007/978-1-62703-493-7_10, © Springer Science+Business Media, LLC 2013

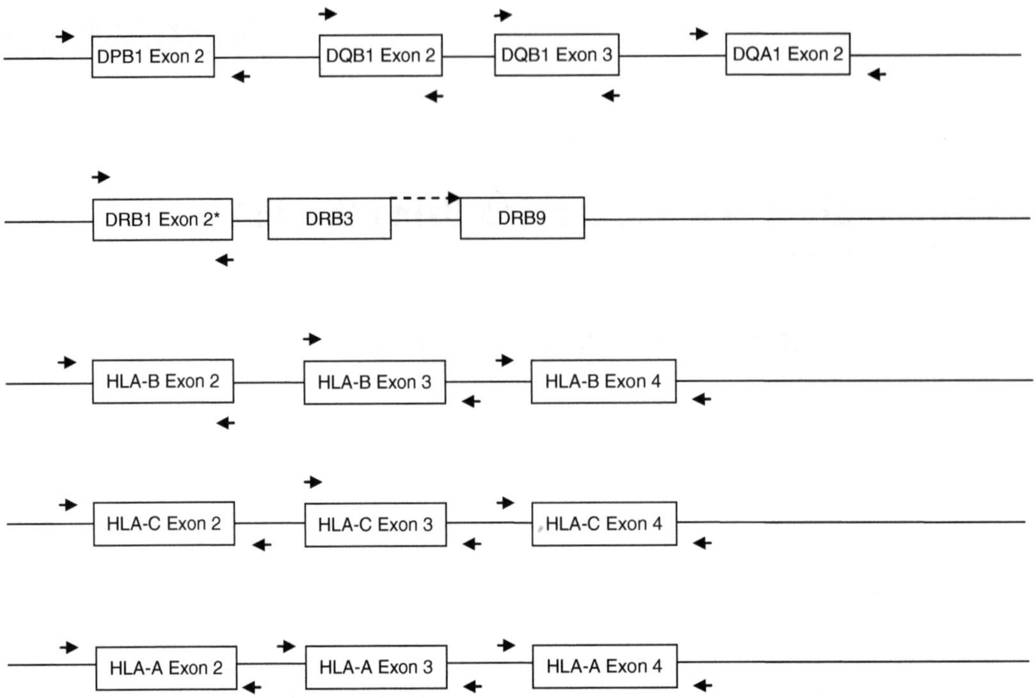

Fig. 1 HLA primer positions. Primer positions capturing coding and noncoding regions for genotyping HLA class I and II loci using the 454 Life Sciences GS GType HLA MR and HR primer sets are illustrated. *Notes*: Primers for DRB1 Exon 2 are generic and also amplify DRB3, DRB4, and DRB5 loci, and other related pseudogenes. *Boxes* in schematic indicate exons; *lines* indicate introns; *arrows* indicate primer positions. Not drawn to scale

1.1 Protocol Overview

In this protocol, an amplicon-based, clonal pyrosequencing strategy is used for HLA genotyping. 454 Life Sciences GS FLX [1] Titanium chemistry and primers are used to sequence the HLA class I and II genes, HLA-A, HLA-B, HLA-C, DRB1/3/4/5, DQA1, DQB1, and DPB1 [2, 3]. To begin, genomic DNA samples are amplified with 14 HLA primer pairs to amplify the sequences, including exon and noncoding regions as illustrated in Fig. 1. Each primer includes a 5′ 26 base pair (bp) adaptor (A or B), and 4 bp library key and a 10 bp multiplex identifier (MID), used to identify the sample, in addition to the HLA primer sequence. The adaptor sequence serves to bind the genomic-target portion of the amplicon to the complimentary A or B capture beads for recovery of forward and reverse sequence reads, respectively (Fig. 2). Following PCR amplification, nonspecific and primer-dimer artifact products are removed from the amplicons, which are quantified, diluted, and pooled for the secondary "clonal" amplification, or emulsion PCR (emPCR) step. The emPCR step includes sepharose beads that carry oligonucleotides complementary to either the A or B adaptor sequence. The primary amplicons are mixed with the beads in a ratio that will yield,

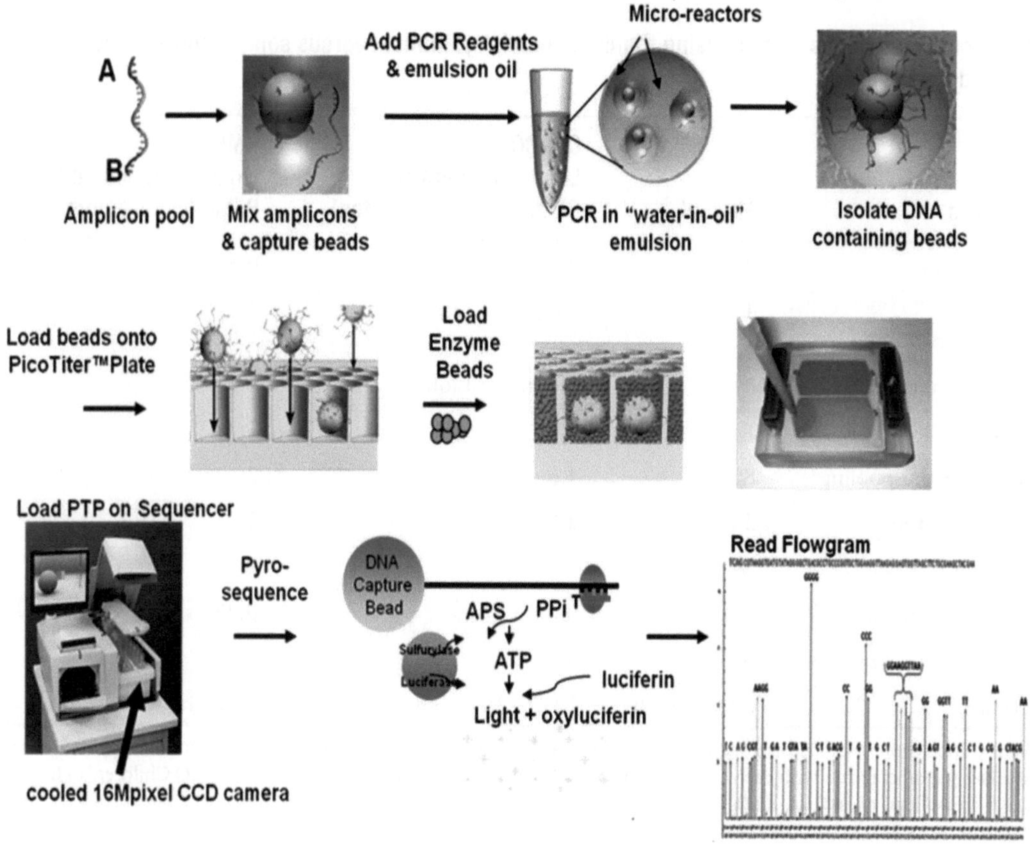

Fig. 2 The 454 Life Sciences GS FLX System Sequencing Procedure. Initial amplifications of HLA loci use primers with 454 Life Sciences Titanium 5′ A or B adapters to allow for the recovery of forward and reverse sequence reads, and a multiplex identifier (MID) sample tags to allow for up to 44 samples to be sequenced per run. Following the primary PCR amplification, the amplicons are purified, quantified, diluted, and pooled (yielding the "amplicon library") for the emulsion PCR (emPCR) step. In this step, the amplicon library is mixed with the appropriate A or B complimentary beads in a ratio designed to generate beads which, on average, have a single DNA fragment bound. These bead-bound sequences are emulsified with amplification reagents in an oil–water mixture to yield aqueous "microreactors," within which, each DNA is amplified to give millions of identical (i.e., "clonal") DNA molecules per bead. Beads that lack amplified DNA are washed away. The DNA containing beads, DNA polymerase and pyrosequencing enzymes are then loaded onto the PicoTiterPlate (PTP) for sequencing on the GS FLX, which generates runs with, on average, 600,000 high-quality reads (reproduced with permission from 454 Life Sciences, a Roche Company: http://www.454.com)

on average, one DNA molecule bound per bead. These bead-bound sequences are emulsified with amplification reagents in an oil–water mixture. Each "microreactor" contains a single bead with a bound DNA fragment. After emPCR, each bead contains millions of identical DNA molecules. These beads, along with DNA polymerase and enzyme beads for the pyrosequencing reaction, are loaded onto a PicoTiterPlate™ (PTP). Each well contains a single bead with a clonally amplified sequence attached.

Table 1
HLA sequencing hands on time using titanium chemistry: Manual versus semi-automated systems at two different sites

Process	Manual	CHRCO: Liquid handlers and REMe (semi-automated)	RMS: Liquid handlers and REMe (semi-automated)
PCR setup	2	2	0.5
AMPure Amplicon cleanup	4	3 (Qiagen Liquidator)	1
DNA quantitation	3–4	3 (Qiagen Liquidator)	1.5
Quality check	1	1	1
Dilution and pooling	8	4.5	3
emPCR setup	2.5–3	2.5	2.5
Emulsion break	3	3	2
Bead enrichment	8	0.25	0.25
Pyrosequencing setup	3–3.5	3	3
Total	34.5–36.5 h	22.25–24 h	14.75 h

Note: Comparison of hands-on time using manual versus semi-automated methods reveals an approximately10 h difference per sequencing run with each increase in robotic sophistication in our laboratories. *CHRCO* Children's Hospital & Research Center Oakland, *RMS* Roche Molecular Systems

The Titanium PTP enables runs with an average of 600,000 high quality reads for amplicon sequencing. The MID tags in the GS GType HLA primer plates allow up to 44 samples to be sequenced at all 8 HLA loci (including DRB3/4/5) in one PTP. The GS FLX generates raw sequencing image files that are processed into sequence text files (.fna files in FASTA format). Next, sequence text files are transferred from the server to a PC for genotyping using Conexio Assign ATF 454 software (developed by Dr. Damian Goodridge, Conexio Genomics, Perth), which compares the sequence files to the most current, curated HLA sequence database (IMGT/HLA Database: http://www.ebi.ac.uk/ipd/imgt/hla/) and assigns HLA genotypes. In general, consensus sequences from 50 or more sequence reads per amplicon are considered "high-confidence" as are the genotype assignments based on these consensus sequences.

1.2 Experience with the System

In the Children's Hospital & Research Center Oakland (CHRCO) laboratory, our hands on time to perform the Titanium chemistry is ~24 h for semi-automated versus ~35 h for manual (Table 1). Assay setup and run time for sequencing all HLA loci in 44

Table 2
Percent of two field (four digit) allelic HLA calls and percent of calls with >1 potential genotype

Genotype	% Class I			% Class II			
Calls	HLA-A	HLA-B	HLA-C	DRB1	DQB1	DQA1	DPB1
(a)							
1	12	9	12	50	51	19	10
2	44	3	26	39	24	0	36
3	4	19	6	2	20	27	29
4	40	5	24	8	5	0	11
5+	0	64	32	1	0	54	14
(b)							
1	93	8	12	50	51	19	10
2	7	8	27	39	24	37	36
3	0	17	5	5	20	22	29
4	0	3	25	5	5	8	11
5+	0	64	31	1	0	14	14

For a given locus, the percentage of genotype calls that are unambiguous at the two field level (previously known as "four digit level") (labeled 1) versus those that are composed of an ambiguity string of two through five or more genotype calls (labeled 2 through 5+) using the 454/Roche Applied Science HLA primers and GS FLX sequencing system in a study on 1,000 Caucasians [4, 5]. (a) Call percentages when expression variants are considered (as would be required for hematopoietic stem cell transplantation). (b) Call percentages when expression variants are not considered (as is often the case in a research study). The inclusion of supplementary coding and noncoding regions in future versions of the typing method would significantly enhance the ability to resolve ambiguous sequences

samples is 40 h (24 h hands-on) plus 1 h analysis time. Using robotics the assay and analysis time takes about 1/4 the time of Sanger sequencing. The average amplicon read depth of the GS FLX system is between ~250 and 650 reads in our hands. In an international alpha-trial testing of 20 blinded samples, the 454 Life Sciences GS FLX System sequencing method demonstrated 98 % concordance with known genotypes between eight participating labs [2]. In our other studies, using at least one control per PTP region per run, 100 % of control sample genotypes (previously characterized by Sanger Sequencing with ambiguity reduction) were concordant [4, 5]. The average rate of detection of novel alleles was ~0.04 % (8/19,069 loci) in Caucasoid study populations [4, 5].

Using this system, class I and II genotype calls are significantly reduced to a single allelic genotype call or to shorter allelic ambiguity strings than expected using traditional Sanger sequencing. Table 2 illustrates the fraction of unambiguous genotype calls and of genotype calls that consist of ambiguity strings of varying lengths observed using 454/Roche Applied Science primers for sequencing class I (exons 2–4) and class II DQB1 (exon 2 and 3) and DRB1, DQA1, DPB1 (exon 2) in a study of 1,000 samples [4, 5]. Note that non-Caucasoid populations would be expected to have fewer ambiguous genotypes, due to unique HLA sequences in these regions. Note also that when expression variants (e.g., null alleles) are taken into consideration (Table 2a versus b) there is little difference for most of the loci except for HLA-A and DQA1 (shaded); this illustrates the need to include additional exons, and in some cases noncoding sequence to further resolve the ambiguities. The inclusion of supplementary coding and noncoding regions in future versions of the typing system will significantly enhance the ability to resolve ambiguous sequences. In conclusion, HLA genotyping utilizing next-generation sequencing (NGS) methods provides a significant improvement in throughput with reduction of ambiguity afforded by clonal analysis of amplicons. The 454 GS FLX System, Titanium chemistry and HLA primers, and the Conexio Assign ATF 454 genotyping software are excellent for high resolution, high throughput analysis of samples for the HLA class I and II loci.

2 Materials

Prepare all solutions using analytical grade reagents and molecular biology grade water.

Follow all waste disposal regulations when disposing of waste materials. Prior to opening any tubes or microwell plates, solutions should be mixed by gentle vortexing and then spun down in a centrifuge to avoid loss of contents and cross-contamination. All disposable supplies including tubes, pipette tips (*see* **Note 1**) and microwell plates are DNase free and sterile. Facilities should allow for separation of prePCR functions from postPCR functions as well as pre-emulsion PCR (emPCR) functions from post-emulsion PCR functions. Throughout the entire protocol all TE (Tris–EDTA) buffer should be low EDTA as described under Genomic PCR Components. All quantities indicated are sufficient to genotype 40 samples and 4 negative controls (*see* **Note 2**) for 8 loci at high resolution. These samples are run on one GS FLX run using a four region PicoTiterPlate (PTP).

2.1 Sample Preparation Components

DNA may be purified from any of a variety of sources using any of the commercially available kits. At the end of the procedure the DNA sample should be in water or TE as described under Genomic PCR Components.

2.2 Genomic PCR Components

1. PCR Workstation (Dead air box): set up in a pre-PCR room (*see* **Note 3**).
2. Vortex: in PCR Workstation.
3. Minifuge: in PCR Workstation.

4. Pre-PCR multichannel pipettes (one of each): 8-channel multipipette, 20–200 μl, 8-channel multipipette, 1–10 or 2–20 μl, 12-channel multipipette, 2–20 μl.
5. Pre-PCR single channel pipettes: various.
6. Pipetting reservoirs.
7. 96-well plate cooler (Eppendorf, Hamburg, Germany) or ice: if plate coolers are used, a quantity of at least four is advisable.
8. PCR primers dried on plates: to obtain high resolution typing, purchase both GS GType HLA MR and HR plates (1 box of each, Roche Applied Science, Indianapolis, IN, USA).
9. DNA sample in water or TE (*see* **Note 4**).
10. 10× PCR Buffer II w/o$MgCl_2$ (Applied Biosystems), 6 ml.
11. 25 mM $MgCl_2$ (Applied Biosystems), 3 ml.
12. 80 % (w/v) Glycerol (*see* **Note 5**), autoclave, cool, and store at room temperature.
13. 100 mM dNTP blend, 25 mM each of dATP, dCTP, dGTP, dTTP (Applied Biosystems) GeneAmp dNTP mix in 350 μl.
14. Plate thermoseals: BioRad microseal "B′ film" recommended.
15. Film sealing roller (or similar tool).
16. AmpliTaq Gold, 5 U/μl (Applied Biosystems), 1.3 ml.
17. Plate centrifuge in pre-PCR environment.
18. Thermal cyclers: the preferred model is the ABI GeneAmp™ PCR System 9700 with 96-well gold-plated silver block (Foster City, CA) (*see* **Note 6**). Four thermal cyclers run simultaneously provide adequate throughput, although eight provide maximum throughput. The thermal cycler should be in a post-PCR environment.

2.3 Amplicon Cleanup Components

1. Plate centrifuge in post-PCR environment.
2. Agencourt SPRIPlate 96R magnet plate (Beckman Coulter, Indianapolis, IN).
3. Pipetting reservoirs.
4. Post-PCR multichannel pipettes (one of each): 8-channel multipipette, 20–200 μl, 8-channel multipipette, 1–10 or 2–20 μl, 12-channel multipipette, if preferred over 8-channel.
5. Agencourt AMPure XP Kit (Beckman Coulter), 60 ml.
6. 70 % Ethanol, 600 ml (*see* **Note 7**).
7. TE (Tris–EDTA buffer) (*see* **Note 4**).
8. Heat block.

2.4 Amplicon Quantification Components

1. Quant-iT™ PicoGreen® dsDNA Assay Kit (Invitrogen, Carlsbad, CA), 1 kit.
2. Pipetting reservoirs.
3. Post-PCR multichannel pipettes (one of each): 8-channel multipipette, 20–200 μl, 8-channel multipipettor, 1–10 or 2–20 μl, 12-channel multipipette, if preferred over 8-channel.
4. Post-PCR single channel pipettes: various.
5. 96-well Flat Bottom Black Polystyrene 96-well plates, 8 (*see* **Note 8**).
6. 50 ml BD Falcon tube.
7. Microplate fluorimeter, 96 wells.

2.5 Amplicon Quality Check Components

1. 96-well E-gels, or 2 % Agarose (Invitrogen).
2. Post-PCR 12-channel multipipette (non-electronic).
3. 10× Blue Juice Gel Loading Dye (Invitrogen), 150 μl.
4. E-gel 96-well mother base + daughter base (Invitrogen).
5. Digital imager (e.g., AlphaImager HP, Protein Simple, Santa Clara, CA) or transilluminator and digital camera.

2.6 Amplicon Dilution and Pooling

1. Pipetting reservoirs.
2. 2 ml deep, square well plates.
3. TE (*see* **Note 4**).
4. Post-PCR single channel pipette: various.
5. 1–20 μl 8 or 12 channel multipipette. (Optional) Rainin Liquidator 96 or Liquid handler (e.g., BioMek).
6. 1.5 ml microfuge tubes.
7. 1.5 ml tubes with O-ring cap.

2.7 Emulsion PCR Setup and Thermal Cycling

1. PCR Workstations (dead air boxes) designated for emPCR set up, in a post-genomic PCR, pre-emPCR room/space: one for emulsion preparation, one for emulsion dispensing (*see* **Note 9**).
2. Vortex: 2, one in each PCR workstation.
3. Minifuge: 2, one in each PCR workstation.
4. TissueLyser or TissueLyser II (QIAGEN, Valencia, CA).
5. MV Tube rack adapters matched to TissueLyser or TissueLyser II (Roche Applied Science).
6. LabQuake Roller (Thermolyne).
7. Pre-emPCR multichannel pipettes (one of each): 8-channel multipipettor, 20–200 μl, 8-channel multipipettor, 1–10 or 1–20 μl, 12-channel multipipettor.
8. Pre-emPCR single channel pipettes: various.

9. Repeat pipette (Eppendorf): to accommodate 1 ml Combitips®.
10. Heat block, set at 65 °C (LabNet Accublock Digital DryBath).
11. emPCR Lib A MV Kit (Roche Applied Science).
12. 1.0 ml Combitips® plus tips (Eppendorf).
13. Thermal cyclers, 4 (*see* **Note 10**).

2.8 Emulsion Breaking

1. Vented hood or ductless fume hood: designated for emulsion breaking, in a post-PCR room (*see* **Note 11**).
2. Disposable lab coats (*see* **Note 12**).
3. GS FLX Titanium emPCR Breaking Kit, LV/MV, 12 pcs (Roche Applied Science).
4. Vacuum source with liquid trap.
5. Conical tubes with caps: 50 ml, quantity 4.
6. Post-PCR multichannel pipettes: 8-channel multipipette, 20–200 μl (Rainin EDP3-Plus; Eppendorf "Repeater Plus" pipettes).
7. Post-PCR pipette: 100–1,000 μl.
8. 100 % Isopropanol, 200 ml.
9. 100 % Ethanol, non-denatured, 100 ml.
10. 1.7 ml tubes, eight siliconized.
11. Centrifuge and rotor with two swinging buckets and 2–50 ml tube adaptors (*see* **Note 13**).
12. Minifuge.
13. Vortex.
14. Serological pipettes: 5, 10, 25 ml (Rainin Glassmaster and Greiner Bio-One Cellstar serological pipettes).

2.9 Bead Washing, Enrichment, Counting, and Sequencing Primer Annealing

1. Vortex (for preparation of enrichment beads).
2. Minifuge (for preparation of enrichment beads).
3. 10 N Sodium hydroxide.
4. Serological pipettes: 5, 10, 25 ml (Rainin Glassmaster and Greiner Bio-One Cellstar serological pipettes).
5. Post PCR pipettes: 1–20 μl, 20–100 μl, 100–100 μl.
6. Magnetic Particle Concentrator (Invitrogen) or REMe unit (Roche Applied Science) and liquid handler (*see* **Note 14**).
7. LabQuake Roller (Thermolyne).
8. Heat block, set at 65 °C for manual; or the REMe unit (Roche Applied Science).
9. Ice if performing without REMe.
10. Bead Counter: CC Size Standard L10, 15 ml (Beckman Coulter, Carlsbad, CA).

11. Isoton II: 20 ml (Beckman Coulter).
12. Accuvettes: 4 (Beckman Coulter) (1 per sequencing pool per region).

2.10 Sequencing

1. 454 Life Sciences Genome Sequencer GS FLX Instrument (*see* **Note 15**).
2. GS FLX Titanium Sequencing Kit XLR70.
3. GS FLX Titanium PicoTiterPlate Kit 70×75, including the four region gasket.
4. Bead Deposition Device (70×75).
5. Bead Deposition Device Counterweight.
6. Microplate Centrifuge: Beckman Coulter Allegra X-15 and rotor, with microplate carriers and covers.
7. Microcentrifuge.
8. Lens paper.

2.11 HLA Genotyping

1. Conexio Genomics Assign ATF 454 software and PC (Windows XP or Windows 7).

3 Methods

3.1 Sample Preparation

Prepare high quality DNA (40–150 ng) in water or TE. We recommend 10 ng of DNA per genomic PCR with a minimum of 2 ng if DNA is limiting.

3.2 Genomic PCR

Note that high resolution typing is achieved only by typing a given sample using both the medium resolution (MR) and the high resolution (HR) GS GType HLA primer plates. One "set" of plates is defined as 1 MR plate plus 1 HR plate (*see* Table 3). Genomic target specific primers are arranged in rows, while Multiplex Identifiers (MIDs) that allow identification (or "tagging") of samples are arranged in columns. Column 12 is intentionally left blank on each plate to make liquid handling easier when performing quantitation of amplicons. Rows G and H are blank on the HR plates.

1. Wipe the pre-PCR dead air box work surface, pipettes, minifuge and vortex with a laboratory wipe moistened with mild detergent solution, then 10 % bleach, then 10 % ethanol.
2. Turn on the UV light for 10′ in the dead air box, with all equipment, including pipettes within. After this decontamination is complete, turn off the light.
3. Label one set of GS GType HLA primer plates as MR-1 and HR-1. Label a second set as MR-2 and HR-2, and two additional

Table 3
GS GType HLA primer plates

MR	HR
HLA-A Exon 2	HLA-A Exon 4
HLA-A Exon 3	HLA-B Exon 4
HLA-B Exon 2	HLA-C Exon 4
HLA-B Exon 3	DPB1 Exon 2
HLA-C Exon 2	DQA1 Exon 2
HLA-C Exon 3	DQB1 Exon 3
DQB1 Exon 2	
DRB Exon 2	

sets as MR-3 and HR-3, and MR-4 and HR-4. Arrange the plates so that MR-1 and HR-1 plates are adjacent to one another with columns aligned. Likewise, MR-2 and HR-2 should have their columns aligned. Remove the seals carefully (*see* **Note 16**).

4. Using a 12 channel micropipette and working by rows, add 10 μl of water to well 1–11, rows A–H on the MR plates and rows A–F on the HR plates. Use different pipette tips each time so as not to cross-contaminate the wells. Let the plates sit at room temperature for 10′ (*see* **Note 17**). Place the plates on ice.
5. While the plates in **step 4** are incubating at room temperature, prepare enough PCR master mix for eight plates: To a 15 ml tube on ice, add in order: 3,618 μl of water, 2,250 μl of 80 % glycerol, 1,800 μl of 10× PCR buffer without Mg^{2+}, 108 μl of 100 mM dNTP blend (25 mM each dA, dC, dG, dT), 288 μl of AmpliTaq Gold DNA polymerase (5 U/μl), 1,296 μl of 25 mM $MgCl_2$ (*see* **Note 18**).
6. To Column 11 of each plate add 2 μl of TE for a negative control (*see* **Notes 19–20**).
7. To each well of columns 1–10 of plates MR-1 and HR-1 (rows A–F only for the latter), add 2 μl of DNA sample numbers 1–10, respectively. DNA should be at a concentration of 5 ng/μl (*see* **Note 21**). Use a fresh tip for each sample to avoid cross-contamination of samples.
8. Repeat **step 7** three times. Pipetting 2 μl of DNA samples numbers 11–20, 21–30, and 31–40 into MR-2 and HR-2, MR-3 and HR-3, and MR-4 and HR-4, respectively.

9. Using a 12-channel multipipette, pipet 23 μl of PCR master mix into each well of the first 11 columns of the MR and HR plates (only rows A–F of the latter). It is important to use a fresh set of tips for each set of plates in order to avoid cross-contamination of primers and samples (*see* **Note 22**)
10. Cover each plate with a fresh seal and seal very tightly (*see* **Note 23**). Vortex gently.
11. Centrifuge the plates for 30 s at 900 × *g*.
12. Place each plate in a thermal cycler block and run the following PCR thermal cycler program: 95 °C—10′; 31 cycles of 95 °C—15″, 60 °C—45″, 72 °C-15″; 72 °C—5′, 4 °C—hold (*see* **Note 24**).
13. If you are not proceeding with the next step immediately, store the plates on ice (for processing the same day) or at −20 °C.

3.3 Amplicon Purification by AMPure

Processing plates two at a time is recommended, multiples are possible if you have multiple Agencourt SPRIPlate 96R magnet plates. Be sure to change pipette tips after transfers (*see* **Note 25**).

1. Thaw the plate with the PCR products (if necessary), vortex gently and centrifuge for 30 s at 900 × *g*.
2. Using an 8-channel multipipette and working by row, transfer 20 μl PCR product (*see* **Note 26**) from the PCR plate to each well of a new 96-well PCR plate keeping the layout the same for each of the eight plates. Change tips after each transfer.
3. Add 20 μl of water and pipet up and down to mix. Change tips after each transfer/mix.
4. Mix the Agencourt AMPure XP beads thoroughly by shaking the bottle to resuspend.
5. Transfer 6.3 ml (enough for one plate) or 12.4 ml (enough for two plates) of the Agencourt AMPure XP beads to a reagent reservoir.
6. Using an 8-channel multipipette and working by row, add 64 μl of SPRI beads to each well and mix thoroughly by pipetting up and down at least ten times until the SPRI bead/PCR mixture is homogeneous. Change tips after each transfer/mix.
7. Incubate the plate for 10 min at room temperature.
8. Place the plate on a 96-well ring magnet plate and incubate for 5 min at room temperature until supernatant is clear.
9. With the plate still on the ring magnet plate, use an 8 or 12-channel micropipette to carefully remove and discard the supernatant without disturbing the beads.
10. Using an 8 or 12-channel multipipette, add 200 μl of freshly prepared 70 % ethanol.

11. Incubate 30 s at room temperature while still on the magnetic ring plate.
12. While the plate is still on the magnetic ring plate, carefully remove and discard the clear supernatant without disturbing the beads.
13. Repeat **steps 7–9**. Remove as much of the supernatant as possible.
14. Place the 96-well plate and magnetic ring plate together on a heat block set at 40 °C until all pellets are completely dry (10–20 min). Do not leave the plate on the heat block longer than necessary.
15. Keep the plate on the magnetic ring stand while removing it from the heat block.
16. Using the 8 or 12 channel multipipette, add 25 μl of TE to each well (*see* **Note 27**). Remove the 96-well plate from the magnetic plate and tap the 96-well plate containing the samples until all pellets are dispersed (about ten times).
17. Place the 96-well plate briefly on the magnetic ring plate, remove and tap again until all pellets are dispersed. This ensures efficient elution of PCR products from the beads.
18. Place the 96-well plate on the magnetic ring plate and incubate for 2 min.
19. Using the multichannel pipette, pipet 20 μl of the supernatant from each well into a fresh 96-well plate (*see* **Note 28**).
20. Cover the plate with a plate seal and store at −20 °C until ready to proceed to E-gel quality check and quantification by Fluorometry using Quant-iTTMPicoGreen® dsDNA Assay Kit.

3.4 E-Gel Check for Amplicon Generation and Removal of Primer Dimer

Dilution of loading dye

1. Place approximately 50 ml of TE in a 50 ml Falcon tube.

   Add 125 μl of "10 X" Blue Juice.

E-gel loading and running

1. Remove the 96-well E-gel from the pouch, and snap it into place on the E-gel mother base (*see* **Note 29**). If you have daughter bases or additional mother bases you may run four gels simultaneously.
2. Using a non-electronic 12 channel multipipette, place 9 μl of each AMPure purified sample into the corresponding well on the E-gel.
3. Add 11 μl diluted loading dye to each well.
4. Press the start button and set time for 7–8 min.

5. Press the start button until the run indicator light turns green.

Digital imaging of the agarose gels

1. Image the E-gels with a digital imager or digital camera equipped with a transilluminator and a filter appropriate for ethidium bromide stained gels. Save the image for analysis (*see* **Note 30**).

3.5 Choosing the Amplicons for the Final Emulsion PCR Pool

For each sample a total of 14 amplicons are generated, each of which, ideally, should be mixed in equimolar amounts for the emPCR reaction. Not all amplicons are generated with equal efficiency and very occasionally there is very little amplicon made but a large amount of primer dimer. To achieve optimal sequencing results it is important to only use well-quantified and relatively pure amplicons for the final mix for each sample.

1. Determine which amplicons to use based on the following criteria:
   (a) If the amplicon detected on the E-gel is much smaller than expected, it is primer-dimer. DO NOT use it for the emPCR pool.
   (b) If the molar ratio of primer-dimer to amplicon is estimated to be 3:1 or more (bands of roughly equal intensity on an E-gel). DO NOT use it in the emPCR pool. Repeat the AMPure procedure on these samples as in Subheading 3.3, **steps 2–18** except: use 10 μl of sample (already AMPure purified once) diluted with 10 μl of water, with the addition of 32 μl of SPRI beads. Reanalyze the product by E-gel as in Subheading 3.4 and determine if it should be included in the amplicon pool as described in Subheading 3.5.
   (c) If a full-length amplicon is completely undetectable on the E-gel and no product is detected by quantification with PicoGreen when performed as in Subheading 3.6, assign this amplicon a concentration value of 0.1 ng/μl and include this reaction in the amplicon pool (see Note 31). This is the treatment that should be applied to negative controls as long as primer dimer has been successfully removed.

3.6 Quantification by PicoGreen Fluorescence

Preparation of DNA serial dilution standard

This procedure makes enough standards for quantification of four plates of amplicons (*see* **Note 32**).

1. Thaw an aliquot of the DNA standard provided with the PicoGreen reagent (100 ng/μl)
2. Transfer TE to ten 1.5 ml microcentrifuge tubes as follows:

   Tube 1: 1,188 μL TE

   Tubes 2–10: 600 μL TE

Table 4
DNA quantification standards

Tube #	Well #	Concentration
1	N/A	50
2	N/A	25
3	A12	12.5
4	B12	6.25
5	C12	3.125
6	D12	1.5625
7	E12	0.78125
8	F12	0.396
9	G12	0.1953
10	H13	0

3. Prepare a 1:100 dilution of the standard by transferring 12 μl of DNA standard to Tube 1 and vortexing for 10 s.
4. Transfer 600 μL from Tube 1 to Tube 2 and vortex for 10 s.

   Complete a dilution series by transferring 600 μL from tube 2 to tube 3, and vortexing for 10 s, then transferring 600 μl from tube 3 to tube 4 and vortexing and so on until Tube 9 has been vortexed. Tube 10 is the no DNA control (*see* **Note 33**).
5. For dilutions from tubes 3–10, transfer 100 μL to the wells of column 12 in a 96-well fluorimeter plate. Since samples are diluted 1:50 in the final assay plate, the values of the standards on the axis of the linear regression plot will take this calculation into account as shown in Table 4.

Preparation of DNA samples

Process no more than two amplicon plates at a time.

1. Using a multichannel pipette, transfer 98 μL of TE to the appropriate columns and rows of the 96-well black fluorometer plate already containing standards; one well for each DNA sample to be measured, i.e., for an MR plate this will be columns 1–11, all rows; for an HR plate this will be columns 1–11, rows A–F.
2. Add 2.0 μL of DNA sample to wells containing the TE and mix by pipetting up and down.

Preparation and addition of diluted PicoGreen reagent

Only make enough PicoGreen reagent to perform the assay on two plates at a time. Protect the second plate from light while reading the first plate.

1. Remove PicoGreen reagent from 4 °C storage and let thaw at room temperature protected from light (*see* **Note 34**).
2. Transfer 24.875 ml TE to a 50 ml Falcon tube.
3. Add 125 μL PicoGreen stock solution to the TE and mix by vortexing. This produces a 1:200 dilution of the original PicoGreen stock. Keep solution protected from light until ready to use (*see* **Note 35**).
4. Darken the room and, using a multichannel pipette, transfer 100 μL of diluted PicoGreen solution to each well containing reference standard or sample dsDNA.

Fluorimetry

1. Turn on the fluorimeter to warm up for 10 min and load the appropriate software application (*see* **Note 35**).
2. Place the 96-well plate on the instrument and start the protocol.
3. Read the second plate immediately after the first.
4. Construct two standard curves to cover the entire range of concentrations. The first curve should include concentrations from 0 to 0.78125 ng/μl. The second curve should include 1.5625–12.5 ng/μl and the blank.
5. Ensure that the standard curve has an R^2 value of each curve is 0.98 or greater and that each point for which there is a visible band on the E-gel gives a positive value. If not, redo dilution of standards and samples and repeat fluorimetry.
6. Ensure that sample readings fall within the range of the standard curve. If any sample readings exceed the highest standard curve value, dilute those samples, re-assay them and take the dilution factor into account when calculating the final concentration.
7. Use the appropriate standard curve (as determined by the Relative Fluorescence reading) to calculate the concentration of each amplicon.

3.7 Amplicon Dilutions and Pooling for emPCR

Initial dilution

1. Use the GS GType HLA Assay Amplicon Dilution Calculator available at http://www.454.com/my454 to calculate "custom" dilutions of amplicons. This tool allows the input of PicoGreen data and will output the amount of TE and amplicon

necessary for the normalization of each sample, i.e., the dilution of each sample to 1×10^9 molecules/µl (*see* **Note 36**).

2. To a 2 ml deep well plate, add the specified amount of TE to each well, maintaining the MR and HR plate layout.
3. Add the specified amount of amplicon to each well, being sure to use a clean tip for each amplicon.
4. Perform dilutions for all plates.

Pooling

1. In a 1.5 ml microfuge tube, with an O-ring cap, make emPCR Pool 1 (initial dilution) by mixing 5 µl of each diluted amplicon from plate MR-1 plus HR-1. Vortex well.
2. As in **step 1** above, make emPCR Pool 2 (initial dilution) by mixing 5 µl of each diluted amplicon from plate MR-2 plus HR-2. Likewise, construct emPCR Pools 3 and 4 (initial dilution) using MR-3 plus HR-3 and MR-4 plus HR-4, respectively

Final dilutions

1. Pipet 495 µl of TE into a new 1.5 ml microfuge tube with an O-ring cap. Add 5 µl of the emPCR Pool 1 (initial dilution) made in **step 1**. Dilute emPCR Pools 2, 3 and 4 (initial dilutions) in a like manner to make these intermediate dilutions (1×10^7 molecules/µl).
2. Dilute the intermediate dilution pools one final time by pipetting 495 µl of TE into a new 1.5 ml microfuge tube with an O-ring cap. Add 5 µl of the emPCR Pool 1 (intermediate dilution) to make the final dilution. Dilute emPCR intermediate Pools 2, 3, and 4 in a like manner to make the final dilutions. Store these final dilutions (1×10^6 molecules/µl) at −20 °C in a 1.5 ml tube with an O-ring cap (*see* **Note 37**).

3.8 Emulsion PCR, Emulsion Breaking, Sequencing and Genotyping Guidelines

1. For *each* of the four final pools, make 8 A and 8 B emulsions, each with 0.4 cpb (copies per bead) i.e., 3 µl of the above dilution per emulsion (6.8×10^6 beads) following the directions in the GS FLX emPCR Method Manual—LibA MV from 454 (*see* **Note 38**).
2. After enrichment and processing for sequencing, following the GS FLX Sequencing Method Manual, load 590,000 beads per region (*see* **Note 39**) on a 70×75 PTP fitted with a four-region gasket. Load Pool 1 in region 1, Pool 2 in region 2, and similarly for Pools 3 and 4.
3. Place the PTP in the GS-FLX instrument and start the amplicon sequencing process.
4. Following sequencing genotyping can be performed by use of various software. We particularly recommend use of Conexio

Genomics Assign ATF 454 which is available directly from Conexio Genomics (Perth Australia).

5. Information critical to high quality genotyping is found in the FAQ document that accompanies the GS GType HLA primer sets and is available at http://www.454.com/my454.

4 Notes

1. To avoid contamination with small amounts of DNA that can result from handling, pipette tips should be purchased already in racks.
2. For some applications, it may be sufficient to have one negative control per run on the GS FLX. In such cases, one negative control and 43 samples can be run. It is also advisable to have one or more samples be a positive control (for example a well-characterized cell line with known genotypes) for each run.
3. The work surface of all dead air boxes (both pre- and post-PCR and pre- and post-emPCR) and hoods should be wiped down with a mild detergent solution, followed by 10 % bleach, followed by 70 % ethanol and then 15′ of UV light both before and after each use. This procedure should be followed for the vortex, minifuge, and pipettes that are used in each dead air box. Gloves and lab coats should be changed when moving between any of the following areas: pre-PCR, post-PCR, pre-emPCR, post-emPCR areas.
4. We highly recommend that the TE solution used throughout the entire sequencing procedure have a low concentration of EDTA (10 mM Tri, 0.1 mM EDTA pH 8.0 ± 0.1). This assures the presence of adequate Mg^{2+} in PCR steps.
5. The manufacturing source of glycerol is important. Aged or impure glycerol can cause general failure in PCR. Glycerol stock should be 100 %, Molecular Biology grade from Sigma Aldrich. To make 80 % (w/v) Glycerol: Place a 100 ml graduated cylinder with a stir bar in the bottom on a balance. Tare the balance. Slowly pour add 80 g of glycerol into the cylinder. Add water to 100 ml. Stir until homogeneous. Remove the stir bar. Add water to 100 ml. Cover with Parafilm® (SPI Supplies, West Chester, PA, USA) and mix. Transfer to a bottle with 150 ml volume. Only 6 ml is required but it is most convenient to make a larger volume for autoclaving.
6. Use of other thermal cyclers *may* be possible. However, it is well known that performance of different brands/models of thermal cyclers vary even if the thermal profile is programmed to be the same.

7. Dilute 420 ml of 100 % non-denatured alcohol to 600 ml with water.
8. The specific type of plate required will depend on the fluorimeter used, see specific fluorimeter manual for details. For Molecular Devices Spectra MAX: Costar or VWR plates are suitable.
9. Since emulsion dispensing may produce aerosols, emulsions may be dispensed in a dead air box separate from the one in which the emulsions are made. These dead air boxes can be in the same post-genomic PCR room. This room is pre-emPCR. At CHRCO, one post-genomic PCR room dead air box is used for making the emulsions, and the emulsions are carefully dispensed on a bench.
10. We have used both the Bio-Rad Tetrad DNA Engine with four Alpha unit reaction modules (i.e., one Tetrad has four blocks and is equivalent to four individual thermal cyclers) and the ABI GeneAmp™ PCR System 9700 with 96-well gold-plated silver block, set on the ABI 9600 simulation mode. Use of other thermal cyclers is not recommended as the performance of different brands/models of thermal cyclers does vary, even if the thermal profile is programmed to be the same.
11. If possible, emulsion breaking should take place in a post-PCR room separate from the post PCR room where emulsion preparation takes place.
12. Since emulsion breaking can produce aerosols, disposable lab coats should be used.
13. We use the Beckman Coulter X-12 or X-15, the Allegra X-15R centrifuge, or the Eppendorf Centrifuge 5430 for this step.
14. Performing bead washing and enrichment manually, employing the Magnetic Particle Concentrator, is laborious. We recommend the use of the robotic enrichment module, i.e., REMe (Roche Applied Science), which requires a liquid handler for use. The REMe is compatible with numerous liquid handlers including, but not limited to, Hamilton Star or Starlet, Biomek Fx, Tecan Genesis, HP Multiprobe. Some liquid handlers may require modification of the deck to accommodate the REMe's height while still allowing use of 1 ml tips to pipette the large volumes involved. Our first hand experiences have been with the HP Multiprobe, the Biomek Fx, and the Tecan Genesis robots.
15. The GS FLX Plus or GS Junior may also be used. In the latter case, the appropriate reagents and equipment (e.g., Bead Deposition Device) must be used and 5–6 samples may be genotyped per run.

16. This genomic PCR procedure is for processing eight plates; it is assumed there are eight thermal cycler blocks available. If there are fewer, adjust the procedure accordingly.
17. This step helps to solubilize the primers, which are dried down in the microwell plates. It helps to reduce the number of amplicon dropouts and the amount of primer dimer formed.
18. The formulation nominally makes enough for 720 reactions. The difference from the GS GType HLA protocol is as follows: (1) less water is used in the master mix due to the pre-solubilization of the primers in the previous step, and (2) we use a 100 mM dNTP blend (each nucleotide at 25 mM) rather than a 40 mM dNTP blend (each nucleotide at 10 mM). If the 40 mM dNTP solution is substituted, be sure to make the appropriate adjustment.
19. While it is desirable to include at least one negative sample per plate when beginning to perform runs, thereafter it is sufficient to include one negative sample per run. Column 11 can then, instead, be used for a sample; there is no qualitative or quantitative difference in the primers in column 11 that make them especially suitable for a negative control. In fact, it is preferable in successive runs, to rotate the position that will be occupied by the negative control. This will make it more likely that any contamination (while extremely rare in our hands) can be detected.
20. We recommend inclusion of at least one positive control (e.g., a cell line of known HLA genotype). This can be placed in any column of a plate set (MR+HR). We recommend rotating its position from run to run.
21. If the amount of DNA available is limiting, much less can be used for each well. We have observed robust amplification using 2 ng. If necessary, you may increase the number of PCR cycles to 35. With less DNA, more primer dimer may initially be formed but can be removed by the PicoGreen procedure described in this protocol. Be sure the DNA is added to the master mix in a 2 μl volume.
22. If an 8-channel micropipette is used to pipette by columns (instead of rows), it is imperative that tips be changed after each transfer to avoid cross-contamination of samples.
23. It is of utmost importance to seal plates tightly. If this is not achieved, evaporation will occur in the wells during thermal cycling and amplicons may drop out. Pay strict attention to the recommendations made regarding brand of seals to use.
24. Note that, compared to the thermal cycling protocol in the GS GType HLA primer manual we recommend use of a modified thermal profile. We have decreased the number of cycles to

reduce the amount of DRB crossover products generated, and added a 72 °C extension step during cycling. The latter changes are useful for more robust generation of long amplicons. The DRB crossover products are a minor in vitro PCR artifact that is revealed by NGS; the ability to detect this readily identifiable population of sequences increases with clonal sequencing because we can detect very minor sequence populations [5].

25. It is of utmost importance, during handling amplicons, to avoid cross-contamination between plates (e.g., contamination of MR-1 with MR-2) because the same MIDs are used for sample identification on each MR plate and each HR plate. ALWAYS change tips between plates.

26. The GS GType protocol specifies use of 22.5 μl. We recommend a slightly smaller volume since less AMPure XP reagent can be used, giving a cost savings.

27. We prefer elution with this larger volume, rather than the 10 μl specified in the GS GType HLA primer protocol, since it assures that the pellets on the magnetic ring stand are fully covered and, thus, complete elution is favored. In addition, a greater volume of eluent makes handling in successive steps easier.

28. A small amount of transfer of pellet in some of the wells is difficult to avoid and is acceptable. In subsequent steps, including gels, quantification and dilution, take care to avoid, as best as possible, any beads that may have carried through.

29. Alternatively, you may perform gel electrophoresis of the amplicons on a standard agarose gel set-up. However, since E-gels are very thin we find them to be much more sensitive. Additionally, the buffer-less system is neat and convenient.

30. This purpose of these gels is only to determine if amplicon has been made and if it is free of primer dimer (not to estimate the size of amplicons). The amplicons run approximately to the top of the well in the adjacent lane. Primer-dimer runs substantially below this.

31. Sometimes, even if no band is visible on a gel, it is possible to detect the amplicon in sequencing since only an extremely small amount of amplicon is necessary.

32. Although it is advisable to make batches of standards in these quantities, do not process more than two amplicon plates at a time because the PicoGreen reagent is light sensitive.

33. Compared to the GS GType HLA protocol, we recommend making two lower concentration standards and, since the concentration of amplicons is generally well below 12 ng/μl, tubes 1 and 2 are not used. You may save the remainder in them to make a smaller amount of the more dilute standards in case a repeat assay of some samples is necessary.

34. Thawing may take greater than 30 min if the vial is full.
35. In order to minimize deterioration of the light sensitive PicoGreen dye, be sure the fluorimeter has been warmed up prior to dilution of the PicoGreen stock.
36. Careful normalizations assure more closely balanced read depths during sequencing. Care should be taken in pipetting. This step can be performed by a liquid handler with a span-eight head that allows for "cherry picking." If such an instrument is available, a file that enumerates the quantities of TE and each amplicon necessary for appropriate dilution can be generated using Microsoft Excel. This file, in turn, can be read by numerous brands of liquid handlers.
37. It is good to store initial, intermediate, and final dilutions for future use as these pools are of sufficient quantity for many emulsions.
38. The GS FLX emPCR Method Manual—LibA MV from 454 recommends the general use a much higher number of copies per bead [4–6]. In our experience, use of such high cpb with this HLA system gives an undesirably high percentage of dot and mixed reads during sequencing.
39. We load 75 % of the number of beads recommended in the GS FLX Sequencing Method Manual (v. Nov 2010). This lower bead density yields favorable numbers of sequence reads which is reflected in the percent passed filter. Our Percent Passed Filter ranges from approximately 28–55 %. Within this range (or higher), acceptable genotyping is obtainable using Conexio Assign ATF 454 v34 software.

Acknowledgments

The authors would like to thank Henry Erlich, Martha Ladner, David Noonan, and Melinda Rastrou for their thoughtful reading of the manuscript. We would also like to acknowledge Damian Goodridge for the development of the genotyping software, and Kazu Osoegawa, Martha Ladner, Franziska Cohen, Sherry Hawbecker, David Noonan for setting this system up and sequencing all the samples in the CHORI lab. We would also like to acknowledge Priscilla Moonsamy and Bryan Hoglund for their contributions to initial development of primers and protocols. E. Trachtenberg is supported in part by NIH grants 2UO1AI067068 and 2P01CA111412.

References

1. Margulies M, Egholm M, Altman WE, Attiya S, Bader JS, Bemben LA, Berka J, Braverman MS, Chen YJ, Chen Z, Dewell SB, Du L, Fierro JM, Gomes XV, Godwin BC, He W, Helgesen S, Ho CH, Irzyk GP, Jando SC, Alenquer ML, Jarvie TP, Jirage KB, Kim JB, Knight JR, Lanza JR, Leamon JH, Lefkowitz SM, Lei M, Li J, Lohman KL, Lu H, Makhijani VB, McDade KE, McKenna MP, Myers EW, Nickerson E, Nobile JR, Plant R, Puc BP, Ronan MT, Roth GT, Sarkis GJ, Simons JF, Simpson JW, Srinivasan M, Tartaro KR, Tomasz A, Vogt KA, Volkmer GA, Wang SH, Wang Y, Weiner MP, Yu P, Begley RF, Rothberg JM (2005) Genome sequencing in microfabricated high-density picolitre reactors. Nature 437:376–380
2. Holcomb CL, Hoglund B, Anderson MW, Blake LA, Bohme I, Egholm M, Ferriola D, Gabriel C, Gelber SE, Goodridge D, Hawbecker S, Klein R, Ladner M, Lind C, Monos D, Pando MJ, Proll J, Sayer DC, Schmitz-Agheguian G, Simen BB, Thiele B, Trachtenberg EA, Tyan DB, Wassmuth R, White S, Erlich HA (2010) A multi-site study using high-resolution HLA genotyping by next generation sequencing. Tissue Antigens 77:206–217
3. Bentley G, Higuchi R, Hoglund B, Goodridge D, Sayer D, Trachtenberg EA, Erlich HA (2009) High-resolution, high-throughput HLA genotyping by next-generation sequencing. Tissue Antigens 74:393–403
4. Skibola CF, Akers NK, Conde L, Ladner M, Hawbecker SK, Cohen F, Ribas F, Erlich HA, Goodridge D, Trachtenberg EA, Smith MT, Bracci PM (2012) Multi-locus HLA class I and II allele and haplotype associations with follicular lymphoma. Tissue Antigens 79:279–286
5. Trachtenberg E, Ladner M, Osoegawa K, Cohen F, Hawbecker S, Ribas F, Noonan D, White S, Graham K, Agraz J, Mohr K, Vinson M, Goodridge D (2011) Want a good read? Next-generation HLA sequencing using the Roche 454 GS FLX platform for five NIH projects. Hum Immunol 72:S124
6. Rastrou M, Holcomb CL, Williams TC, Goodridge D, Lazaro AM, Tilanus M, Erlich HA. (2012) In vitro generated PCR crossover products identified by next-generation sequencing correspond to SOM. Human Immunology, Supplement, 12-OR

References

Chapter 11

Chimerism Testing by Quantitative PCR Using Indel Markers

Ketevan Gendzekhadze, Laima Gaidulis, and David Senitzer

Abstract

Engraftment monitoring is critical for patients after Hematopoietic Stem Cell Transplantation (HSCT). Complete donor chimerism is the goal; therefore, early detection of rejection and relapse is crucial for guiding the patient post HSCT treatment. Quantitative PCR for chimerism testing has been reported to be highly sensitive. In this chapter we discuss the quantitative PCR (qPCR) method using 34 Indel (Insertion and Deletion) genetic markers spread over 20 different chromosomes.

Key words Chimerism, Quantitative PCR, Informative markers, Engraftment

1 Introduction

In Greek mythology, the Chimera was a monstrous hybrid creature composed of several different animals: lion, goat, and snake. A human chimera would contain two or more genetically distinct types of cells. A chimera can be the result of blood transfusions, pregnancy, fraternal twin transfer in utero, solid organ transplant, or hematopoietic stem cell transplantation (HSCT). In the latter case the origin of the cells circulating in the blood or populating the bone marrow is useful to determine the chimeric state of the recipient. The recipient should have only donor cells. Early detection of recipient cells can be indicative of graft-versus-host disease (GVHD), rejection, and/or recurrent malignancy. Chimerism testing can be useful for the detection of donor cell engraftment in HSCT regardless of the source of the stem cells, i.e., bone marrow, mobilized peripheral blood stem cells (PBSC), or umbilical cord blood stem cells.

This is accomplished by the identification of genetic markers that are unique to the patient and those that are unique to the donor. Prior to transplantation, samples from the patient and the donor are evaluated using blood, buccal swab, or saliva. The chimeric state of

Andrea A. Zachary and Mary S. Leffell (eds.), *Transplantation Immunology: Methods and Protocols, Second Edition*, Methods in Molecular Biology, vol. 1034, DOI 10.1007/978-1-62703-493-7_11,

the recipient is described as "microchimerism" when the amount of recipient cells is <1 %; while "full Chimerism" indicates the complete lymphohematopoietic replacement with donor cells; if host cells are detected at >1 %, then the term "mixed chimerism" is used [1].

In HSCT the interaction of donor T-cells with host-derived antigen-presenting cells (APC) is essential not only for GVHD, but also in graft versus leukemia (GVL) effect [2]. The picture is more abstruse taking into consideration the use of T cell depleted donors and pre-transplant conditioning regimens. Non-myeloablative or reduced intensity conditioning regimens, together with post-transplant immunosuppressive treatments, emphasize the importance of documenting the source of the chimerism: either myeloid and/or lymphoid chimerism [3]. Lineage-specific chimerism can be performed using purified subsets of peripheral blood cells as $CD3^+$, $CD4^+$, $CD8^+$, $CD19^+$, $CD34^+$, $CD56^+$ [4–6]. "Split chimerism" is used when one lineage is host and the other is of donor origin, e.g., myeloid cells are 100 % host and T cells are 100 % donor.

The set of guidelines for chimerism testing after HSCT has been published in 2001 [1]. The technique used should be sensitive and informative; should be checked at 1, 3, 6, and 12 months post-transplant; and the source of sample is very important (bone marrow and/or peripheral blood). The lineage-specific chimerism should be considered for non-myeloablative and reduced-intensity conditioning.

Chimerism testing is used to detect donor cell engraftment in HSCT as a routine, and to check identity of the engrafted cells after multiple cord transplantation. Patients with inadequate marrow function, candidates for donor lymphocyte infusion (DLI), or for second transplant should be closely evaluated for chimerism.

The number of tested loci, and/or alleles per locus must be sufficient so that informative markers for donor and recipient can be identified. Numerous genetic markers have been tested to determine chimerism, e.g., blood group antigens (ABO, NM, Rh, Kell, Kidd, Duff, Ss, P), immunoglobulin isotypes, sex chromosome markers, Human Leukocyte Antigens (HLA); polymorphic loci with variable number of tandem repeats (VNTR), short tandem repeats (STR); single nucleotide polymorphisms (SNP) and insertion and/or deletion (Indel) variations. Detection methods have also varied, e.g., mixed agglutination, flow cytometry, fluorescent in situ hybridization (FISH), restriction fragment length polymorphism (RFLP), Southern blot, and several PCR based methods, including quantitative PCR. The ideal genetic marker system is comprised of a high number of polymorphic loci, with both frequent alleles per loci in different ethnic groups, not restricted to gender, easily detectable using highly sensitive laboratory technique. STR-PCR is currently the most widely used technique, due its high informativity and reliability. STR sequences are microsatellites of two to eight base pairs, which are repeated numerous times in a tandem in the genome, therefore, each STR locus has several alleles and the use of different loci can discriminate nearly any recipient and donor pair, regardless of sex [7]. Pre-transplant recipient, donor and post-transplant samples are first amplified in multiplex PCR reactions, using extremely small amounts of starting material, a big advantage for patients with severe leucopenia. The fluorescently labeled PCR amplicons are detected using capillary electrophoresis with an allelic ladder as a reference. The fluorescence intensity of the informative markers is used to calculate the percentage of the recipient cells in the post-transplant samples. The major problems with this method are low sensitivity (1–5 %) and difficult interpretation steps, including the existence of stutter bands (amplicons containing one less repeat than the normal allele).

Early detection of rejection and relapse post-HSCT may influence the therapeutic strategies for patient management. Quantitative PCR (qPCR) for chimerism testing has been reported to demonstrate a sensitivity of 0.1 %. In this chapter, we discuss a qPCR chimerism method using Indel (Insertion and deletion) genetic markers. Since each Indel locus is bi-allelic, a large number of loci should be analyzed to reach a similar discrimination rate of STR-PCR. The method uses a panel of 34 Indel loci, distributed on 20 different chromosomes. The test is comprised of two major steps, screening and quantification. The amount of DNA for each reaction is much higher compared with STR-PCR. Also, to insure accuracy of qPCR, each quantification reaction uses a pre-transplant DNA sample. There are no stutter bands to complicate the interpretation. We think that the ability to detect early changes in chimerism with greater accuracy would be beneficial in monitoring and predicting of post-transplant adverse clinical events.

2 Materials

1. Sample requirements:
   Whole blood (10 ml), buccal swab, saliva, or bone marrow (in ACD or EDTA tubes) sample from the patient pre-transplantation is required for the identification of patient-specific markers. Donor peripheral blood, buccal swab, or saliva can be used to identify informative markers for the donor(s). The amount of DNA required is 1 μg from each source.
2. Laboratory equipment:
   A standard complement of equipment is required including calibrated pipettes, single and repeating (dispensing 0.5–20 μl; 20–200 μl, 200–1,000 μl), aerosol resistant tips, gloves, a vortex mix, and a microcentrifuge for 1.5 ml tubes, as well as a centrifuge with microtiter plate assembly. Applied Biosystems 7500 Sequence Detection System (SDS Software Version 1.4) and

AlleleSEQR® Suite Chimerism Analysis Software (#5002696 Celera-Version 1.2 Build 1) are used for the analysis.

3. Plasticware:
   1.5 ml microcentrifuge tubes, MicroAmp Optical 96-well Reaction Plate (ABI #N801-0560), MicroAmp Optical Adhesive Film (ABI #4311971), MicroAmp Adhesive Film Applicator (ABI#433183), AlleleSEQR® Chimerism Screening Plate (#5002645 Celera (15–30 °C)).

4. PCR reagents:
   5× PCR Master Mix (#F78885X25, Celera (−15 °C)).
   Positive control marker CA999 which contains two pair of primers and one dual-labeled probe to a segment of the RNase P gene (#F79995X25, Celera (−15 °C)).
   Molecular Grade Water (Sigma).
   34 CR Primer-probe mixes (#F70015X25 to #F0345x25 Celera (−15 °C)).

3 Methods

Summary: AlleleSEQR® chimerism detection of engraftment is a quantitative PCR assay based on a panel of 34 insertion/deletion (Indel) markers. Recipient pre-transplant (PRE) and donor (DON) DNA samples are first screened against the 34 Indel marker panel. A list of recipient-specific and a list of donor-specific informative markers are identified by the screening assay. Quantitation of the recipient cells in the post-transplant sample is performed by qPCR on recipient pre-transplant and post-transplant DNA samples using recipient-specific informative markers. A cycle threshold (ΔΔCT) relative quantitation formula is used to calculate the percentage of the recipient cells in the post-transplant sample by the AlleleSEQR® Suite beta program as shown in Fig. 1 [8] (*see* **Note 1** in case AlleleSEQR® is not available).

3.1 Cell Separation

When lineage-specific chimerism is ordered, enriched cell subsets are prepared by positive selection using magnetic beads. Sorted cells also can be used. Whole Blood (WB) Micro Beads from Miltenyi for CD3 (#130-090-874), CD4 (#130-090-877), CD8 (#130-090-878), CD14 (#130-090-879), CD15 (#130-091-058) and CD19 (#130-090-880) were incubated with peripheral blood (PB) or bone marrow (BM) and separated by AutoMACS Separator according to the manufacturer's instructions. A single-cell suspension devoid of dead cells and cell debris is the prerequisite for efficient cell separation; therefore, it is highly recommended to filter the bone marrow specimen before cell subset separation or DNA isolation.

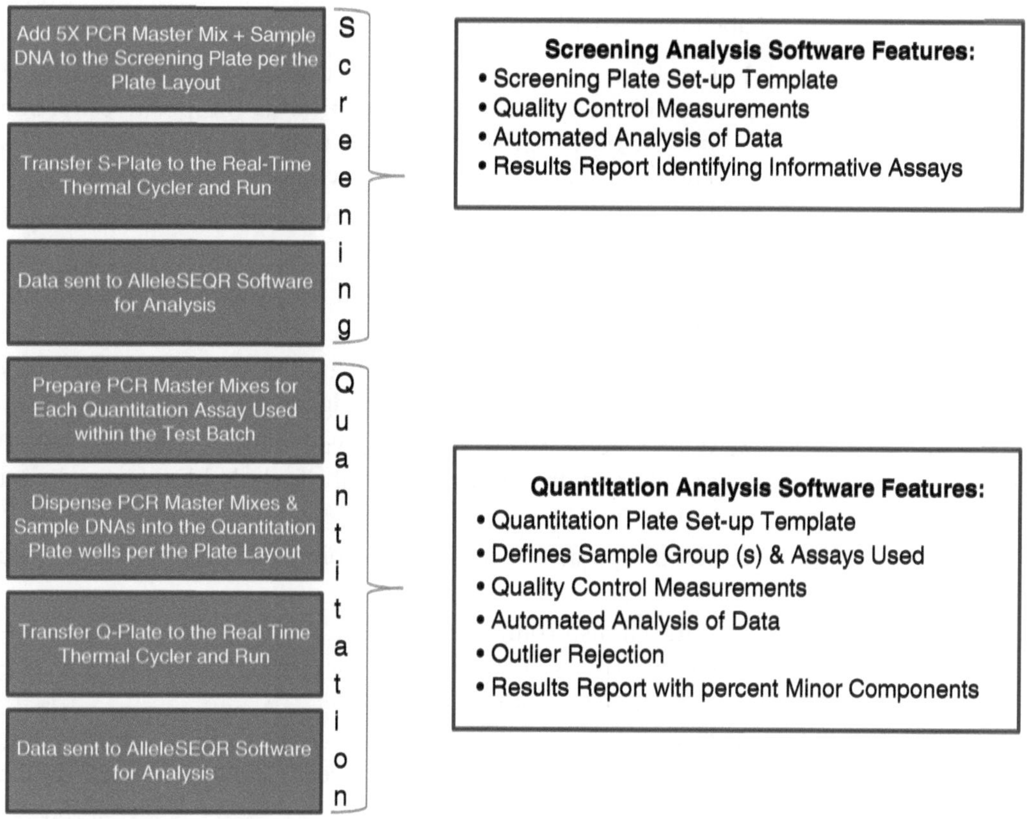

Fig. 1 Assay workflow. The test consists of two steps: screening and quantification. The screening identifies informative markers in PRE and DON samples, which are selected for quantification

Steps for filtering Bone Marrow:

1. Place 30 nm nylon Pre-Separation Filter (AutoMACS #130-041-407) on a 15 ml conical tube labeled with the patient information.
2. Wet Pre-Separation Filter by vigorously pipetting 500 μl running buffer (autoMACS Pro Running Buffer #130-091-221) into reservoir. Discard effluent.
3. Pipet bone marrow suspension (minimum 500 μl, maximum 3,500 μl) into reservoir of Pre-Separation Filter.
4. Allow cell suspension to run through and wash with 2–3× 500 μl running buffer.
5. Spin sample for 10 min at 280 × *g* (no brake). Remove supernatant. If needed, concentrate cells to 1–2 ml before proceeding below. Bone marrow specimen is ready for CD3 cell population or DNA isolation.

Labeling cells with magnetic beads:

1. Label three 15 ml conical tubes with the patient information and subset type. Label one conical as the positive fraction and the other as the negative fraction, e.g., CD3+ and CD3–. The third tube is the "working" conical.
2. Mix ACD tube well and add 2 ml whole blood to conical #1 (working conical)
3. Add 100 μl MACS Whole Blood Microbeads per 2 ml anticoagulated whole blood.
4. Mix well on vortexer (speed 7) and incubate in an open rack for 15 min at 4–8 °C (in the refrigerator).
5. With a sterile transfer pipette, wash cells by adding 5–10 ml of cold running buffer per 1 ml of whole blood; cap, invert to mix.
6. Centrifuge at 280 × *g* for 10 min at room temperature, no brake.
7. Without disturbing the cell pellet, carefully pipet off the supernatant. To avoid cell loss, leave a residual volume of supernatant (approx. 1–2 mm in height).
8. Resuspend cell pellet by making a 1:2 dilution with running buffer. Vortex gently. Do not invert. The final volume should not exceed 3.5 ml.
9. Proceed to the magnetic separation step using the AutoMACS separator. This last step can also be done manually.

3.2 DNA Isolation

Both recipient pre-transplant and donor samples are required for the screening test to identify the informative markers. Genomic DNA is extracted from PB or BM using Qiagen EZ1 DNA Blood 350 μl Kit (#951054) with the EZ1 Workstation. Genomic DNA is extracted from cell subsets using QIAamp DNA Blood Mini Kit (#51106). The whole genome amplification (WGA) technique is used to increase the quantity of DNA whenever needed. DNA is first amplified by Qiagen REPLI-g Midi-Kit (#150045) with Multiple Displacement Amplification (MDA) technology then purified with Qiagen QIAamp DNA Mini Kit (#51304). DNA concentrations are determined using the NanoDrop ND-1000 Spectrophotometer.

3.3 DNA Dilution for Screening Test

The goal of the screening is to identify patient pre-transplantation (PRE) and donor (DON) specific informative markers. Two DNA samples, donor and patient pre-transplant, are screened against panel of 34 primer pairs called CA001-034. Each AlleleSEQR® Chimerism Screening plate (Fig. 2), already contains marker specific primers that accommodate one pair of donor and patient samples; rows A, B, C contain Patient DNA; E, F, G—donor DNA; D and H remain empty. It is recommended to add from 1 to 10 ng of DNA per well

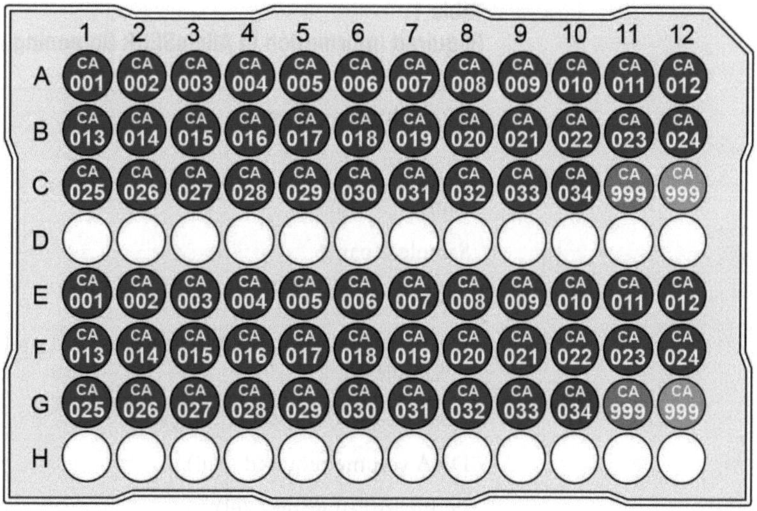

Fig. 2 Layout of screening plate. The 96-well screening plate contains 34 primer pairs located A1–C10 and E1–G10, Wells C11, C12, G11, G12 have primers called CA999 for internal controls. PRE and DON DNA are added in rows: A, B, C for PRE and E, F, G for DON; D, H stays empty. Negative controls, which do not contain DNA are wells C12 and G12

of the screening plate. Volume for samples 1 (PRE) and 2 (DON) is calculated for 37 wells. 25 μl mix containing diluted DNA and 5× PCR Buffer, is dispensed per well. Calculations are facilitated using the AlleleSEQR® software; based on DNA concentration, the program estimates proportions for each component of the PCR reaction. The software of AlleleSEQR® Screening Module is comprised of four windows: Test information, Test preparation, Start test, Test analysis. Following the basic instructions and filling in all the information asked for in **step 1**, the software automatically calculates proportions for DNA dilutions and provides a detailed procedure protocol for **step 2**.

1. Enter all required information in AlleleSEQR Screening module as shown in Table 1.

   Calculations are based on the formula, using:

   Υ ng of DNA per well,

   X ng/μl DNA

   Required DNA volume is $Z = (\Upsilon / X) \times 37$ μl

   For example 10 ng/μl DNA concentration, using 5 ng per well, Z would = 18.5 μl.

2. Label three 1.5 ml microcentrifuge tubes as:

   (1) Patient DNA ID

   (2) Donor DNA ID

   (3) NTC (No Template Control)

Table 1
Required information in AlleleSEQR Screening module

Screening test name	
Operator ID	
Sample 1 name	Patient DNA
Sample 2 name	Donor DNA
Plate lot number	
DNA concentrations (ng/μl) for Sample 1 and Sample 2	Varies
Amount of DNA per well (ng)[a]	1, 2, 5, or 10 ng
DNA volume required (/μl)	Automatic calculation
PCR certified water (/μl)	Automatic calculation
Modified TE buffer/water lot number	

[a]We use 5 ng DNA/well

Table 2
Example calculations of proportions for DNA dilutions using 5 ng of 10 ng/μl PRE and DON DNA

PCR master mix/DNA sample reaction	Patient DNA (μl)	Donor DNA (μl)	NTC
PCR certified water	721.5	721.5	60 μl
5× PCR Master Mix	185	185	15 μl
DNA sample (μl)[a]	18.5	18.5	NA
Total volume of sample reaction mix	925	925	75 μl

[a]Z = 18.5 μl for 10 ng/μl DNA concentration, using 5 ng per well

Each PCR Master Mix/DNA sample reaction includes:

*Z*μl DNA + (740 − *Z*) μl water + 185 μl of 5× PCR Buffer = 925 μl Total. Negative Controls (NTC) mix contains = 60 μl water + 15 μl of 5× PCR Buffer = 75 μl total volume, as shown in the table provided by the software setup protocol. Table 2 illustrates examples of calculations using 5 ng of 10 ng/μl PRE and DON DNA.

3. Dispense 25 μl of the reaction Mix for Sample 1 into wells A1-C11 of the screening plate and 25 μl of the reaction Mix for Sample 2 into wells E1-G11.
4. Dispense 25 μl of the Reaction Mix for NTC to wells C12 and G12 (Fig. 2).

Assay	Chrom	PRE	DON	Result
CA001	8	-	-	Not Informative
CA002	14	+	-	Informative for PRE
CA003	18	+	+	Not Informative
CA004	13	+	+	Not Informative
CA005	13	-	+	Informative for DON

Fig. 3 Analysis view. Only 5 markers are shown from 34 total. *First column*—Primer marker name, *second column*—chromosome location, *third and fourth columns* indicate if the marker was Present (+) or Absent (–) in each sample (PRE and DON), and the *last column* shows the outcome

5. Seal the plate with adhesive film using applicator, vortex, and centrifuge to collect the contents at the bottom of the wells and load into RT-PCR Instrument.
6. Power on the instrument and make sure the plate orientation is correct, well A1 is oriented to the back left corner, then click *Run Test* button.
7. After the run is done, click the *Analyze Screening test* Data button to analyze the screening test data and display the results window.

The screening report includes four different views:

1. *Analysis view* (Fig. 3)—list of markers, chromosome location, presence or absence in patient (PRE) and donor (DON) sample.

   Informative PRE markers are those present in PRE sample, but absent in DON (+/–) (CA002). Informative DON markers are those present in DON sample, but absent in PRE (–/+) (CA005).

   Non-informative marker are those present or absent in both PRE/DON samples (+/+) or (–/–) respectively (CA001, CA003, CA004). Donor informative markers are especially useful for double cord transplant chimerism interpretation (*see* **Note 2**).
2. *Plate view* of the report (Fig. 4) shows the location of informative markers on the screening plate.
3. *Data view* (Fig. 5) includes raw data, delta C_T, and informative marker information.
4. *Report view* (Fig. 6) contains the Summary of Screening results.

3.4 Quantification Test

The goal of this part is to quantify at least two genetic markers identified in screening process.

	Sample	1	2	3	4	5	6	7	8	9	10	11	12
A	PRE		CA002										
B	PRE												
C	PRE												
D													
E	DON					CA005							
F	DON												
G	DON												
H													

Fig. 4 Plate view. The 96-well layout only shows the location of informative markers. For PRE and DON. In this example, Informative marker CA002 for PRE sample is in well A2, and informative marker CA005 for DON sample is in well E5

Well	Sample	Assay	Start	End	CT	Delta CT	Marker State	Informative	Well Type
1	PRE	CA001	3	15	40	13.6	Negative	NO	Normal
49	DON	CA001	3	15	40	13.6	Negative	NO	Normal
2	PRE	CA002	3	15	29	2.7	Positive	YES	Normal
50	DON	CA002	3	15	40	13.6	Negative	NO	Normal
5	PRE	CA005	3	15	40	13.6	Negative	NO	Normal
53	DON	CA005	3	15	28	2.3	Positive	YES	Normal

Fig. 5 Data view. An example of six wells is shown. The table contains the information from previous views (Figs. 3 and 4). Sorted by Assay is shown here. Wells 1 and 49 of screening plate contain both CA001 marker for PRE and DON, CT raw data is included, and Delta CT is calculated for each marker. Presence and Absence are called here as Negative and Positive, and NO and YES indicate if the marker is informative. Well types can be Normal and Control

3.4.1 Informative Marker Selection

Generally, any informative markers can be used for the quantitation. It is recommended to select two markers from two different chromosomes for the quantitative testing (*see* **Note 3**).

3.4.2 Quantification Set-Up

Quantification module of AlleleSEQR® software also contains four windows:

Step 1—Quantification test information

Step 2—Test preparation

AlleleSEQR Chimerism Screening Plate Report			
Screening test name: TEST			
Operator ID: INITIALS			
Informative Markers for CON10-00592 EMO-11-R PRE			
		Marker:	Chromosome:
		CA002	14
		CA016	17
	Quality Measurments:		
		Amp Control:	Pass
		NTC:	Pass
		Atypical Count:	0
Informative Markers for CON10-00593 EMO-12-D DON			
		Marker:	Chromosome:
		CA005	13
		CA015	5
	Quality Measurments:		
		Amp Control:	Pass
		NTC:	Pass
		Atypical Count:	0
AlleleSEQ	For Research Use Only. Not for use in diagnostic procedures.		
\\fs2\Histotrac\Instrument Interfaces\Q-PCR\Chimerism\ScreeningTests\TEST			
Tuesday, March 20, 2012 11:54:42 AM			

Fig. 6 Report view. This view contains the summary of screening results

Step 3—Start test

Step 4—Test analysis. Each quantification test needs Reference Sample (PRE using patient informative markers or DON, using donor specific markers) and post-transplant sample (s). You can set up several patients (up to four pairs) on the same PCR plate.

3.4.3 Calculation Number of Wells

Each PRE/POST pair needs 20 wells; 2 wells are for PRE informative markers, and 1 well is for internal control, because each sample is run in triplicate number of wells is: $3 \times (2+1) = 9$ for PRE and the same number for POST, 18 wells. 2 additional wells are for Negative Controls of two markers.

Each PCR plate should include Negative Control for CA999 and Negative control for each of the informative markers used in the plate. A maximum of four patient pairs (PRE and POST) can be accommodated in one 96-well PCR plate.

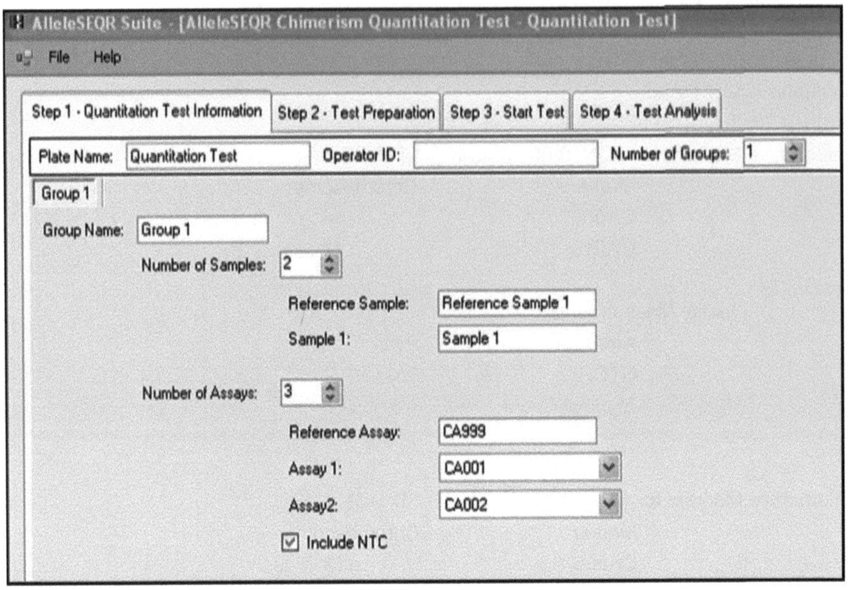

Fig. 7 Quantification test information menu

Each step of the process is described below:

1. Add information about reference and post-transplant samples in Quantification Test Information Menu (Fig. 7):
   (a) Select number of patients in "Number of Group" drop-down menu. If you only have 1 PRE/POST pair, the number of patients is equal to 1. We recommend running two informative markers for PRE, therefore the "number of assays" field equals 3 (two for informative markers and one for internal control CA999).
   (b) Select which Informative Markers you desire to run in drop-down menu, "Assay 1 and Assay 2".
   (c) If you have two post-transplant samples, number of samples will equal 3 (REF, POST 1, and POST 2).
2. Test preparation step:

   Information is taken from **step 1** to prepare three plate layout views:
   (a) For each sample pipet 15 μl of diluted DNA to each well. A sample plate layout is shown in Fig. 8a.
   (b) *DNA dilutions*: DNA quantity used for 10(9+1) reactions is 500 ng. If there is not enough DNA, a minimum of 200 ng DNA should be used for ten reactions (PRE, POST) or we should proceed with Whole Genome Amplification (*see* Subheading 3.2).

   In case of 500 ng and *X* ng/μl DNA, add *Z* = 500/*X* μl DNA + (150 − *Z*) μl water.

   For example, for 20 ng/μl DNA concentration, Mix = 25 μl DNA + 125 μl Water.

a

	1	2	3	4	5	6	7	8	9	10	11	12
A	REF1	REF1	REF1	REF1	REF1	REF1	REF1	REF1	REF1	POST1	POST1	POST1
B	POST1	POST1	POST1	POST1	POST1	POST1	NTC	NTC	NTC			

b

	1	2	3	4	5	6	7	8	9	10	11	12
A	CA999	CA999	CA999	CA001	CA001	CA001	CA002	CA002	CA002	CA999	CA999	CA999
B	CA001	CA001	CA001	CA002	CA002	CA002	CA999	CA001	CA002			

Fig. 8 (**a**) Sample well plate layout. Only rows A and B are shown for the Pre1 and Post1 samples. (**b**) Assay well plate layout. Only A and B rows shown for PRE1/POST1 sample, informative marker CA001 and CA002)

Pipet 15 μl of diluted DNA per well following Sample Well Plate Layout pattern and 15 μl of water in NTC wells.

(c) *Assay-guide for Informative marker pipetting*, 10 μl of each diluted marker (pair of primers). An example of an assay well plate layout is shown in Fig. 8b for pre- and post-samples with the informative markers, CA001 and CA002.

(d) *Informative marker dilutions*: Using Assay Well Plate Layout record the total number of wells (n) needed for each assay. In this example, each marker needs 7 wells. Make dilutions for $n+2$ reaction, in that case, number of reactions would equal 9 (7+2).

Informative Marker Dilution for $(n+2)$ reaction = 5 $(n+2)$ μl marker + 5 $(n+2)$ μl of 5× PCR Buffer.

Example: Using 9 (7+2) reactions, the marker dilution = 45 μl marker + 45 μl of 5× PCR Buffer. Pipet 10 μl of diluted marker into appropriate wells designated in the Assay Well Plate Layout.

3. Start test step:
   Seal the plate with MicroAmp Adhesive Film and spin at 400 × *g* for 1 min and load into Real-Time PCR Instrument.
4. Test analysis:
   Analyzes the quantitation test data and displays the results. The software calculates the average from the triplicates for each informative marker, and % is calculated as an average from both markers (*see* **Note 4** for Interpretation of the results and **Note 5** for using Donor Specific Informative markers).

3.5 Data Analysis Algorithms

The algorithms implemented in AlleleSEQR® Suite Chimerism Analysis Software are hard-coded and warning flags are triggered when the result is outside of recommended range. To be able to troubleshoot and interpret the chimerism test results we will discuss the details of the algorithm.

A. *Screening test algorithm (wells 36 (C12) and 84 (G12)*: NTC is determined as Pass/Fail per sample. The C_T threshold is 38, if $C_T < 38$, the software displays message: "Warning: NTC Quality Measurement Indicates Possible DNA contamination".

B. *Amplification control quality measurement (wells 35 (C11) and 83 (G11)*: The amplification Control well has a C_T value of less than 34, then Amplification Control is determined as Pass. If $C_T > 34$, Amplification control is determined as Failed and displays following warning message: "Warning: Amp Control Quality Measurement indicates input DNA copy number below recommended level". When Amplification control well fails, assays for that sample, having C_T <38 are called "Atypical".

C. *Negative results*: C_T great than 38.

D. *Positive results*: If $C_T < 30$ for the Amplification Control well (CA999), positive ΔC_T range is of −2.0 to +3.5, otherwise the call is "Atypical". If C_T for the Amplification Control (CA999) is less than 34, but greater or equal than 30, positive Δ C_T range is of −2.0 to +2.0, outside of the range is considered "Atypical". High C_T (36–38) means low DNA copy number, and the results are not reliable.

E. *Quantitation Test Algorithm*: Each reaction was setup in triplicate and the mean C_T was applied in the formula for accurate quantitation. The calculations are performed by the AlleleSEQR® Quantitation Software based on the relative quantitation $\Delta\Delta C_T$ method [8]. To simplify the explanation, consider only one marker, e.g., CA001 as an REF (usually patient) informative marker (run in triplicate). Therefore;

Each sample (POST) has 6 C_T values: 3 for CA001, 3 CA999 (POST/CA001; POST/CA999).

REF sample also generates 6 C_T values: 3 for CA001, 3 for CA999 (REF/CA001; REF/CA999).

Formula uses 4 mean C_T: $C_{T\ POST}$/CA001, POST/CA999, REF/CA001, and REF/CA999.

Each Mean C_T generates Standard Deviation. For each POST/CA001 combination:

$\Delta\Delta C_T = (C_{T\ POST}$/CA001 − C_T POST/CA999) − (Mean C_T REF/CA001 − Mean C_T REF/CA999).

Second and third $\Delta\Delta C_T$ are obtained with the same formula, where (Mean C_T REF/CA001 − Mean C_T REF/CA999) is the same number all three times.

Using three $\Delta\Delta C_T$, Mean Minor Component DNA percent (%R) = Mean of three $2^{-\Delta\Delta CT} \times 100$ %.

F. *No Amplification*: Using the previous example there are four examples of NO AMPLIFICATION state:

1. If the mean C_T for **REF/CA999** is greater than 32, and displays message: "No Amplification in<REF sample name>/CA999", it means not enough REF DNA was used.
2. If the C_T of two or more wells in **REF/CA001** is greater than 37 or the mean C_T for the three replicates is greater than 38, and displays warning: "No amplification in <REF sample name>/CA001", it means not enough REF DNA was used.
3. If the C_T of two or more wells in **POST/CA001** is greater than 37 or the mean C_T for the three replicates is greater than 38, and displays warning: "No amplification in <POST sample name>/CA001", it means not enough POST DNA was used.
4. If the C_T of two or more wells in **POST/CA999** is greater than 37 or the mean C_T for the three replicates is greater than 38, and displays warning: "No amplification in <POST sample name>/CA999", it means not enough POST DNA was used.

4 Notes

1. It is possible to use the real-time PCR instrument software, e.g., ABI Sequence Detection System (SDS) software, if AlleleSEQR® is not available. Detector Manager, Reporter Dye and Quencher Dye should be selected. Cycling parameters are as follows:

   10 min at 95 °C, 40 cycles of 10 s at 95 °C and 35 s at 63 °C.

2. *Double Cords transplant or second transplant using different donor.*

   Screening: two screening tests are run: PRE vs. Donor 1 (D1) and PRE vs. Donor 2 (D2).

   Informative Marker Selection: Shared PRE informative markers from Screening 1 and Screening 2 should be selected. Unique D1 markers should be absent in D2 and vice versa. Quantitation for double cords: set up three groups.

	Informative marker	Reference sample	Post sample	Result
Group 1	PRE	PRE	POST	% Patient (R)
Group 2	D1	D1	POST	% Cord 1 (D1)
Group 3	D2	D2	POST	% Cord 2 (D2)

Ideally %R+%D1+%D2=100 %.

Because the test is accurate to detect microchimerism, if the % of reference component is high, %R+%D1+%D2 could be more than 100 %. In this case use the following formula:

$$\%R = \%R / (\%R + \%D1 + \%D2)$$

$$\%D1 = \%D1 / (\%R + \%D1 + \%D2)$$

$$\%D2 = \%D2 / (\%R + \%D1 + \%D2)$$

If the reportable recipient obtained is between 30 and 60 % recipient, repeat the quantitative test with the donor sample as the reference sample (pre). The value obtained should be reported rather than the measurable recipient percentage from the first assay.

3. If only one informative marker is available, cancel Q-PCR tests and order STR instead. The % of recipient is reported as an average. We had reported cases where two markers differ by more than 15 %, explained by cytogenetics results. Those discrepancies should be confirmed using more informative markers or STR. Whenever possible, it is recommended to use the same two markers to follow a patient post transplant.
4. Interpretation
   PRE specific percentage is reported. The report comment changes based on value.

0 %	Complete chimerism; no amplification
<0.1 %	Microchimerism
0.1–5.0 %	Weak chimerism
5.1–10 %	Mixed chimerism
10.1–100 %	Rejection or relapse

5. Check donor specific markers if the % PRE DNA >30 %. qPCR test is more sensitive to detect microchimerism. DON specific markers are also used to detect possible GVHD in organ transplantation, e.g., liver transplant. For Donor Lymphocyte Infusion (DLI) it is also recommended to quantify DON specific markers. The STR test should be used to detect monozygotic twins, because Indels are biallelic; therefore, the probability to have identical alleles in unrelated persons is higher than when using microsatellite markers.

Acknowledgments

Many thanks to Trakulboon, Surathep, Wong, David, and Bost Doug for their critical review of the manuscript.

References

1. Antin JH, Childs R, Filipovich AH, Giralt S, Mackinnon S, Spitzer T, Weisdorf D (2001) Establishment of complete and mixed donor chimerism after allogeneic lymphohematopoietic transplantation: recommendations from a workshop at the 2001 Tandem Meetings of the International Bone Marrow Transplant Registry and the American Society of Blood and Marrow Transplantation. Biol Blood Marrow Transplant 7:473–485
2. Mapara MY, Sykes M (2005) Induction of mixed vs full chimerism to potentiate GVL effects after bone-marrow transplantation. Methods Mol Med 109:469–474
3. Mickelson DM, Sproat L, Dean R, Sobecks R, Rybicki L, Kalaycio M, Pohlman B, Sweetenham J, Andresen S, Bolwell B, Copelan EA (2011) Comparison of donor chimerism following myeloablative and nonmyeloablative allogeneic hematopoietic SCT. Bone Marrow Transplant 46:84–89
4. Montero A, Savani BN, Kurlander R, Read EJ, Leitman SF, Childs R, Solomon SR, Barrett AJ (2005) Lineage-specific engraftment and outcomes after T-cell-depleted peripheral blood stem cell transplant with Flu/Cy/TBI conditioning. Br J Haematol 130:733–739
5. Jaksch M, Uzunel M, Remberger M, Sundberg B, Mattsson J (2005) Molecular monitoring of T-cell chimerism early after allogeneic stem cell transplantation may predict the occurrence of acute GVHD grades II-IV. Clin Transplant 19:346–349
6. Scheffold C, Kroeger M, Zuehlsdorf M, Tchinda J, Silling G, Bisping G, Stelljes M, Buechner T, Berdel WE, Kienast J (2004) Prediction of relapse of acute myeloid leukemia in allogeneic transplant recipients by marrow CD34+ donor cell chimerism analysis. Leukemia 18:2048–2050
7. Senitzer D, Gaidulis L (2001) Short tandem repeat (STR) analysis of engraftment in allogeneic stem cell transplantation. ASHI Q 25:49–53
8. Livak KJ, Schmittgen TD (2001) Analysis of relative gene expression data using real-time quantitative PCR and the 2(-Delta Delta C(T)) method. Methods 25:402–408

Chapter 12

Gene-Specific PCR Typing of Killer Cell Immunoglobulin-Like Receptors

Raja Rajalingam and Elham Ashouri

Abstract

By interacting with specific HLA class I molecules, the killer cell immunoglobulin-like receptors (KIR) regulate the effector function of natural killer (NK) cells and subsets of CD8 T cells. The KIR receptors and HLA class I ligands are encoded by unlinked polymorphic gene families located on different human chromosomes, 19 and 6, respectively. The number and type of KIR genes are substantially variable between individuals, which may contribute to human diversity in responding to infection, malignancy and allogeneic transplants. PCR typing using sequence-specific primers (PCR-SSP) is the most commonly used method to determine KIR gene content. This chapter describes a step-by-step protocol for PCR-SSP typing to identify the presence and absence of all 16 known KIR genes. Moreover, the chapter provides the basic rules to verify the accuracy of KIR genotyping results and explains specific methods for the data analysis.

Key words Killer-cell immunoglobulin like receptors, KIR receptors, Natural killer (NK) cell receptors, KIR genotyping, KIR typing, Innate immune receptors, Leukocyte receptor complex (LRC)

1 Introduction

Killer cell immunoglobulin-like receptors (KIR) that recognize certain HLA class I molecules are expressed on natural killer (NK) cells and on subsets of T lymphocytes, mostly CD8 cells with memory phenotype [1–4]. Therefore, KIR receptors have the potential to contribute to both innate and adaptive immune responses against infections, tumors, and allogeneic transplants [5–7]. A family of 16 homologous genes clustered at the leukocyte receptor complex on chromosome 19q13.4 encodes KIR receptors [8–10]. Fourteen of which are functional genes encoding receptors that trigger either inhibition (3DL1-3, 2DL1-3, 2DL5) or activation (3DS1, 2DS1-2DS5) or both (2DL4) and two are pseudogenes (2DP1 and 3DP1) that do not encode a cell-surface receptor.

Andrea A. Zachary and Mary S. Leffell (eds.), *Transplantation Immunology: Methods and Protocols, Second Edition*, Methods in Molecular Biology, vol. 1034, DOI 10.1007/978-1-62703-493-7_12, © Springer Science+Business Media, LLC 2013

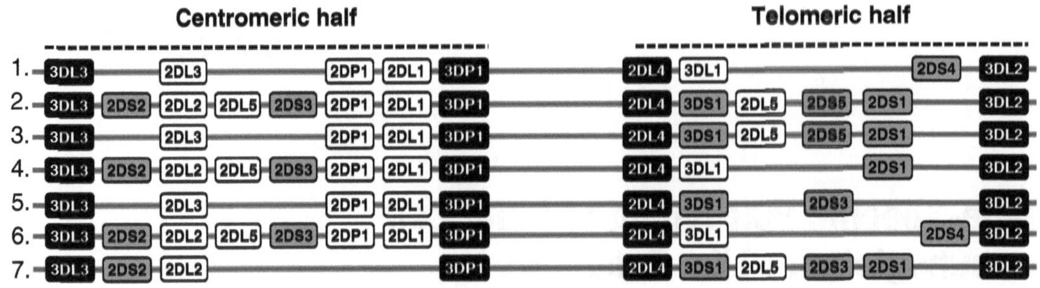

Fig. 1 KIR haplotypes have variable gene content. Map of selected KIR haplotypes is shown. Haplotype 1 represents group-A KIR haplotype and the remainder are the representative of over 30 known group-B haplotypes. The framework genes present in all haplotypes are shown in *black boxes*; genes encoding activating KIR are in *gray boxes*; and those for inhibitory receptors are in *white boxes*. KIR2DP1 and KIR3DP1 are pseudogenes that do not encode functional receptors. Inheritance of two distinct gene content haplotypes, one from each parent, produces substantial diversity in humans that may contribute to the individual's immunity

The number and type of KIR genes differ substantially between haplotypes, which are further diversified by the allelic polymorphism of most KIR genes [8, 11–16] (*see* Fig 1). Over 30 KIR haplotypes with distinct gene content have been characterized to date by sequencing genomic clones and haplotype segregation analysis in families [8, 13, 15–19]. They are broadly classified into two groups [8, 19, 20]: group A and B. Group-A haplotypes have relatively fixed gene content comprising KIR3DL3-2DL3-2DP1-2DL1-3DP1-2DL4-3DL1-2DS4-3DL2 (*see* Fig 1: haplotype 1). In contrast, group-B haplotypes have variable gene content comprising several genes and alleles that are not part of the A haplotype (*see* Fig 1: haplotypes 2–7). Particularly, KIR2DS1, 2DS2, 2DS3, 2DS5, 2DL2, 2DL5, and 3DS1 are associated only with group-B haplotypes, and thus B haplotypes generally encode more activating KIR receptors than the A haplotype that encodes a single activating receptor, KIR2DS4. The gene content varies dramatically between different group-B haplotypes. Only four KIR genes (KIR2DL4, 3DL2 and 3DL3, 3DP1) are invariably present on all KIR haplotypes (therefore ubiquitously present in all individuals) and thus they are referred to as "framework" genes [8]. Inheritance of paternal and maternal haplotypes comprising different KIR gene content generates substantial diversity between humans in their KIR gene profile. For example, homozygotes for group-A haplotypes (*see* Fig 1: haplotype 1) have only seven functional KIR genes, while heterozygotes for group-A and group-B haplotypes (*see* Fig 1: haplotypes 1 + 2) may have all 14 functional KIR genes.

The combined variation in gene content and allelic polymorphism results in unrelated individuals always having different KIR genotypes, which may individualizes immune response and thus contribute to human health and disease. KIR genotyping has increasingly been used for epidemiological studies to show links between select KIR genes and the risk of developing certain human diseases [21]. Furthermore, donors with group-B KIR haplotypes are found to have improved relapse-free survival after unrelated hematopoietic cell transplantation for acute myelogenous leukemia [22]. Moreover, the absence of donor HLA class I ligands for recipient inhibitory KIR was shown to be associated with reduced long-term graft survival in HLA-A, B, DR compatible kidney transplants [23–25].

Uhrberg et al. developed the first KIR genotyping method in 1997 using sequence-specific primers-based PCR (PCR-SSP) [20]. Since then, many KIR genotyping methods have been developed that use either the SSP strategy [26–36] or an approach that utilizes sequence-specific oligonucleotide hybridization of PCR-amplified products (PCR-SSO) [37]. The PCR-SSO is an acceptable method for high-volume sample testing, but requires substantial time for extensive post-PCR processing and complex interpretation, thus limiting its utility [37]. The reverse SSO method utilizing Luminex-technology is available from commercial vendors that simplifies the SSO assay but requires expensive reagents and a Luminex instrument [38]. The most commonly used method for KIR genotyping is SSP-PCR amplification because of its simple hands-on-procedure and straightforward interpretation. This chapter describes the step-by-step protocol of PCR-SSP typing method for KIR genotyping. Moreover, using our previously published data set [39], we describe the basic rules to verify the accuracy of genotyping results and approaches for the data analysis.

2 Materials

2.1 Facility

1. It is highly recommended that laboratories performing PCR amplification use physical barriers to prevent the contamination (carry-over) of DNA from previously amplified DNA product. It is ideal to have physically separate locations—one dedicated for pre-PCR work (i.e., DNA isolation and PCR set up), and another for post-PCR detection (i.e., separation of PCR-amplified DNA fragments).
2. Optimally, pre-PCR manipulations should be handled in a laminar flow hood to decrease the possibility of contamination.
3. Pre- and post-PCR work area should be equipped with a separate set of pipettors, lab coats, and other supplies.
4. Utilize disposable gloves and use new/sterile disposable plastic supplies.

2.2 Materials for PCR Amplification

1. *Samples*: High-quality whole genomic DNA sample extracted from peripheral blood or tissues using standard protocols (*see* **Notes 1** and **2**).
2. *Controls*: A panel of reference samples that include DNA standards positive and negative for each variable KIR gene (*see* **Note 3**).
3. *Primers*: Oligonucleotide primers for each KIR gene and for the internal positive control gene (*see* Table 1 for primer sequences) (*see* **Note 4**).
4. *Taq* DNA polymerase (5 U/μL) (*see* **Note 5**).
5. 10× PCR buffer II (10 mM Tris–HCl, 50 mM KCl) (*see* **Note 5**).
6. 100 μM of each dNTP mix.
7. 25 mM of $MgCl_2$.
8. Ultrapure PCR grade water.
9. Thermal cycler with 96-well block.
10. 96-well PCR plates.
11. Strips of eight PCR reaction tubes (0.2 mL volume).
12. Electronic single and multichannel (8 and 12 channel) repetitive pipettors and compatible tips to dispense multiple aliquots of the desired volume following a single aspiration.
13. Sterile disposable tubes (1.5 mL).
14. Vortex mixer.
15. Centrifuges capable of holding 1.5 mL tubes and 96-well PCR plates.

2.3 Materials for Gel Electrophoresis

1. Electrophoresis-grade agarose.
2. 10× TAE electrophoresis buffer (400 mM Tris, 200 mM acetic acid, 10 mM EDTA).
3. Orange G gel loading buffer (0.5 % Orange G, 20 % Ficoll, 100 mM EDTA).
4. 100 bp DNA ladder.
5. Ethidium bromide solution (10 mg/mL) (*see* **Note 6**).
6. Horizontal gel electrophoresis instrument with high-voltage power supply.
7. Gel-casting tray and 25-well combs with teeth appropriately separated for use with multichannel pipettors.
8. Gel-photo documentation system.
9. Microwave or heating apparatus to dissolve the agarose.

Table 1
Oligonucleotide primers used for KIR genotyping

Name	Sequence (5′–3′)
Forward primers	
2DL1F	CCATCAGTCGCATGACG
2DL2F2	ACTTCCTTCTGCACA(C/G)AGAA
2DL3F3	CTTCATCGCTGGTGCTG
2DL4F1	CTGCATGCTGTGATTAGGTA
2DL5F	TGCCTCGAGGAGGACAT
3DL1F1	AT(C/T)GGTCCCATGATGCT
3DL2F1	TGCAGGAACCTACAGATGTTAT
3DL3F1	CACTGTGGTGTCTGAAGGAC
3DS1F	GGCAGAATATTCCAGGAGG
2DS1F1	CTCCATCAGTCGCATGAG
2DS1F2	CTCCATCAGTCGCATGAA
2DS2F	TGCACAGAGAGGGGAAGTA
2DS3F	TCACTCCCCCTATCAGTTT
2DS4F1	TCCTGCAATGTTGGTCG
2DS5F	AGAGAGGGGACGTTTAACC
2DP1F	TCTGTTACTCACTCCCCCA
3DP1F1	AGAGTATTCCGAAACACCG
PIC-F	ATGATGTTGACCTTTCCAGGG
Reverse primers	
2DL1R1	CCACTCGTATGGAGAGTCAT
2DL1R2	AATGTTCCGTTGACCTTGGT
2DL2R1	CCCTGCAGAGAACCTACA
2DL3R1	CAGGAGACAACTTTGGATCA
2DL4R1	CTGTTGAGGGTCTCTTGCT
2DL5R1	TCATAGGGTGAGTCATGGAG
3DL1R1	CTGAGAGAGAAGGTTTCTCATATG
3DL2R1	CTTGAGTTTGACCACACGC
3DL3R1	TCTCTGTGCAGAAGGAAGC
3DS1R1	GGCACGCATCATGGA
2DS1R	AGGGCCCAGAGGAAAGTT
2DS2R1	CGCTCTCTCCTGCCAA
2DS3R	GCATCTGTAGGTTCCTCCT
2DS4R1	ACGGAAACAAGCAGTGGA
2DS5R	GGAAAGAGCCGAAGCATC
2DS5RD	CAGAGGGTCACTGGGC
2DP1R	GGAAAGAGCCGAAGCATC
3DP1R1	CTGACAACTGATAGGGGGAA
PIC-R	ATTGTGTAACTTTTCATCAGTTGC

3 Methods

3.1 PCR Amplification Procedure

1. Determine the quality and quantity of DNA by UV spectrophotometry or other standard methods, and adjust the concentration of the DNA to ~100 ng/μL (*see* **Note 7**).
2. *Primer solution preparation.* The stock oligonucleotide primers are generally obtained in salt-Free lyophilized form. Before opening, spin the tube at 111,8 ×*g* for 2 min to ensure that the oligonucleotides are at the bottom of the tube. Oligonucleotides should be resuspended in a sterile buffered solution (e.g., TE at pH 7.0) (*see* **Note 8**). Vortex oligonucleotides thoroughly after resuspension.
3. For optimal long-term use, it is recommended to prepare stock (100 μM) and working (10 μM) solutions of primers (*see* **Note 9**). For instance, if the lyophilized oligonucleotide primers are received at 59.68 nM (or 59,680 pM) add 596.8 μL water to prepare 100 μM stock solution. To make 500 μL of 10 μM working solution of KIR primer, mix 50 μL of 100 μM stock solution, and add to 450 μL water. Similarly, to make 500 μL of 5 μM working solution of internal positive control primer, mix 25 μL of 100 μM stock solution, and add to 475 μL water.
4. For routine use, prepare 16 distinct primer mixes as shown in Table 2 by combining working solution of four distinct primers in 1.5 mL tubes (*see* **Note 10**). Vortex to mix well and transfer 100 μL of each primer mix into 0.2 mL PCR tubes (or strips of eight tubes). Arrange them in the first two vertical rows of a 96-well PCR tube holder in the following order: well 1A (Mix-1), well 1B (Mix-2), well 1C (Mix-3), well 1D (Mix-4), well 1E (Mix-5), well 1F (Mix-6), well 1G (Mix-7), well 1H (Mix-8), well 2A (Mix-9), well 2B (Mix-10), well 2C (Mix-11), well 2D (Mix-12), well 2E (Mix-13), well 2F (Mix-14), well 2G (Mix-15), and well 2H (Mix-16). This allows the use of 8-channel repetitive pipettors to dispense the primers into the 96-well PCR plate.
5. Six DNA samples (one control and five test samples) can be typed using one 96-well PCR plate (*see* Fig 2). Using an 8-channel multiple repeating pipettor, dispense 3.6 μL of each primer mix as shown in Fig 2.
6. Prepare 193.8 μL of PCR master-mix for each DNA sample by adding the following components in a 1.5 mL tube: 108.46 μL of ultrapure PCR grade water, 25.5 μL of 10× PCR buffer II (final concentration 1×), 2.04 μL of 100 μM dNTP mix (final concentration 200 μM each), 30.6 μL of 25 mM $MgCl_2$ (final concentration 3.0 mM), 25.5 μL of

Table 2
Primer mix composition for KIR genotyping

Primer mix	KIR gene	Gene-specific primers working solution (10 μM)		Positive internal control (PIC) primers working solution (5 μM)		Genomic PCR product size (bp)	Missing sequences[a]
		Forward	Reverse	Forward (PIC-F)	Reverse (PIC-R)		
1	2DL1	150 μL of 2DL1F	75 μL of 2DL1R1 + 75 μL of 2DL1R2	30 μL	30 μL	1,903 and/or 1,818	
2	2DL2	150 μL of 2DL2F2	150 μL of 2DL2R1	30 μL	30 μL	1,877	004, 009
3	2DL3	150 μL of 2DL3F3	150 μL of 2DL3R1	30 μL	30 μL	816	0010, 00102
4	2DL4	150 μL of 2DL4F1	150 μL of 2DL4R1	30 μL	30 μL	695	
5	2DL5	150 μL of 2DL5F	150 μL of 2DL5R1	30 μL	30 μL	1,151	
6	3DL1	150 μL of 3DL1F1	150 μL of 3DL1R1	30 μL	30 μL	1,661	037, 040, 054
7	3DL2	150 μL of 3DL2F1	150 μL of 3DL2R1	30 μL	30 μL	1,882	031, 048
8	3DL3	150 μL of 3DL3F1	150 μL of 3DL3R1	30 μL	30 μL	1,905	019 , 030, 031
9	3DS1	150 μL of 3DS1F	150 μL of 3DS1R1	30 μL	30 μL	1,847	
10	2DS1	75 μL of 2DS1F1 + 75 μL of 2DS1F2	150 μL of 2DS1R	30 μL	30 μL	1,922 and/or 1,897	008
11	2DS2	150 μL of 2DS2F	150 μL of 2DS2R1	30 μL	30 μL	1,781	00104
12	2DS3	150 μL of 2DS3F	150 μL of 2DS3R	30 μL	30 μL	1,812	
13	2DS4	150 μL of 2DS4F1	150 μL of 2DS4R1	30 μL	30 μL	2,050	
14	2DS5	150 μL of 2DS5F	75 μL of 2DS5R+ 75 μL of 2DS5RD	30 μL	30 μL	1,952 and/or 180	003, 009, 011
15	2DP1	150 μL of 2DP1F	150 μL of 2DP1R	30 μL	30 μL	1,825	
16	3DP1	150 μL of 3DP1F1	150 μL of 3DP1R1	30 μL	30 μL	1,900	

[a]Missing sequences are based on KIR allignment from IPD-KIR database available at http://www.ebi.ac.uk/ipd/kir/ (Release 2.4.0., 15 April 2011)

	1	2	3	4	5	6	7	8	9	10	11	12
A	Mix-1	Mix-9	Mix-1	Mix-9	Mix-1	Mix-9	Mix-1	Mix-9	Mix-1	Mix-9	Mix-1	Mix-9
B	Mix-2	Mix-10	Mix-2	Mix-10	Mix-2	Mix-10	Mix-2	Mix-10	Mix-2	Mix-10	Mix-2	Mix-10
C	Mix-3	Mix-11	Mix-3	Mix-11	Mix-3	Mix-11	Mix-3	Mix-11	Mix-3	Mix-11	Mix-3	Mix-11
D	Mix-4	Mix-12	Mix-4	Mix-12	Mix-4	Mix-12	Mix-4	Mix-12	Mix-4	Mix-12	Mix-4	Mix-12
E	Mix-5	Mix-13	Mix-5	Mix-13	Mix-5	Mix-13	Mix-5	Mix-13	Mix-5	Mix-13	Mix-5	Mix-13
F	Mix-6	Mix-14	Mix-6	Mix-14	Mix-6	Mix-14	Mix-6	Mix-14	Mix-6	Mix-14	Mix-6	Mix-14
G	Mix-7	Mix-15	Mix-7	Mix-15	Mix-7	Mix-15	Mix-7	Mix-15	Mix-7	Mix-15	Mix-7	Mix-15
H	Mix-8	Mix-16	Mix-8	Mix-16	Mix-8	Mix-16	Mix-8	Mix-16	Mix-8	Mix-16	Mix-8	Mix-16

Control (1–2) **Sample-1** (3–4) **Sample-2** (5–6) **Sample-3** (7–8) **Sample-4** (9–10) **Sample-5** (11–12)

Fig. 2 The template map of 96-well PCR plate indicating the position of primer mixes 1–16 for each DNA sample. The composition of each primer mix is listed in Table 2

DNA (around 100 ng/μL), and 1.7 μL of Taq DNA polymerase. Vortex and centrifuge briefly.

7. Using a single channel pipettor, add 11.4 μL of PCR mix in each well for each sample (total PCR volume = 15 μL).
8. Cover plates with acetate film and centrifuge briefly to ensure that all the liquid is at the bottom of the wells. Place in the thermal cycler (*see* **Note 11**).
9. Perform PCR amplification under the following thermal cycling conditions: initial denaturation for 3 min at 95 °C; then 5 cycles of 94 °C for 20 s, 65 °C for 20 s, and 72 °C for 90 s; then 35 cycles of 94 °C for 20 s, 61 °C for 20 s, and 72 °C for 90 s; with final extension at 72 °C for 10 min.
10. Once the PCR thermal cycling is complete, remove the PCR plate and proceed with gel electrophoresis.

3.2 Gel Electrophoresis Procedure

1. Prepare 150 mL of 2 % agarose in 1× TAE per gel and heat until the agarose has completely gone into solution.
2. Cool gel mixture to 65 °C, add ~5 μL ethidium bromide, and gently mix to avoid bubble formation.
3. Pour gel mixture into the gel-casting tray, insert four 25-well combs, and allow the gel to solidify for 30 min.
4. Fill the electrophoresis chamber with appropriate volume of 1× TAE buffer and submerge the gel into the chamber. Gently remove the combs.

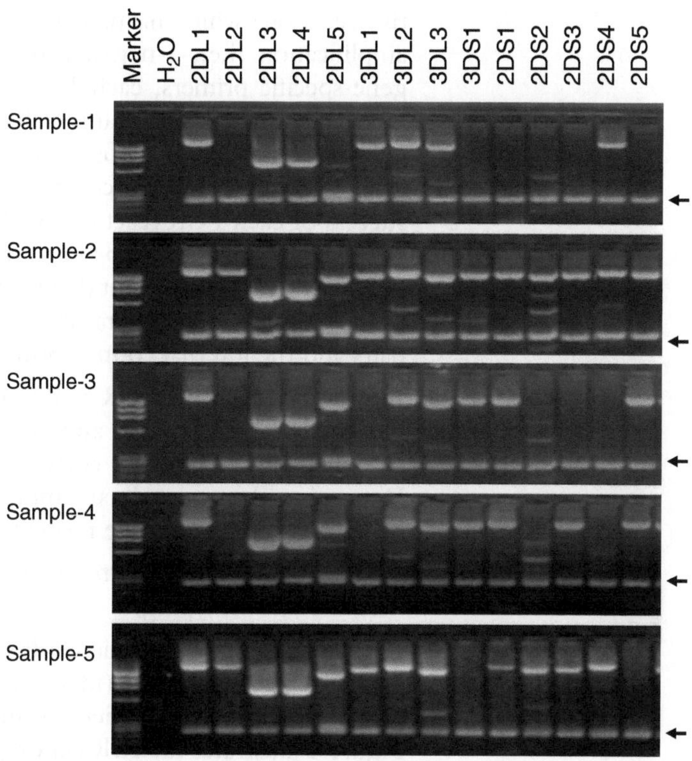

Fig. 3 KIR genotyping by the gene-specific PCR amplification method. Agarose gel pictures showing the PCR typing results of five representative DNA standards obtained from the UCLA KIR Exchange Program. Subject-1 has fewer genes (AA homozygote) and subject-2 has all known KIR genes (AB heterozygote). *Arrows* indicate internal positive control bands specific to an invariant gene

5. Add 5 μL Orange G gel loading buffer to each PCR well, mix, and centrifuge briefly.
6. Load 2 μL of the 100 bp DNA ladder to the first well of each row.
7. Using a 12-channel pipettor, load 10 μL of each PCR product into the gel.
8. Electrophorese for 30 min at 100 V or until the Orange G has migrated 3 cm.
9. Visualize the gel using a UV light source and photograph the gel for a permanent record. The KIR genotyping result of five unrelated samples by our SSP-PCR typing is depicted in Fig 3.

3.3 Interpretation of Gel Results

1. Each PCR well includes a unique set of primers designed to have perfect matches with a single KIR gene and produce a product with a particular known size (*see* Table 2). Under strictly controlled PCR conditions, perfectly matched primer pairs result in the amplification of target sequences (i.e., a posi-

tive reaction) while mismatched primer pairs do not result in amplification (i.e., a negative reaction). In addition to KIR gene-specific primers, each PCR reaction includes a positive internal control primer pair which amplifies a 256 bp fragment from a conserved Polyposis coli gene. The presence of the 256 bp positive internal control band is used to confirm the success of each PCR reaction (*see* Fig 3). In the presence of a positive typing band, the product of the internal control primer pair may be weak or absent due to the differences in concentration and melting temperatures between the specific primer pairs and the internal control primer pair.

2. Interpretation of the PCR-SSP typing results is relatively simple and straightforward, and is done basically detecting an amplified product of the correct size by gel electrophoresis. Determine the approximate molecular weight of each PCR product by comparing the mobility against the DNA ladder.
3. Check if the typing results of the control DNA is consistent with the known typing.
4. Record the results in a Microsoft Excel spreadsheet indicating which genes are present (identified by number 8) and which genes are absent (identified by number 1) for each sample. Figure 4 illustrates the KIR genotyping raw data for a set of 26 samples (S-1 to S-26) that we recently published [39]. We use this data set as an exemplar to describe data analysis methods (hereafter called the exemplar data set).

3.4 KIR Genotyping Data Analysis

1. Rearrange the order of columns (data of different KIRs) using the cut and paste option in Microsoft Excel to sort genes that are associated with group-A haplotypes (2DL1, 2DL3, 3DL1, and 2DS4), group-B haplotypes (2DS2, 2DL2, 2DS3, 2DL5, 3DS1, 2DS5, and 2DS1), then framework/pseudogenes (2DP1, 3DP1, 2DL4, 3DL2, and 3DL3) as shown in Fig 5. Then, using the custom sort option in Microsoft Excel, sort the rows (data of different samples) to select samples with similar KIR genotypes. *See* Fig 5 for the sorted raw data for exemplar data set presented in Fig 4.
2. *Verification of raw data.* False-negative results are a common problem associated with the gene-specific PCR amplification-based KIR genotyping. We recommend reviewing the raw data vigorously to verify if it agrees to the following basic rules:
   (a) Four framework genes (KIR3DL3, 3DP1, 2DL4, and 3DL2) must be present in each sample.
   (b) KIR2DL3 and 2DL2 behave as alleles of same locus, and thus subjects negative for both 2DL3 and 2DL2 are questionable.

Sample I.D.	2DL1	2DL2	2DL3	2DL4	2DL5	3DL1	3DL2	3DL3	3DS1	2DS1	2DS2	2DS3	2DS4	2DS5	2DP1	3DP1
S-1	8	1	8	8	1	8	8	8	1	1	1	1	8	1	8	8
S-2	8	1	8	8	8	8	8	8	8	8	1	1	8	8	8	8
S-3	8	1	8	8	1	8	8	8	1	1	1	1	8	1	8	8
S-4	8	1	8	8	8	1	8	8	8	8	1	1	8	8	8	8
S-5	8	8	8	8	1	8	8	8	1	1	8	1	8	1	8	8
S-6	8	1	8	8	8	8	8	8	8	8	1	1	8	8	8	8
S-7	8	1	8	8	8	8	8	8	8	8	1	1	8	8	8	8
S-8	8	1	8	8	8	1	8	8	8	8	1	1	1	8	8	8
S-9	8	1	8	8	8	8	8	8	8	8	1	8	8	1	8	8
S-10	8	1	8	8	8	8	8	8	8	8	1	1	8	8	8	8
S-11	8	1	8	8	1	8	8	8	1	1	1	1	8	1	8	8
S-12	8	1	8	8	8	1	8	8	8	8	1	8	8	1	8	8
S-13	8	1	8	8	8	8	8	8	8	8	1	1	8	8	8	8
S-14	8	1	8	8	8	8	8	8	8	8	1	1	8	8	8	8
S-15	8	8	8	8	8	1	8	8	1	8	8	1	8	1	1	8
S-16	8	1	8	8	1	8	8	8	1	1	1	1	8	1	8	8
S-17	8	1	8	8	1	1	8	8	1	1	1	1	8	1	8	8
S-18	8	1	8	8	8	8	8	8	8	8	1	1	8	8	8	8
S-19	8	1	8	8	8	8	8	8	8	8	1	1	8	8	8	8
S-20	8	1	8	8	1	8	8	8	1	1	1	1	8	1	8	8
S-21	8	8	8	8	8	8	8	8	8	8	8	1	8	8	8	8
S-22	8	1	8	8	8	8	8	8	8	8	1	8	8	1	8	8
S-23	8	1	8	8	1	8	8	8	1	1	1	1	8	1	8	8
S-24	8	1	8	8	1	1	8	8	1	1	1	1	8	1	8	8
S-25	8	1	8	8	1	8	8	8	1	1	1	1	8	1	8	8
S-26	8	1	8	8	1	8	8	8	1	1	1	1	8	1	8	8

Fig. 4 Microsoft Excel spreadsheet indicating which genes are present (identified by number 8) and which genes are absent (identified by number 1) for a set of 26 exemplar samples (S-1 to S-26) that we have recently published [39]

(c) KIR3DL1 and 3DS1 behave as alleles of same locus, and subjects negative for both of these KIRs are extremely infrequent.

(d) KIR2DS4 negatives are generally negative for KIR3DL1 (likely BB genotype carriers).

(e) KIR2DS2 has strong linkage disequilibrium with 2DL2, and therefore genotype with $KIR2DS2^{Pos}$ but $KIR2DL2^{Neg}$ is rare.

Genotyping results of any samples that do not confirm these basic rules, as well as those with ambiguous and uncertain typing results must be retyped using an alternative typing method. Since the KIR gene family has been the subject of rapid evolution [40, 41], several genotypes with unusual gene content and recombinant genes are reported as the consequence of unequal cross-overs [42–44]. Therefore, it is critical to retype using an alternative typing method to confirm if a sample carries an unusual/rare KIR genotype.

	Group-A haplotype associated KIR				Group-B haplotype associated KIR							Framework/Psuedogenes					Genotype	
Sample I.D.	2DL1	2DL3	3DL1	2DS4	2DS2	2DL2	2DS3	2DL5	3DS1	2DS5	2DS1	2DP1	3DP1	2DL4	3DL2	3DL3	Number	Haplogroup
S-11	8	8	8	8	1	1	1	1	1	1	1	8	8	8	8	8	1	AA
S-16	8	8	8	8	1	1	1	1	1	1	1	8	8	8	8	8	1	AA
S-20	8	8	8	8	1	1	1	1	1	1	1	8	8	8	8	8	1	AA
S-23	8	8	8	8	1	1	1	1	1	1	1	8	8	8	8	8	1	AA
S-25	8	8	8	8	1	1	1	1	1	1	1	8	8	8	8	8	1	AA
S-26	8	8	8	8	1	1	1	1	1	1	1	8	8	8	8	8	1	AA
S-1	8	8	8	8	1	1	1	1	1	1	1	8	8	8	8	8	1	AA
S-3	8	8	8	8	1	1	1	1	1	1	1	8	8	8	8	8	1	AA
S-17	8	8	1	8	1	1	1	1	1	1	1	8	8	8	8	8	2	AA
S-24	8	8	1	8	1	1	1	1	1	1	1	8	8	8	8	8	2	AA
S-4	8	8	1	8	1	1	1	8	8	8	8	8	8	8	8	8	3	AB
S-2	8	8	8	8	1	1	1	8	8	8	8	8	8	8	8	8	4	AB
S-6	8	8	8	8	1	1	1	8	8	8	8	8	8	8	8	8	4	AB
S-7	8	8	8	8	1	1	1	8	8	8	8	8	8	8	8	8	4	AB
S-10	8	8	8	8	1	1	1	8	8	8	8	8	8	8	8	8	4	AB
S-13	8	8	8	8	1	1	1	8	8	8	8	8	8	8	8	8	4	AB
S-14	8	8	8	8	1	1	1	8	8	8	8	8	8	8	8	8	4	AB
S-18	8	8	8	8	1	1	1	8	8	8	8	8	8	8	8	8	4	AB
S-19	8	8	8	8	1	1	1	8	8	8	8	8	8	8	8	8	4	AB
S-21	8	8	8	8	8	8	1	8	8	8	8	8	8	8	8	8	5	AB
S-8	8	8	1	1	1	1	1	8	8	8	8	8	8	8	8	8	6	BB
S-9	8	8	8	8	1	1	8	8	8	1	8	8	8	8	8	8	7	AB
S-22	8	8	8	8	1	1	8	8	8	1	8	8	8	8	8	8	7	AB
S-12	8	8	1	8	1	1	8	8	8	1	8	8	8	8	8	8	8	BB
S-15	8	8	1	8	8	8	1	8	1	1	8	1	8	8	8	8	9	BB
S-5	8	8	8	8	8	8	1	1	1	1	1	8	8	8	8	8	10	AB
Number of carriers	26	26	20	25	3	3	3	15	14	11	15	25	26	26	26	26		
% of carriers	100	100	76.9	96.1	11.5	11.5	11.5	57.7	53.7	42.3	57.7	96.1	100	100	100	100		

Fig. 5 The raw data shorted on genes associated with group-A haplotypes (2DL1, 2DL3, 3DL1, and 2DS4), group-B haplotypes (2DS2, 2DL2, 2DS3, 2DL5, 3DS1, 2DS5, and 2DS1), framework/pseudogenes (2DP1, 3DP1, 2DL4, 3DL2, and 3DL3) as well as by KIR gene content. The carrier frequency of each KIR gene is determined by dividing the number of individuals positive for the gene by the total number of individuals tested in the panel, and then multiplying by 100 (shown in the *bottom row*). The KIR haplotypes are predicted on the basis of presence and absence of certain KIR genes (*see* **step 5** under Subheading 3.4). The presence of the T4 gene cluster (positive for KIR2DL5-3DS1-2DS5-2DS1) is shaded in *gray*

3. *Determination of KIR gene frequencies.* The percentage of individuals carrying each KIR gene in the study group is determined by direct counting (individuals positive for the gene divided by the individuals tested in the study group × 100). The percent carrier frequencies of each KIR gene within the exemplar data set are provided in the bottom row of Fig 5.
4. *KIR genotype frequency determination.* KIR gene content of a given individual is conventionally called the "KIR genotype,"

which is variable among individuals. Within the exemplar data set, ten distinct KIR genotypes are detected (*see* Fig 5). The percent frequency of each KIR genotype can be determined by direct counting of individuals carrying a particular genotype divided by the total number individuals tested in the study group × 100. For example, genotype #1 in the exemplar data set (*see* Fig 5) is determined to be 30.8 % (i.e., 8/26 × 100).

5. *Prediction of KIR haplogroups from genotyping data.* The group-A and group-B KIR haplotypes can be predicted from the KIR genotyping data (*see* Fig 5). Individuals having only genes of the group-A KIR haplotypes (KIR3DL3-2DL3-2DL1-2DP1-3DP1-2DL4-3DL1-2DS4-3DL2) are considered to be homozygous for the A-haplotype and assigned as AA genotype carriers. Please note that some group-A KIR haplotypes may have deleted one or more of these genes and thus can produce a short KIR genotype. For example, the samples S-17 and S-24 in Fig 5 appear to be homozygous for short A-haplotypes that miss the KIR3DL1 gene. Individuals lacking any of the four A-haplotype associated genes (KIR2DL1, 2DL3, 3DL1 and 2DS4) that have a known function and carry one or more group-B haplotype associated genes are considered to be homozygous for group-B haplotypes, and assigned as the carriers of BB genotypes. All other individuals are regarded to be heterozygous for A and B haplotypes and assigned as AB genotype carriers. The individuals with AB genotypes have all nine genes present on the A-haplotype, as well as one or more B-haplotype specific genes (2DL2, 2DL5, 2DS1, 2DS2, 2DS3, 2DS5, and 3DS1). The AB and BB genotypes are collectively referred together as Bx genotypes [45].
6. *Prediction of group-A and group-B haplotypes.* Frequencies of A and B haplotypes are calculated using the following formula: group-A = $2n\mathrm{AA} + n\mathrm{AB}/2N$ and group-B = $2n\mathrm{BB} + n\mathrm{AB}/2N$, where nAA, nAB, and nBB are the numbers of AA, AB, and BB genotypes and N is the total number of individuals tested within the study group.
7. *Classification of KIR genotypes on the basis of centromeric and telomeric gene-clusters.* Based on the linkage disequilibrium, we discovered two frequently occurring gene-clusters [46]. One cluster comprises KIR2DS2-2DL2-2DS3-2DL5 genes and is located at the centromeric half of the KIR gene complex, while another cluster comprises KIR3DS1-2DL5-2DS1-2DS5 genes and is located at the telomeric half of the complex (*see* Fig 1). For simplicity we call these clusters C4 and T4, in which "C" represents centromeric, "T" represents telomeric, and "4" indicates number of genes. On the basis of the presence and

absence of C4 and T4 clusters, the Bx genotypes are further divided into the following four subsets: C4Tx (presence of C4 and absence of T4), CxT4 (absence of C4 and presence of T4), C4T4 (presence of both C4 and T4), CxTx (absence of both C4 and T4). These Bx subsets are substantially variable in activating KIR gene content, and their frequencies differ significantly between human populations [47].

8. The function of the inhibitory KIR receptors depends on the availability of their specific cognate HLA class I ligands. Given that KIR genes at chromosome 19q13.4 and HLA genes at chromosome 6p21.3 are polymorphic and display significant variations, the independent segregation of these unlinked gene families produce diversity in the number and type of KIR-HLA pairs inherited in individuals [48], which could potentially influence the health and disease status of a given individual [21]. Therefore, it is critical to type for the KIR-binding HLA class I motif to determine if specific combinations of KIR-HLA genes are associated with specific diseases.

4 Notes

1. DNA extraction is the first step in the KIR genotyping method. Preparation of high quality DNA is critical for amplification of KIR genes since the length of the PCR-amplified fragments of most KIR genes is in the range of 2,000 base pairs.
2. Heparin has been shown to inhibit some PCR reactions and therefore heparinized blood should be avoided. EDTA or Citrate (ACD) anticoagulant is preferred.
3. It is critical to include sufficient control DNA standards (controls should represent 10 % of the test samples) to confirm the accuracy and reliability of positive/negative KIR genotyping results. The control panel must include positive and negative DNA standards for each variable KIR gene. The UCLA International KIR Exchange Program provides a comprehensive set of KIR genotyping control standards (http://www.hla.ucla.edu/pdf/KIR_brochure.pdf) that fulfills these requirements.
4. Custom oligonucleotide primers may be purchased from commercial vendors. Each primer is designed to carry a 3′ residue matching a unique position conserved on all known sequences of a given KIR gene. The primers recognize most of the sequences submitted to date in the IPD-KIR database available at http://www.ebi.ac.uk/ipd/kir/ (Release 2.4.0., 15 April 2011). Primer lengths are adjusted to result in annealing temperatures between 59 °C and 67 °C to enable PCR amplification of all KIR genes under the same PCR thermal cycling conditions.

5. We obtained the best results with AmpliTaq DNA polymerase and 10× PCR buffer II (Applied Biosystem, Foster city, California).
6. Ethidium bromide is a carcinogen. Handle with appropriate personal protective equipment including gloves, gown, and eye protection.
7. PCR amplification may fail if the DNA is contaminated with cellular proteins. Since the heme proteins of red blood cells are known to inhibit PCR amplification, many DNA isolation methods, particularly the salting out method [49] requires red cell removal prior to DNA extraction.
8. Oligonucleotides may not readily dissolve in sterile, distilled water. Adding NaOH to the water until the pH rises to 7.0 may help. If the oligonucleotides are resuspended at pH < 7.0 (deionized water may have a pH as low as 5.0), the oligonucleotide could begin to degrade and may lose functionality within a couple of weeks.
9. The 100 μM stock primer solution can be stored long term at −20 °C, while the 10 μM working primer solution can be stored at 4 °C for 3–4 months.
10. If you see too many nonspecific bands with 2DS5 (primer mix 14), re-run the 2DS5 PCR with two different primer combinations, one with 2DS5F and 2DS5R (produce 1,952 bp product) and another with 2DS5F and 2DS5RD (produce 180 bp product).
11. Ensure that the sealer covers the PCR plate properly and the plate fits snugly into the thermal cycler to avoid evaporation and amplification failure.

Acknowledgments

This work was supported by the Translational Research Funds from the UCLA Department of Pathology and Laboratory Medicine to Dr. Rajalingam. The authors have no conflicts of interest.

References

1. Parham P (2005) MHC class I molecules and KIRs in human history, health and survival. Nat Rev Immunol 5:201–214
2. Rajalingam R (2011) Human diversity of killer cell immunoglobulin-like receptors and disease. Korean J Hematol 46:216–228
3. Caligiuri MA (2008) Human natural killer cells. Blood 112:461–469
4. Narni-Mancinelli E, Vivier E, Kerdiles YM (2011) The 'T-cell-ness' of NK cells: unexpected similarities between NK cells and T cells. Int Immunol 23:427–431
5. Biron CA, Nguyen KB, Pien GC et al (1999) Natural killer cells in antiviral defense: function and regulation by innate cytokines. Annu Rev Immunol 17:189–220

6. Lanier LL (2008) Evolutionary struggles between NK cells and viruses. Nat Rev Immunol 8:259–268
7. Ruggeri L, Capanni M, Urbani E et al (2002) Effectiveness of donor natural killer cell alloreactivity in mismatched hematopoietic transplants. Science 295:2097–2100
8. Wilson MJ, Torkar M, Haude A et al (2000) Plasticity in the organization and sequences of human KIR/ILT gene families. Proc Natl Acad Sci USA 97:4778–4783
9. Vilches C, Parham P (2002) KIR: diverse, rapidly evolving receptors of innate and adaptive immunity. Annu Rev Immunol 20:217–251
10. Trowsdale J (2001) Genetic and functional relationships between MHC and NK receptor genes. Immunity 15:363–374
11. Shilling HG, Guethlein LA, Cheng NW et al (2002) Allelic polymorphism synergizes with variable gene content to individualize human KIR genotype. J Immunol 168:2307–2315
12. Martin AM, Kulski JK, Gaudieri S et al (2004) Comparative genomic analysis, diversity and evolution of two KIR haplotypes A and B. Gene 335:121–131
13. Middleton D, Meenagh A, Gourraud PA (2007) KIR haplotype content at the allele level in 77 Northern Irish families. Immunogenetics 59:145–158
14. Hou L, Steiner NK, Chen M et al (2008) Limited allelic diversity of stimulatory two-domain killer cell immunoglobulin-like receptors. Hum Immunol 69:174–178
15. Hsu KC, Liu XR, Selvakumar A et al (2002) Killer Ig-like receptor haplotype analysis by gene content: evidence for genomic diversity with a minimum of six basic framework haplotypes, each with multiple subsets. J Immunol 169:5118–5129
16. Whang DH, Park H, Yoon JA et al (2005) Haplotype analysis of killer cell immunoglobulin-like receptor genes in 77 Korean families. Hum Immunol 66:146–154
17. Uhrberg M, Parham P, Wernet P (2002) Definition of gene content for nine common group B haplotypes of the Caucasoid population: KIR haplotypes contain between seven and eleven KIR genes. Immunogenetics 54:221–229
18. Yawata M, Yawata N, Draghi M et al (2006) Roles for HLA and KIR polymorphisms in natural killer cell repertoire selection and modulation of effector function. J Exp Med 203:633–645
19. Pyo CW, Guethlein LA, Vu Q et al (2010) Different patterns of evolution in the centromeric and telomeric regions of group A and B haplotypes of the human killer cell Ig-like receptor locus. PLoS One 5:e15115
20. Uhrberg M, Valiante NM, Shum BP et al (1997) Human diversity in killer cell inhibitory receptor genes. Immunity 7:753–763
21. Khakoo SI, Carrington M (2006) KIR and disease: a model system or system of models? Immunol Rev 214:186–201
22. Cooley S, Trachtenberg E, Bergemann TL et al (2008) Donors with group B KIR haplotypes improve relapse-free survival after unrelated hematopoietic cell transplantation for acute myelogenous leukemia. Blood 113: 726–732
23. van Bergen J, Thompson A, Haasnoot GW et al (2011) KIR-ligand mismatches are associated with reduced long-term graft survival in HLA-compatible kidney transplantation. Am J Transplant 11:1959–1964
24. Rajalingam R, Gebel HM (2011) KIR-HLA mismatching in human renal allograft transplantation: emergence of a new concept. Am J Transplant 11:1771–1772
25. Rajalingam R (2008) Variable interactions of recipient killer cell immunoglobulin-like receptors with self and allogenic human leukocyte antigen class I ligands may influence the outcome of solid organ transplants. Curr Opin Organ Transplant 13:430–437
26. Gomez-Lozano N, Vilches C (2002) Genotyping of human killer-cell immunoglobulin-like receptor genes by polymerase chain reaction with sequence-specific primers: an update. Tissue Antigens 59:184–193
27. Sun JY, Gaidulis L, Miller MM et al (2004) Development of a multiplex PCR-SSP method for Killer-cell immunoglobulin-like receptor genotyping. Tissue Antigens 64:462–468
28. Vilches C, Castano J, Gomez-Lozano N et al (2007) Facilitation of KIR genotyping by a PCR-SSP method that amplifies short DNA fragments. Tissue Antigens 70:415–422
29. Du Z, Gjertson DW, Reed EF et al (2007) Receptor-ligand analyses define minimal killer cell Ig-like receptor (KIR) in humans. Immunogenetics 59:1–15
30. Martin MP, Carrington M (2008) KIR locus polymorphisms: genotyping and disease association analysis. Methods Mol Biol 415: 49–64
31. Ashouri E, Ghaderi A, Reed EF et al (2009) A novel duplex SSP-PCR typing method for KIR gene profiling. Tissue Antigens 74:62–67
32. Kulkarni S, Martin MP, Carrington M (2010) KIR genotyping by multiplex PCR-SSP. Methods Mol Biol 612:365–375
33. Chainonthee W, Bottcher G, Gagne K et al (2010) Improved KIR gene and HLA-C KIR ligand sequence-specific primer polymerase chain reaction genotyping using whole genome amplification. Tissue Antigens 76:135–143

34. Alves LGT, Rajalingam R, Canavez F (2009) A novel real-time PCR method for KIR genotyping. Tissue Antigens 73:188–191
35. Thompson A, van der Slik AR, Koning F et al (2006) An improved RT-PCR method for the detection of killer-cell immunoglobulin-like receptor (KIR) transcripts. Immunogenetics 58:865–872
36. Houtchens KA, Nichols RJ, Ladner MB et al (2007) High-throughput killer cell immunoglobulin-like receptor genotyping by MALDI-TOF mass spectrometry with discovery of novel alleles. Immunogenetics 59:525–537
37. Crum KA, Logue SE, Curran MD et al (2000) Development of a PCR-SSOP approach capable of defining the natural killer cell inhibitory receptor (KIR) gene sequence repertoires. Tissue Antigens 56:313–326
38. Nong T, Saito K, Blair L et al (2007) KIR genotyping by reverse sequence-specific oligonucleotide methodology. Tissue Antigens 69(Suppl 1):92–95
39. Levinson RD, Okada AA, Ashouri E et al (2010) Killer cell immunoglobulin-like receptor gene-cluster 3DS1-2DL5-2DS1-2DS5 predisposes susceptibility to Vogt-Koyanagi-Harada syndrome in Japanese individuals. Hum Immunol 71:192–194
40. Khakoo SI, Rajalingam R, Shum BP et al (2000) Rapid evolution of NK cell receptor systems demonstrated by comparison of chimpanzees and humans. Immunity 12:687–698
41. Abi-Rached L, Moesta AK, Rajalingam R et al (2010) Human-specific evolution and adaptation led to major qualitative differences in the variable receptors of human and chimpanzee natural killer cells. PLoS Genet 6:e1001192
42. Shilling HG, Lienert-Weidenbach K, Valiante NM et al (1998) Evidence for recombination as a mechanism for KIR diversification. Immunogenetics 48:413–416
43. Martin MP, Bashirova A, Traherne J et al (2003) Cutting edge: expansion of the KIR locus by unequal crossing over. J Immunol 171:2192–2195
44. Gomez-Lozano N, Estefania E, Williams F et al (2005) The silent KIR3DP1 gene (CD158c) is transcribed and might encode a secreted receptor in a minority of humans, in whom the KIR3DP1, KIR2DL4 and KIR3DL1/KIR3DS1 genes are duplicated. Eur J Immunol 35:16–24
45. McQueen KL, Dorighi KM, Guethlein LA et al (2007) Donor-recipient combinations of group A and B KIR haplotypes and HLA class I ligand affect the outcome of HLA-matched, sibling donor hematopoietic cell transplantation. Hum Immunol 68:309–323
46. Du Z, Sharma SK, Spellman S et al (2008) KIR2DL5 alleles mark certain combination of activating KIR genes. Genes Immun 9:470–480
47. Ashouri E, Farjadian S, Reed EF et al (2009) KIR gene content diversity in four Iranian populations. Immunogenetics 61:483–492
48. Nonaka M, Kuroda N, Naruse K et al (1998) Molecular genetics of the complement C3 convertases in lower vertebrates. Immunol Rev 166:59–65
49. Miller SA, Dykes DD, Polesky HF (1988) A simple salting out procedure for extracting DNA from human nucleated cells. Nucleic Acids Res 16:1215

Chapter 13

Complement-Dependent Cytotoxicity Crossmatch

Jeremy Ryan Peña, Donna Fitzpatrick, and Susan L. Saidman

Abstract

The complement-dependent cytotoxic crossmatch is an informative test that detects alloantibodies in pre- and post-transplant patients, which may dictate clinical management of transplant patients. While challenging to perform, the cytotoxic crossmatch represents the only assay that provides direct evidence for the presence of potentially pathologic (i.e., cytotoxic) alloantibodies. The cytotoxic crossmatch combines patient (recipient) serum and donor cells. If donor-reactive alloantibodies are present in patient serum, these antibodies can bind donor cells. Antibody-antigen complexes, in turn, can activate the complement cascade, leading to complement-mediated cytotoxicity. Two commonly performed cytotoxic crossmatches, using donor lymphocytes as target cells, are described.

Key words Cytotoxicity, Complement, Antihuman globulin (AHG), Crossmatch, Histocompatibility testing, HLA antibody

1 Introduction

Cytotoxic crossmatch testing has been an important assay in histocompatibility/tissue typing laboratories to establish graft and host compatibility. At its most basic concept, the cytotoxic crossmatch seeks to address the question: "Does a recipient have alloantibodies against an allograft that may lead to graft rejection and/or dysfunction?"

Except in syngeneic cases, donor grafts will have varying degrees of antigen mismatch compared with patient/recipient. This mismatch can result in sensitization following transplantation. Alloantibodies against the HLA antigens, the human major histocompatibility complex, are the most important alloantibodies associated with graft rejection and dysfunction [1]. In pre-transplant patients, preformed anti-HLA antibodies can be due to prior pregnancy (including unrecognized conception), blood transfusion or a previous transplant. However, the mere presence of preformed allo-antibodies with reactivity to HLA epitopes in a (potential) recipient does not imply that anti-HLA antibodies will injure a

Andrea A. Zachary and Mary S. Leffell (eds.), *Transplantation Immunology: Methods and Protocols, Second Edition*, Methods in Molecular Biology, vol. 1034, DOI 10.1007/978-1-62703-493-7_13, © Springer Science+Business Media, LLC 2013

potential graft. The graft itself needs to express the specific HLA molecules that the anti-HLA antibody targets. Such graft reactive antibodies targeting HLA molecules are termed donor-specific alloantibodies (DSA). The presence of HLA DSA, in the recipient, against a potential donor is associated with poor graft survival when transplantation occurs [2] and thus, is generally a contraindication to transplantation.

A number of methods have been developed to identify anti-HLA alloantibodies and to determine if they are donor specific. The traditional method performed by Histocompatibility/Tissue Typing/HLA laboratories to detect DSA is the complement-dependent cytotoxicity (CDC) assay. The basic CDC crossmatch is performed by isolating donor cells (usually lymphocytes from peripheral blood, spleen or lymph node) and exposing donor cells to recipient serum with the addition of exogenous complement. When DSA are present in patient serum, these antibodies can bind HLA molecules expressed by donor lymphocytes. If DSA are complement-fixing isotype(s) and are present in sufficient titer, donor lymphocytes then undergo complement-mediated damage and death.

The CDC assay can be technically challenging to perform, requiring laboratories to develop and/or determine optimal reagents and conditions to be used [3]. In particular, the scoring and interpretation of crossmatch results requires significant expertise. Due to the multiple biologic reagents used in CDC, it is important to include appropriate controls to determine if cytotoxic effects are truly from DSA binding target antigen and fixing complement, which further complicates performing the CDC. These include positive- and negative-control sera (i.e., sera with known anti-HLA antibody and sera with no known anti-HLA antibody).

The American Society for Histocompatibility and Immunogenetics (ASHI) has published protocols that make it possible for laboratories to perform and interpret the cytotoxic crossmatch tests [4, 5]. Additionally, investigators have made modifications to the CDC, which have resulted in varying improvements in sensitivity. Substituting total lymphocytes (which in the periphery are mostly T cells) with B cells has been shown to improve sensitivity [6]. However, because B cells occur in fewer numbers than T cells in peripheral blood [7], it can be difficult to acquire a sufficient number of B cells. Currently, cytotoxicity assays usually use separated B cells and T cells versus a total lymphocyte population, which can be helpful in determining the presence of Class I and/or Class II alloantibodies. Increasing incubation times [8] and addition of washing steps prior to addition of complement in the standard CDC (also called the Amos modified CDC) [9] have been shown to increase sensitivity.

The most useful modification of the CDC for increasing sensitivity of alloantibody detection is the addition of antihuman globulin (AHG) [6]. In the AHG-enhanced or -augmented CDC (AHG-CDC), a secondary exogenous antibody, usually against immunoglobulin light chain, is added to the reaction well containing patient serum, donor cells and complement. The addition of the second antibody allows complement fixation to occur maximally by providing multiple antibody Fc portions in closer proximity [10].

An oft-cited advantage of the CDC or AHG-CDC is that various isotypes of anti-HLA alloantibodies can be detected (e.g., IgM) with concurrent information regarding the ability of DSA to fix complement. The use of donor cells also allows interrogation of the complete donor antigen repertoire against which a recipient is or may become allo-sensitized. Antibody reactivity, in part, is dependent on three-dimensional conformation of the antigen [11]. Indeed, some target HLA molecules may require secondary (and possibly, higher) molecular conformation changes for appropriate recognition by an anti-HLA antibody [12]. However, a disadvantage of the technique is that non-HLA alloantibodies may also be detected by CDC as long as the non-HLA antigen, to which the patient is alloreactive, is also expressed by or adsorbed onto the surface of donor lymphocytes. Such antibodies are not usually associated with graft dysfunction [13] but can result in ruling out a donor as incompatible unnecessarily. Since non-HLA antibodies are often auto-antibodies, an auto-crossmatch can be helpful [14]. They are also often IgM, which can be reduced by treating serum with dithiothreitol (DTT), dithioerythritol (DTE), or 63° for 10 min and are usually low affinity, so the multiple washes of the Amos modified or AHG assays may result in less frequent interference.

The flow cytometry crossmatch (FCXM) also utilizes donor lymphocytes to detect DSA but with reported greater sensitivity compared to CDC [15] and is slightly more sensitive than T cell AHG-CDC [16, 17]. However, determination of the clinical significance of DSA detected by FCXM over DSA detected by AHG-CDC is not without controversy. A positive FCXM is has been associated with increased risk of early graft loss in some reports [18, 19]. However, a positive FCXM may not be an absolute contraindication to transplantation [20, 21] and other studies have shown the FCXM offers no advantage for patients who have a negative AHG-CDC crossmatch [22, 23]. Techniques for both AHG-CDC and FCXM can be variable, resulting in variable sensitivities, which may account for the differences. In general, both CDC and FCXM suffer from "false positive" reactions due to auto or non-HLA antibody, so determining if reactivity is due to HLA antibody is important when interpreting any cell based crossmatch assay.

Solid phase assays utilize purified or recombinant HLA molecules and with certain exceptions, detect only IgG antibodies. They are helpful in determining if a patient's antibody is HLA specific and thus if a positive CDC or FCXM is relevant. The single antigen bead assay performed on the Luminex® platform has been shown to be the most sensitive [24] method for DSA detection. Detection of anti-HLA antibodies in kidney transplantation has been reported to have a concordance rate of 85 % between bead assays and total lymphocyte CDC [25]. However, there are problems with these assays. In general, the solid phase assays do not yield information regarding complement binding activities (except for a new complement-binding bead-based test). Also, the presence of a positive DSA by bead assays can be perplexing when the same specimen is negative by AHG-CDC and FCXM. It has been suggested that sensitivity and concordance of fluorescent microspheres with other crossmatching methods can be affected because of variability in antigen density on the beads [26]. As laboratories gain more experience, concerns about oversensitivity of these assays have arisen. Low-level allo-antibodies may not be clinically relevant [27]. Importantly, because HLA molecules on beads may not be in their native form, neo- or cryptic antigens may become available, leading to nonspecific reactivity. Such reactivities may also not be clinically relevant [28]. Finally, these newer assays also have non-standardized result interpretation and it is unclear if "detection" equals pathologic antibodies [29], whereas with CDC and AHG-CDC, there is cytotoxicity ascribed to the presence of alloantibodies.

There is no "perfect" assay for detection of DSA prior to transplantation. Although new technologies have been introduced, the CDC crossmatch continues to provide valuable information to clinicians and laboratorians working in histocompatibility testing and transplantation.

2 Materials

2.1 Reagents

1. Acetone: *caution*: Acetone is volatile and toxic. Please read Material Safety Data Sheet (MSDS) and follow safety precautions. Store in a flammable cabinet.
2. Anti-human globulin (AHG): Goat anti-human globulin (kappa light chain). Upon receipt, aliquot into 1–2 mL volumes (if needed) and freeze undiluted at −80 °C. Whenever AHG is thawed, it must be used within 60 min and never refrozen. Each new lot of AHG must be carefully evaluated for reactivity and optimal dilution prior to use and once a year thereafter (*see* Subheading 3.12).
3. AHG and complement (AHG-C′) mix: Just prior to use, remove AHG and complement stock solutions from −80 °C and gently thaw. Dilute complement with Veronal buffered saline (VBS) (*see* **Note 1**) to current dilution in use then add appropriate amount of stock AHG to achieve the desired dilution of both AHG and C′.

4. T cell positive control: Use a monoclonal antibody specific for a monomorphic determinant on all HLA-A, -B, and -C molecules (e.g., W6/32); or any antibody known to cause cytotoxicity with T lymphocytes in a complement-dependent manner. Test to determine optimal dilution, aliquot to prevent repeated freeze–thaw cycles, and store at −80 °C.
5. B cell positive control: Use a monoclonal antibody specific for a monomorphic determinant on HLA-DR molecules (e.g., Ia7.2); or any antibody known to cause cytotoxicity with B cells in a complement-dependent manner. Test to determine optimal dilution, aliquot to prevent repeated freeze–thaw cycles, and store at −80 °C.
6. Carboxyfluorescein diacetate (CFDA): Make a 10 mg/mL stock solution of CFDA resuspended in acetone. Use glassware only. Mix and store at −70 °C in capped tube, indefinitely. To make a working solution of CFDA, add 5 μL stock CFDA to 5 mL PBS, or use appropriate dilution as determined by titration for each new stock solution. Working solution must be made daily. Both stock and working CFDA need to be protected from light.
7. Complement (C′): Pooled rabbit serum complement is labile. To minimize loss of activity, rapidly thaw stock bottle (received from vendor) in a 37 °C water bath with gentle swirling and remove from bath once thawed. Do not vortex and do not leave thawed C′ in the water bath. Aliquot the stock solution into 1–2 mL volumes while keeping the thawed complement on ice (or while working in a cold room). Store aliquots at −80 °C. Each new lot of C′ should be carefully evaluated for reactivity and optimal dilution prior to use (*see* Subheading 3.11).
8. Distilled water (dH_2O).
9. Deoxyribonuclease (DNase): Add 250 mg DNase to 100 mL filter-sterilized distilled H_2O to make a 2.5 mg/mL solution. Mix gently, store on ice water bath for 60 min to fully solubilize enzyme. Aliquot into 200 μL volumes, freeze, and store at −80 °C. Stable indefinitely at −80 °C, 4 h at room temperature. Original DNase powder must be stored in desiccator at −20 °C.
10. 0.2 M Dithiothreitol (DTT): For each 0.3086 g of DTT powder (MW = 154.3 g/L), add 10 mL 1× VBS and pH to 7–8. Filter (0.8 μm) and dispense into 200 μL aliquots and store at −80 °C. Stable for 4 months. Store stock DTT powder in a desiccator at −20 °C. *Caution*: DTT can be toxic. Please read MSDS and follow safety precautions
11. EDTA: EDTA disodium salt (Mallinckrodt 4931 or equivalent). Store at room temperature.
12. Ethidium bromide (EB): 10 mg/mL solution. Store per manufacturer's recommendations. *Caution*: EB is *carcinogenic*.

Please read MSDS and follow proper institutional/local safety and disposal guidelines.

13. EB diluent (5 % EDTA-RPMI): Dissolve 10 g EDTA in 150 mL RPMI at 37 °C. Adjust pH to 7.2 with 1 N NaOH, Q.S. to 200 mL with RPMI. Filter-sterilize and divide in two 100 mL sterile bottles. Stable indefinitely at 2–6 °C in the dark, unless there is significant color change or microbial growth.
14. Heat-inactivated complement (HIC): Any rabbit serum complement that has been heat-inactivated for 30 min in a 56 °C water bath.
15. HEPES buffer: *N'*-2-Hydroxyethylpiperizine-*N'*-ethanesulfonic acid buffer, 1 M, store at 2–6 °C. Stability as labeled.
16. Human serum albumin (HSA): Aseptically mix one part of a 25 % (w/v) human serum albumin solution with 2.3 parts normal saline to make a 7.5 % HSA solution. Dispense in 10 or 50 mL volumes and store at −20 °C. Stable for 2 years.
17. Immunomagnetic selection beads: Dynabeads® (Invitrogen/ Life Technologies) for Class I (#219.02) and CD19 pan B cell (#111.43D).
18. Mineral Oil, Heavy.
19. Normal Human Serum (NHS): Heat-inactivate at 56 °C for 30 min if not already done by manufacturer. Prescreen to ensure there are no Class I or II cytotoxic antibodies. Aliquot in small volumes to avoid repeated thawing and refreezing. Check for debris and aggregates, filter if necessary. Stability: 2 years at −20 °C. Filter-sterilize (0.22 μm) before use.
20. Normal saline (0.9 % NaCl, sterile).
21. Phosphate buffered saline, 1× (PBS): To 200 mL 10× PBS (without calcium and magnesium), add dH_2O to almost 2 L. pH to 7.4, then Q.S to 2 L. Filter-sterilize and store at 2–6 °C for up to 6 months.
22. PBS with 0.6 % citrate (PBS/citrate): Dissolve 12 g Na Citrate ($Na_3C_6H_5O_7{\cdot}2H_2O$ in 1×PBS). When fully dissolved, Q.S. to 2 L with PBS. Filter (0.8 μm) and store at 2–6 °C for up to 6 months.
23. RPMI 1640, 1× with L-Glutamine (RPMI): (with calcium and magnesium). Store at 2–6 °C. Stability as labeled by manufacturer. Changes in color or any turbidity may indicate media is contaminated—always check before use and discard if contaminated.
24. RPMI with 2 % NHS: Add 1 part NHS to 49 parts RPMI. Filter-sterilize. Make fresh daily and keep on ice while not in use.
25. RPMI with 20 % NHS: Add 1 part NHS to 4 parts RPMI. Filter-sterilize. Make fresh daily and keep on ice while not in use.

26. RPMI with 20 % HSA (DNAse wash): Add 2 parts 7.5 % HSA to 8 parts RPMI. Make fresh daily as needed. Keep on ice when not in use.
27. 10% Sodium azide (NaN_3): Make a 10 % NaN_3 stock solution (w/v) by dissolving 10 g NaN_3 in 100 mL dH_2O. Store at room temperature indefinitely. To use as a preservative, add 1.0 mL of 10 % NaN_3 stock per 100 mL of solution (to get a final concentration of 0.1 % NaN_3). *Caution*: NaN_3 can be explosive when in contact with copper. Do not combine with acids. Please read MSDS and follow safety precautions. Follow proper institutional and local disposal guidelines.
28. Sodium citrate: $Na_3C_6H_5O_7{\cdot}2H_2O$.
29. Trypan blue: 0.4 % solution. Store at RT. Dilute in half with normal saline to make a 0.2 % solution for cell count and viability testing. Stability of 0.4 % solution as labeled. Discard 0.2 % solution after 2 weeks.
30. Veronal Buffered saline stock, 5×: Store at room temperature, stability as labeled.
31. Veronal Buffered saline 1× (VBS): Combine 20 mL 5× VBS and 80 mL dH_2O. Adjust pH to 7.4 + 0.2. Filter-sterilize and store in 50 mL aliquots at 2–6 °C for up to 1 month.
32. VBS with 1 % HSA and 0.1 % NaN_3 (VBS/HSA/NaN_3): Combine 95 mL 1× VBS, 4 mL 25 % HSA solution and 1 mL 10 % sodium azide. Stable for 1 month at 2–6 °C or indefinitely at −20 °C.
33. WBC Diluent (for cell counting): 5 mL 1N HCl, Q.S. to 50 mL with dH_2O. Add three drops Wright's Stain. Store at room temperature. Stability: 1 year.

2.2 Equipment and Supplies

1. 100 mm Petri dish, plastic (sterile).
2. 50 mL centrifuge tubes.
3. 96-well microtiter plate.
4. Centrifuges that are compatible with microtest trays (aka microwell plates, Terasaki plates) and various tube sizes.
5. Dissecting scissors and forceps.
6. Filter sets (0.22 μm pore size for filter sterilization, etc.).
7. Fluorescent microscope, inverted.
8. Freezers (−20 and −85 °C).
9. Hemocytometer, Neubauer 1/10 mm deep.
10. Microliter syringe, 6-channel, handheld, to deliver 1 or 5 μL volumes (e.g., syringe dispenser with fixed needles, Hamilton or equivalent).

11. Needles (20–25 gauge).
12. Nylon wool.
13. Pipettors (including micropipettors, 9″ Pasteur pipettes).
14. Personal protective equipment (including face mask/goggles or plastic shielding).
15. Rare earth magnet (Dynal MPC-1 #12001 or MPC-6 #12002).
16. Sterile gauze.
17. Syringes, 3 and 10 mL volumes (sterile).
18. Microtest trays (72-well).
19. Tubes, various (50 mL conical tubes, 10 mL glass with cap, 1.5 microfuge tube).
20. Yellow-top blood collection tubes (ACD anticoagulant).
21. Automatic cell/serum dispenser (optional).

3 Methods

3.1 Preparation of Patient Serum

1. Thaw patient sera to be tested. If sera are to be DTT treated for crossmatching, perform DTT treatment just prior to plating (*see* Subheading 3.2; **Note 2**).
2. Plan a layout for samples location in microtest trays keeping in mind the number of patient specimens and dilutions (*see* **Note 3**). *See* Fig. 1 for examples of tray layouts.
3. Label and oil microtest trays by dispensing 5–10 μL of heavy mineral oil into each well (*see* **Note 4**).
4. Make twofold serial dilutions of each serum (commonly up to 1:8) using RPMI with 20 % NHS in a 96-well microtiter plate (*see* **Note 5**). Use NHS as a negative control and appropriate T and/or B cell positive controls. For AHG crossmatches, serum with broad reactivity (so it is positive with most cells) but that reacts only in the presence of AHG should be used as an AHG control. If testing DTT-treated sera, untreated sera should also be tested as a comparison (*see* **Note 6**).
5. Transfer 1 μL of each serum and each dilution into microtest trays (*see* Fig. 1 for suggested layout), in duplicate, using a 6-channel microliter syringe. Cover trays.
6. Use microtest trays with patient sera immediately or store at −70 to −80°C until ready to use (*see* **Note 7**).

3.2 DTT Treatment of Patient/Recipient Sera

1. Thaw aliquot of frozen 0.2M DTT. Use a fresh aliquot of DTT daily.
2. Treat 0.39 mL of serum with 0.01 mL of 0.2M DTT and incubate in a 37 °C water bath for 30 min. You may use a different

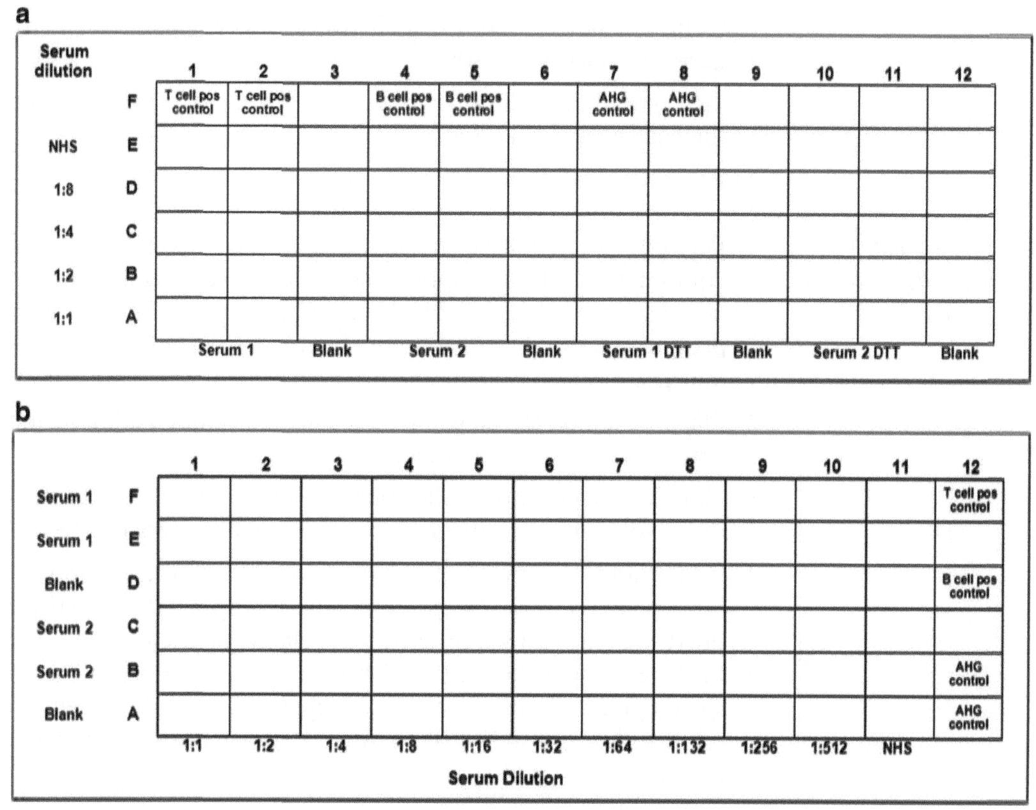

Fig. 1 Examples of crossmatch tray layouts. (**a**) For testing two sera with DTT. (**b**) For testing high titer sera

volume of serum (if serum specimen is limited) and 0.2M DTT provided a final concentration of 0.005M DTT is achieved (*see* **Note 8**).

3. Centrifuge the DTT-treated serum at high speed (approximately 15,000×*g*) for 5 min to clarify the serum. The supernatant is now ready for testing. An untreated serum control should also be tested. For the untreated control, combine 0.39 mL of serum with 0.01 mL PBS.

3.3 Preparation of Donor Cells from Whole Blood

1. Donor cells to be used for crossmatching can be prepared from peripheral blood, lymph nodes or spleen. Follow the protocols listed for lymph node or spleen in Subheadings 3.4 and 3.5, respectively.
2. Collect whole blood in 10 mL yellow-top (YTT) (ACD) Vacutainer® tubes and mix well (*see* **Note 9**).
3. Prechill PBS and PBS/citrate on ice.
4. Centrifuge YTT at 1,150×*g* for 10 min.
5. Remove as much plasma as possible from all tubes without disturbing buffy coat and discard. Carefully remove the buffy coat.

Combine buffy coats from all tubes into a separate, 10 mL glass tube (*see* **Note 10**).

6. Add chilled PBS/citrate up to a final volume of 5 mL and keep the cell suspension on ice.
7. Proceed to Subheading 3.7 to isolate T and B cells.

3.4 Preparation of Donor Cells from Spleen

1. Perform spleen dissection and flushes using personal protective equipment (PPE) and appropriate safety measures. In particular, dissections should be done behind plastic shielding to prevent splashing and care must be taken to avoid needle-stick injuries.
2. Place spleen on sterile gauze and trim off as much adipose and connective tissue as possible.
3. Cut the spleen into smaller pieces and gently place in a Petri dish. Add sufficient normal saline to partially cover the pieces.
4. While holding a piece of spleen with sterile forceps, carefully introduce a 19- or 20-gauge needle (using a 10 mL syringe filled with normal saline), into the splenic parenchyma. Gently flush cells from the spleen with normal saline. Puncture each spleen piece in multiple sites and repeat flushing. Blanching of tissue indicates a well-flushed piece. Perform flushing on all the pieces.
5. Collect the cell suspension from the petri dish and transfer into sterile 9″ Pasteur pipettes packed with a small tuft of nylon wool (*see* **Note 11**). Allow the cell suspension to pass through (under gravity) to remove tissue debris.
6. Centrifuge the cell suspension at 800 × *g* for 5 min at room temperature. Remove supernatant and resuspend cell pellet in 2–3 mL fresh normal saline.
7. Proceed to Subheading 3.6 to determine cell count.

3.5 Preparation of Donor Cells from Lymph Nodes

1. Perform lymph node (LN) dissection and flushes under aseptic techniques, using PPEs and appropriate safety measures. In particular, dissections should be done behind plastic shielding to prevent splashing and care must be taken to avoid needle-stick injuries.
2. Place the lymph node on sterile gauze and trim off as much adipose and connective tissue as possible.
3. Bisect the lymph node (for larger nodes, you may cut them into smaller pieces) and gently place it in a sterile Petri dish. Add sufficient normal saline to partially cover the LN.
4. While holding a piece of lymph node with sterile forceps, carefully introduce a 22-gauge needle or smaller, with a 3 mL syringe filled with normal saline, into the node. Gently flush cells from the LN with normal saline. Puncture each lymph node piece in multiple sites and repeat flushing.

5. Collect the cell suspension from the petri dish and transfer into sterile 9″ Pasteur pipettes packed with a small tuft of nylon wool (*see* **Note 11**). Allow the cell suspension to pass through (under gravity) to remove tissue debris.
6. Centrifuge the cell suspension at 800 × *g* for 5 min at room temperature. Remove supernatant and resuspend cell pellet in 2–3 mL fresh normal saline.
7. Proceed to Subheading 3.6 to determine cell count.

3.6 Cell Counting and Viability Determination

1. Mix lymphocyte suspension well, but gently, and prepare a 1:20 dilution by adding 50 μL of cells to 950 μL of 0.2 % Trypan blue. Mix well.
2. Load a hemocytometer per manufacturer's recommendations.
3. Allow cells to settle for 3 min and count cells contained within the two large 1 mm squares that are diagonal to one another. Note the number of viable cells (no dye) and nonviable (blue) cells as separate counts.
4. If cell suspension has a large number of red cells, use WBC diluent to make the 1:20 dilution, which will lyse the red cells.
5. Calculate the total number of viable cells harvested (*see* **Note 12**).
6. If viability of cells from blood is ≥90 %, proceed to **step 6**. If viability is <90 %, or if using spleen or LN cells, treat the cell suspension with DNAse to remove dead cells as follows:
   (a) Pellet cells and resuspend cells in 1 mL RPMI to achieve a cell concentration not to exceed 10^7 cells/mL (add more RPMI if needed).
   (b) Thaw an aliquot of DNase solution and add 0.1 mL of DNase solution per mL of cell solution. Mix and incubate in a 37 °C water bath for 15 min.
   (c) Add 2 mL of DNase wash solution for every mL of treated cell solution. Centrifuge at 400 × *g* for 5 min at room temperature. Remove supernatant.
   (d) Resuspend cell pellet in 4 mL of DNase wash and centrifuge to pellet. Remove supernatant. Repeat.
7. Resuspend cells to a final concentration of approximately 3.5×10^6 cells/mL using PBS/citrate in preparation for T and B cell isolation.

3.7 Isolation of T and B Cells by Immunomagnetic Selection

1. If using cells isolated from whole blood (Subheading 3.3), continue with **step 2**. If using cells from spleen or lymph nodes (Subheading 3.4 or 3.5), centrifuge $15–20 \times 10^6$ cells at 800 × *g* for 5 min. Decant the supernatant and resuspend cell pellet in 2.5 mL chilled PBS/citrate. Frozen cells that have been thawed and DNAse treated may also be used. Keep on ice until ready for **step 3** (*see* **Note 13**).

2. Resuspend Class I Dynabeads® by swirling gently. Add 5 μL of Class I beads to 5 mL PBS into a sterile 10 mL glass tube. Place tube on the rare earth magnet for 30 s. Gently aspirate out supernatant then remove tube from the magnet.
3. Transfer chilled cells into 10 mL tube with beads. Cap tube and mix gently.
4. Place tube on rotator in the cold for 5 min, avoiding end-over-end rotation. Ideally, the rotator should be in a cold room/ refrigerator.
5. Place tube on the rare earth magnet for 3 min. Aspirate the supernatant and transfer to a fresh 10 mL tube and set aside on ice. This supernatant contains B cells as well as other CD8 negative cells and will be used in **step 14**. Alternatively, B cells can also be isolated from a separate 10 mL YTT. Be careful not to disrupt the selected cells that are along the side of the test tube while it is on the magnet.
6. Remove the tube from the magnet and add 5 mL chilled PBS/ citrate. Gently swirl to resuspend beads and cells.
7. Place the tube on the rare earth magnet for 30 s. Aspirate and discard supernatant. Remove tube from magnet and add 5 mL chilled PBS and gently swirl.
8. Repeat **step 7** three more times.
9. Place tube on the rare earth magnet for 30 s. Aspirate and discard supernatant.
10. Add 200 μL working solution of CFDA to the tube and gently swirl the tube to mix the beads and cells with the CFDA working solution.
11. Cap and incubate the tube at 37 °C for 15 min in the dark.
12. While incubating T cells with CFDA, isolate B cells. If only HLA Class I testing is to be done using T cells, proceed to **step 17**.
13. Resuspend CD19 Dynabeads® beads by swirling gently. Combine 5 μL of CD19 beads and 5 mL of PBS into a 10 mL glass tube. Place tube on the rare earth magnet for 30 s. Gently aspirate out supernatant and remove tube from the magnet.
14. Add the supernatant from **step 5** (which should contain non-CD8+ cells, including B cells) into the tube with CD19 beads (from **step 13**) and gently mix.
15. Place the B cell tube on a rotator in the cold for 5 min (*see* **step 4**) then place the tube on the rare earth magnet for 3 min. Gently aspirate and discard the supernatant. Remove the tube from the magnet, add 5 mL chilled PBS/citrate and swirl gently.
16. Follow **steps 7–11** for the B cell tube.
17. After incubation with CFDA, add 5 mL of PBS to tubes containing either T or B cells. Place tube(s) on the rare earth

magnet for 30 s. Aspirate supernatant and remove tube(s) from magnet. Repeat.

18. Resuspend cells in 200 μL RPMI with 2 % NHS. Add 1 μL of each cell suspension into a blank well on an oiled microtest tray and view it with the inverted fluorescent microscope. Check for adequate labeling with FDA and if an appropriate number of cells are in the well. Ideal cell concentration is approximately 2,000–3,000/μL (or approximately $2–3 \times 10^6$ cells/mL). If cell concentration is too high, add more RPMI with 2 % NHS as needed. If there are too few cells, resuspend in 5 mL PBS, place on magnet for 30 s, remove supernatant and resuspend in appropriate amount of RPMI with 2 % NHS.

3.8 Standard Complement-Dependent Cytotoxic Crossmatch (CDC)

1. Remove serum trays from freezer, check for frozen serum button in each well and allow trays to equilibrate to room temperature (from Subheading 3.1).
2. Add 1 μL of well mixed, bead-isolated lymphocyte suspension (from Subheading 3.7) to each serum containing well of the microtest trays with a 6-channel microliter syringe using the "dip and wipe" method (*see* **Note 14**).
3. Check that the serum and cell are in contact in each well (*see* **Note 15**). Incubate the trays at room temperature for 30 min in the dark. For reactions using B cells, incubate at 37 °C (*see* **Note 16**).
4. Add 5 μL of the correct dilution of C′ in VBS (*see* Subheading 3.11) using a multi-syringe dispenser. "Dip and wipe" needles between wells. Optional washing of the tray can be performed prior to addition of C′ (*see* **Note 17**).
5. Incubate for 60 min at room temperature, in the dark. Turn on fluorescent scope to warm up instrument, if necessary.
6. Stain cells with ethidium bromide by adding 2 μL EB working solution to each well.
7. Determine cytotoxic results by using a fluorescent inverted microscope with the appropriate filter sets for CFDA and EB. Shield trays from light as much as possible, and read within 1 h (*see* **Note 18**).
8. Go to Subheading 3.10 for scoring and interpretation of results.

3.9 Antihuman Globulin Enhanced Cytotoxicity Crossmatch (AHG-CDC)

1. Remove serum trays (from Subheading 3.1) from freezer, check for frozen serum button in each well and allow trays to equilibrate to room temperature.
2. Add 1 μL of well mixed bead isolated T lymphocyte suspension (from Subheading 3.7, *see* **Note 19**) to each serum containing well of the microtest trays with a 6-channel microliter syringe using the "dip and wipe" method (*see* **Note 14**).

3. Check for serum and cell contact in each well (*see* **Note 15**). Incubate trays at room temperature for 30 min in the dark.
4. Wash the wells by dispensing 5 μL RPMI into each well, making sure to "dip and wipe" in between wells. Inspect trays to ensure that the RPMI goes under the oil overlay.
5. Briefly pulse centrifuge tray(s) to a speed of 190 × *g* for 10 s to ensure that the cells collect to the bottom of each well. Alternatively, the tray can be gently passed over a magnet to pull cells to the bottom of each well, if cells are isolated with magnetic beads.
6. Remove the supernatant by flicking the tray over a biohazard container (*see* **Note 20**).
7. Repeat **steps 4–6** three more times (*see* **Note 21**).
8. Add 5 μL of the appropriately diluted AHG-C′ mix (*see* Subheading 3.12) using a 6-channel microliter syringe. There is no need to "dip and wipe" the syringe between rows. Check wells to ensure mixing of AHG-C′ and cells.
9. Incubate for 60 min at room temperature, in the dark. Turn on fluorescent scope to warm up instrument, if necessary.
10. Add 2 μL EB working solution to each well and view under a fluorescent scope with the appropriate filter sets for CFDA and EB. Shield trays from light as much as possible, and read within 1 h (*see* **Note 18**).
11. Go to Subheading 3.10 for scoring and interpretation of results.

3.10 Scoring and Interpretation of Results of the Complement-Dependent Cytotoxicity Assay (Both Standard CDC and AHG-CDC)

1. Score each well by determining the % nonviable cells. Note that viable cells will retain the CFDA and appear green. Dead/nonviable cells will take up EB and appear red (*see* **Note 22**). Table 1 shows how to score cytotoxicity results.
2. Assess control wells for appropriate results. The negative control (i.e., NHS) should show ≥80 % viability (i.e., score should only be 1 or 2). The positive control (i.e., serum with known class I or II alloantibody) should show ≥80 % cell death

Table 1
Cytoxicity scoring system

% Dead cells	Score	Interpretation
Not readable	0	Invalid (technical issue)
0–10	1	Negative
11–20	2	Doubtful negative
21–50	4	Weak positive
51–80	6	Positive
>80	8	Strong positive

(i.e., score should be 8). If testing for both class I and class II, there should be a positive control for each.

3. Verify that inter-well variability is acceptable. Replicate wells should only be one score apart to be reliable (e.g., if a certain dilution is tested in duplicate, and one well is given a score of 4, to be valid, the duplicate well should have a score of either 2 or 6).
4. Report if the donor is crossmatch compatible or incompatible with a patient. If serologic reactivity of any serum is positive with neat serum, the crossmatch is considered "positive." Usually reactivity will decrease as the titer increases. If serologic reactivity of the serum (at all dilutions) is comparable to the negative control, the crossmatch is considered "negative." If neat serum is negative but higher dilutions are positive, it may be due to very strong antibody (prozone) or due to increased nonspecific cell death as the protein concentration in the well decreases.
5. Dilutions/titers that are consistently scored as 4, 6 or 8 are considered positive. A score of 1 is considered negative. A score of 2 may have variable interpretation depending on the laboratory. When replicate wells have different scores, provided they are all within one score difference of each other, the dilution is called positive if >50 % are positive. If ≥50 % of replicates are negative, then the dilution is called negative (*see* **Note 23**).
6. Determine the endpoint titer. The endpoint titer is the last dilution that is positive. The endpoint can be used to monitor allo-reactivity in a patient as well as response to treatment.
7. If there is a non-reproducible, doubtful, or uninterpretable result, repeat the crossmatch in its entirety (*see* **Note 23**). If similar results occur, or repeat testing is not possible, the findings should be reported as "technically unsatisfactory."
8. Always review the clinical and laboratory history of each patient to aid in the interpretation of the crossmatch. Patients treated with therapeutic antibodies can have anomalous results (*see* **Note 24**).

3.11 Evaluation of Complement

1. When a new lot of complement (C′) is required, multiple lots should be evaluated to identify the best one, and the optimal dilution should be determined. The goal is to find a lot of complement that gives the strongest cytotoxic effect with known anti-HLA antibodies. It is also important to ensure that the lot of C′ does not result in high background cytotoxicity when tested with serum without anti-HLA antibodies. It is often necessary to use different lots of C′ for T versus B cells.
2. Prepare C′ titration trays (1 serum per tray) using two reagent sera (one strong, one weak) with well characterized HLA Class I specificity for testing T cells, and two reagent sera

C' dilution		1	2	3	4	5	6	7	8	9	10	11	12
1:16	F												T cell pos control
1:8	E												
1:4	D												B cell pos control
1:2	C												
1:1	B												AHG control
No C'*	A												AHG control
Serum Dilution**		1:1	1:2	1:4	1:8	1:16	1:32	1:64	1:132	1:256	1:512	NHS	***

*No Complement = VBS with 20% HIC

** It may be necessary to start at a higher dilution if serum titer is >1:512. It's important to include at least one dilution past the endpoint.

*** Add known lot and dilution of C' to serum controls in row 12

Fig. 2 Example of C′ titration tray layout

(one strong, one weak) with well characterized HLA Class II specificity for testing B cells. Also make trays using a negative serum (e.g., NHS). Make multiple serial dilutions of each serum in RPMI w/20 % NHS, including at least one dilution past the titer endpoint (it may be necessary to start at a higher dilution if antibody titer endpoint is ≥1:512). Add diluted serum to oiled microtest trays (1 μL/well using a 6-channel microliter syringe). Include a negative control (NHS) as well as T and/or B cell positive controls on the trays. *See* Fig. 2 for example of a tray layout. Make enough trays to test each reagent serum against each lot of C′ with two cells (i.e., two trays per serum for each C′ to be tested). Make enough NHS trays to test each lot of C′ with one T cell and one B cell (*see* **Note 25**). Making extra trays is recommended.

3. Choose cells that will be positive with each reagent serum. It is best to test both fresh and frozen cells to ensure the C′ is acceptable with both if frozen cells will be used in crossmatch assays. Since frozen cells are more sensitive to C′-mediated cytotoxicity, use frozen cells on the NHS trays. Isolate T and/or B cells as outlined in Subheadings 3.3, 3.6, and 3.7.

4. Perform a CDC assay (Subheading 3.8) with B cells, and perform both CDC and AHG assays (Subheading 3.9) with T cells using the complement titration trays. Thaw each lot of C′ and prepare dilutions during the first incubation (cells + serum). Make C′ dilutions using VBS with 20 % heat-inactivated C′. Make 60 μL of each dilution for each tray. Also prepare VBS with 20 % HIC (no complement) as a control to be added to one row (*see* **Note 26**). Transfer C′ dilutions to the wells of a 96 well tray and keep on ice until added to the trays during the

assay. It is best to have everything for making the dilutions set up before the cells are added to avoid over incubation.

5. When testing by the AHG method, do not mix the C′ and AHG. Instead, after the last wash, add 1 μL of AHG at the appropriate dilution (*see* Subheading 3.12) to each well using a 6-channel microliter syringe in the same order as the C′ will be added. Set a timer for 2 min after the start of the first row. Do not test more than two trays at a time to avoid over incubating. At exactly 2 min, add 5 μL of each C′ dilution using the 6-channel microliter syringe in the same order as the AHG was added.
6. Score and interpret the results (Subheading 3.10). Identify the most dilute titer of C′ that still gives a score of "4" or greater (positive). This titer is the endpoint. The dilution that should be used for subsequent testing should be the dilution just before the endpoint. For instance, if the endpoint for a lot of C′ is 1:4, then for testing, use a dilution of 1:2 for the complement lot (*see* **Note 27**).
7. Do not use lots of C′ that give a high background (i.e., when viability <80 % in control wells containing the lot of C′ being tested with NHS or medium; or when addition of HIC still results in <80 % viability).

3.12 Evaluation of Antihuman Globulin (AHG)

1. When a new lot of AHG is required, lots should be evaluated to identify the best one, and the optimal dilution should be determined (*see* **Note 28**).
2. Prepare AHG titration trays (1 serum per tray) using at least two reagent sera (one strong, one weak) with well-defined HLA Class I antibody specificity, known to have AHG dependent reactivity. Also prepare trays with a negative serum (e.g., NHS). Make multiple serial dilutions of each serum in RPMI w/20 % NHS, including at least one dilution past the titer endpoint. Add diluted serum to oiled microtest trays (1 μL/well using a 6-channel microliter syringe). Include a negative control (NHS) and T cell positive control on the trays. *See* Fig. 3a for example of tray layout. Make enough trays to test each reagent serum against each AHG sample with two cells and to test NHS with one cell only. Making extra trays is recommended. Freeze trays at −80 °C until use.
3. Choose cells that will be positive with the Class I specific serum on each tray. It is best to test both fresh and frozen cells to ensure the AHG is acceptable with both if frozen cells will be used in crossmatch assays. Use a frozen cell on the NHS trays. Isolate T cells as outlined in Subheadings 3.3, 3.6, and 3.7. Perform an AHG-CDC (Subheading 3.9) but do not mix the C′ and AHG.

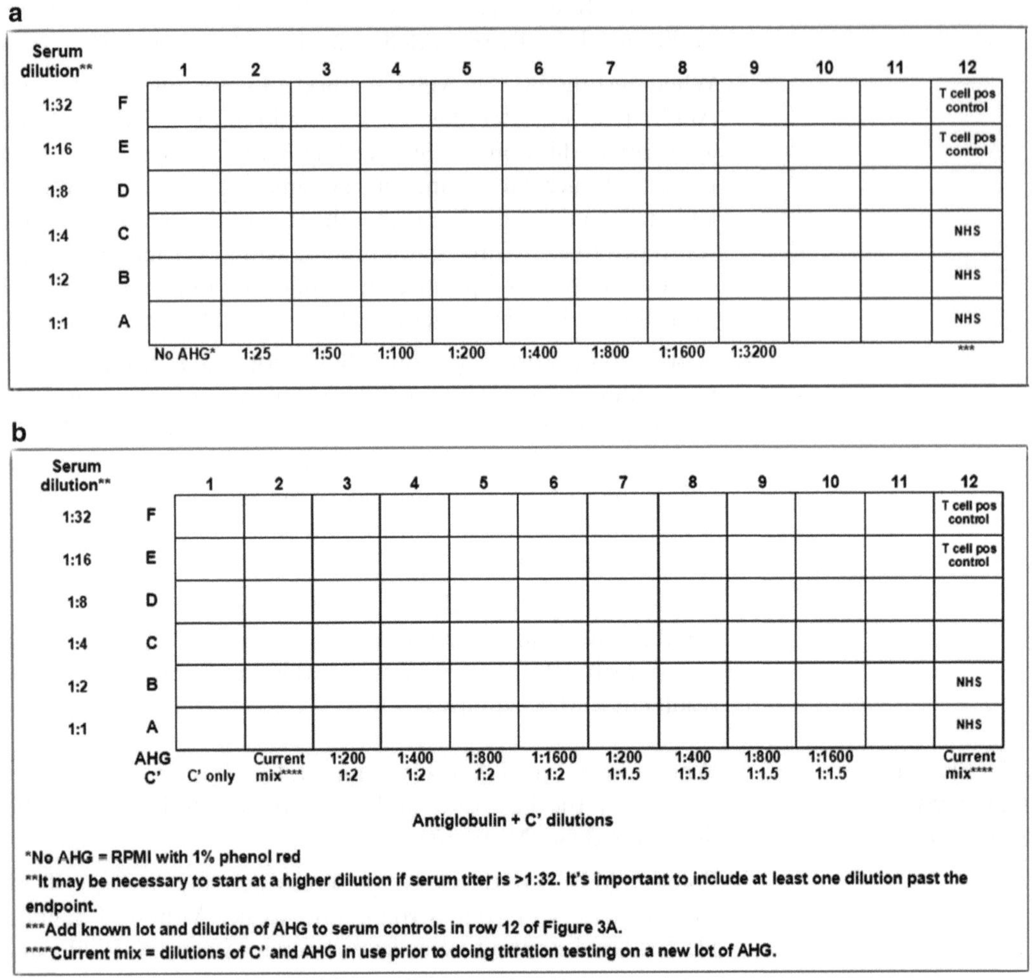

Fig. 3 Examples of AHG titration tray layouts. (**a**) Initial evaluation and titration of AHG. (**b**) Example of tray layout for testing AHG-C′ mix

4. Once cells are added to the trays, prepare serial dilutions of each lot of AHG (1:25 to 1:3,200) using RPMI with 1% phenol red as the diluent (Phenol red provides color to make it easier to see when AHG has been added to a well). Transfer the AHG dilutions to the wells of a 96 well tray and keep on ice. It is best to have everything for making the dilutions set up before the cells are added to avoid over incubation.

5. After the last wash add 1 μL of each AHG dilution to the appropriate wells in the same order as the C′ will be added. Set a timer for 2 min after the start of the first row. Do not test more than two trays at a time to avoid over incubating. At exactly 2 min, add 5 μL of C′ at the appropriate dilution (Subheading 3.11) if known or at 1:1.5 in VBS using the 6-channel microliter syringe in the same order as the AHG was added.

6. Score and interpret the results (Subheading 3.10). Choose the AHG which augments the reactivity the most. Choose the dilution of AHG that is at least one dilution stronger than that which gives maximal augmentation of sensitivity.
7. Once the lot and dilution of AHG are chosen, it must be tested for optimal dilution when premixed with C′ (*see* **Note 29**). Use the same trays and cell(s) used for AHG titration above. *See* Fig. 3b for example of tray layout. Perform an AHG-CDC (Subheading 3.9).
8. Thaw AHG (test both old and new lots if appropriate) once cells are added to the trays. Prepare AHG and complement (AHG-C′) mixes by making multiple dilutions of each lot of AHG (e.g., 1:200, 1:400, 1:800, and 1:1,600) and dilutions of complement in VBS. Test complement dilutions at both the endpoint titer and the dilution just prior to the endpoint determined in Subheading 3.11 (*see* **Note 30**). Also test with a heat-inactivated complement (HIC) control.
9. Identify the dilution of AHG-C′ mix which gives you the maximum positive score. If multiple dilutions have maximum scores use the most dilute AHG-C′ mix for AHG-CDC testing (e.g., if 1:200 and 1:400 AHG in 1:4 C′ both are scored "8" but 1:800 AHG in 1:4 C′ is scored "6," the optimal dilution to use is 1:400 AHG in 1:4 C′).

4 Notes

1. We use VBS for diluting complement, but it can be difficult to find. Many labs successfully use RPMI (with calcium and magnesium) for C′ dilution.
2. Once the sera are removed from freezer, they should be plated the same day to prevent an additional freeze–thaw cycle. After use, keep on ice or at 4 °C until returned to freezer. If a large tube of patient serum is thawed, aliquot in smaller volumes before refreezing to prevent additional freeze–thaw cycles. Test the untreated serum in parallel with the DTT treated serum. DTT treatment is done to inactivate IgM (usually non-HLA) antibodies. However, IgM antibodies may also represent new antibodies so careful review of patient's clinical history is important.
3. We generally make several serum trays with the same sera (in the event duplicates or repeats are needed). This will save time in having to remake the tray and the attendant issues that arise with freeze-thawing sera should the test need to be repeated. We usually test trays in duplicate as well.

4. We prefer to use the automatic oiler since the quantity of oil dispensed is more uniform.
5. To make dilutions, add 50 μL of RPMI with 20 % NHS to wells 2 through 4, in a 96-well microtiter plate. Add 50 μL of undiluted serum to the first well. Add 50 μL of patient serum to the second well which contains serum diluent and mix well. Transfer 50 μL of this to the third well, mix well and transfer 50 μL to the fourth well (1:8). Follow the crossmatch template to place sera in appropriate wells. Add 50 μL of NHS to the fifth row (negative control). Repeat serial dilutions with each of the patient's sera. If there is additional space, dilutions up to 1:256 may be made (*see* Fig. 1b). If a patient is known to have antibody, crossmatch trays can be made initially with further dilutions allowing the endpoint to be reached, eliminating the need to repeat crossmatches. *See* Figure 1 for crossmatch tray layout.
6. If testing DTT-treated sera, leave one empty row or column between the DTT-treated and untreated sera to prevent crossover contamination.
7. Once a microtest tray with sera has been thawed, it should not be refrozen.
8. When utilizing a new batch of 0.2M DTT, treat a known serum with IgM antibody against the cell being tested in parallel as a control. A strong titer IgM antibody may not be completely removed by DTT treatment. If this is suspected, several dilutions of serum may be made and treated with DTT. In addition, ensure that the 0.2M DTT has a pH 7–8. The maximal effects of DTT treatment have been shown to occur when the final concentration is 2.5–5 mM DTT [30].
9. In general, two (2) appropriately collected yellow-top tubes (YTT) are sufficient. Using >3 or more YTT may actually result in lower yield when used with magnetic bead isolation. Only use >3 YTT if white count is <1,000/μL. Blood should be kept at room temperature and ideally processed within 48 h of collection.
10. Taking the very top layer of red cells increases white cell yield, however, taking excess RBC layer can ultimately decrease your yield.
11. Do not use a large quantity of nylon wool or allow the suspension to incubate within the nylon wool for an extended time. Nylon wool can bind B cells which may lead to decreased B cell yield [31]. Alternatively, some labs will draw the cell suspension into a pipette, let the heavy tissue debris briefly settle into the tip of the pipette, and then eject the debris separately from the rest of the cell suspension.

12. The total viable cell harvest is = [number of viable cells in two (2) large squares × 10^5/mL × volume of cell suspension]. Example: If 100 total cells were counted in two squares, then $100 \times 10^5 = 10 \times 10^6$ cells/mL. Suppose you have 2 mL of cell suspension, then you multiply 10×10^6 cells/mL × 2 mL. The total viable cell harvest is 20×10^6 cells. The viable cells should be >90 %. Viability (%) = Total viable (no dye) cell harvest/Total (no dye + dye) cell harvest × 100 %.
13. If separating T and B cells, always isolate the T cells before B cells. Keeping cells cold at all times during the separation is very important, to prevent phagocytic cells from attaching to the beads. Alternative selection methods can be employed to isolate T and B cells. With slight modification of the protocols, both the CDC and AHG-CDC can be performed using alternatively isolated cells.
14. The use of a 6-channel microliter syringe can be maximized by utilizing some tricks. When dispensing between rows/columns, the needles should be dipped in a saline wash then wiped dry on a clean paper towel. The first drop is then ejected on to the paper towel. The subsequent volumes can then be introduced into the next set of wells. This is referred to as "dip and wipe." It is important to do this to optimize uniform volume delivery into wells and to avoid cross-contamination. Ejecting the first drop also removes any solution that may have been diluted while dipping the needle tip in saline. Alternatively, an automated tray dispenser (Lambda Jet, One Lambda Inc.) may be used to optimize uniform volume delivery into wells and to minimize carryover.
15. It may be helpful to look at microtest trays using a light box. If necessary, use a spinal needle stylus for mixing components. Dip stylus in sterile saline and wipe dry before using in another well to avoid contamination.
16. Reactions with B cells can be incubated at room temperature; however, false-positive crossmatches occur frequently. Incubating B cell crossmatches at 37 °C reduces nonspecific antibody binding.
17. Prior to the addition of C′, the plate can be washed as described in Subheading 3.9, **steps 4–7**. This is the Amos-modified CDC, which increases sensitivity for detecting a DSA and may remove low avidity/non-HLA antibodies [9].
18. Although not optimal, trays can be held for a few hours at 4 °C (in the dark) if they cannot be assessed by fluorescent microscopy immediately. An alternative staining method uses trypan blue or eosin exclusion to stain dead cells followed by formaldehyde fixation to prolong the time that scoring can be done [32], but this cannot be used with bead isolated cells.

19. We perform the AHG-CDC with T cells only. The AHG can bind surface immunoglobulin on B cells and may result in false-positive crossmatches. However, because only T cells are used, DSA against HLA class II molecules may not be detected by AHG-CDC. Select laboratories use B cells with AHG-CDC by using a two color fluorescence technique and report the sensitivity of B cell AHG-CDC to approach that of FCXM [33].
20. Take great care not to drop the plate. Grasp the side of the tray (along the long-axis) with just your fingertips making sure that the bottom of the plate is facing your palm (wells should be upright and away from your palm). Rapidly flick out the supernatant by inverting the tray over a biohazard container with a quick snap of the wrist along the long plane of the tray and return to the upright position. Avoid hitting the tray on a hard surface as this may dislodge cells.
21. When performing washes, it is also important not to allow trays to sit too long, which may "dry out" the wells and lead to cell death. Some laboratories use fewer than four washes. In our experience, sensitivity of the AHG-CDC is increased with four washes prior to the addition of AHG and complement.
22. In theory, the actual percentage of dead cells can be calculated by counting the number of red fluorescent cells for every 100 cells. However, in practice, the distribution of cells in each well will not be uniform and enumeration can be unwieldy, especially when many wells are being analyzed. Thus, the % of dead cells can be an estimate based on the ratio of red and green cells. This clearly can lead to subjective scoring. It is sometimes helpful, when there is not a clear-cut estimate, to have more than one person/reader score the reactions independently and reach a consensus. We have found that it is also helpful to directly compare the staining pattern of the negative and positive controls before analyzing patient sera. Assuming that the negative control is >80 % viable and the positive control has >80 % cytotoxicity, this visually allows the scorer to note wells with increased cytotoxicity over the negative control.
23. In general, sera from allo-immunized patients will have distinctly positive reactivities at multiple dilutions. Occasionally, in weakly positive patients, only the neat serum (undiluted) will be positive but the 1:2 dilution will have % viability that is similar to the negative control. In this situation, as long as the neat serum duplicate wells are clearly scored positive (i.e., >4), the serum should be reported as "positive." Another commonly encountered difficulty in interpreting results is when there is discordance among replicate wells. An example of how one could make a decision about reactivity to determine *antibody titer* is shown in Table 2. Other issues arise from control

Table 2
Example of how cytotoxicity scores may be used to determine antibody titer

Scores in replicate wells by reader 1				Scores in replicate wells by reader 2				
1	2	3	4	1	2	3	4	Interpretation
8	6							Positive
6	4							Positive
4	4							Positive
4	2							Reread. Negative, if the same result*
2	2							Negative*
6	2							Reread (by Reader 1 and/or 2)
4	4	4	2					Positive
4	4	2	2					Reread. Negative, if the same result*
4	4			4	2			Positive
4	2			4	2			Negative*
4	4	2	2	4	4	4	2	Positive
4	4	4	2	4	2	2	2	Negative*

Note: The above table is for determining antibody titer. Any of the scoring combinations under the "Interpretation" column and marked by "*" in a well with neat (undiluted) sera should be considered to be *weakly positive* or *suspicious* for positive for crossmatch interpretation. Patient history and antibody specificity information are especially important for determining compatibility in these situations. Also note that the table assumes that a score of "2" is considered to be negative

wells that which are scored incongruently from expected. For instance, if the negative control (serum) has viability <80 %, and the patient serum is scored with 4 and 2, it may be worthwhile repeating the assay.

24. Knowledge about sensitizing events and antibody specificity history are very important when interpreting crossmatch results. Also, patients who are being treated with therapeutic antibodies can pose some challenges for proper interpretation of CDC and AHG-CDC crossmatches. The antibodies in Table 3 have been shown to interfere anywhere from 3 months (polyclonal antibodies) up to 6 months or more (monoclonal antibodies).

25. While antibody, complement and cofactor (e.g., calcium) concentrations are important for complement fixation, a sometimes-ignored aspect of optimizing CDC/AHG-CDC are the target cells being used. The endpoint C′ can be different depending on cell type used (i.e., T cells versus B cells)

Table 3
Therapeutic antibodies that may interfere with the cytotoxicity assay

Antibody	Antigen target	T cell CDC	B cell CDC
Atgam	Multiple, includes HLA	*Positive*	*Positive*
Thymoglobulin	Multiple, includes HLA	*Positive*	*Positive*
Zenopax (Daclizumab)	IL2R/CD25 (activated T cells)	*Positive—if T cells are activated*	*Negative*
Rituxan (Rituximab)	CD20 (B cells)	+/–[a]	*Positive*
Campath (Alemtuzumab)	CD52	*Positive*	*Positive*

[a]CD20 has been detected on some normal T cells [34] so it may be possible for Rituxan, in patient serum, to cause a weakly false positive T cell crossmatch

because each of these cells may have different levels of complement regulatory factors [35, 36] and antigen density [37], which, may impact formation of the complement membrane attack complex. It is often necessary to use different lots of C′ for different cell types (e.g., have a T cell C′ and a B cell C′) since a lot that is strong enough for T cells may cause nonspecific cytotoxicity with B cells.

26. It is essential to include heat-inactivated complement (complement heated at 56 °C for 30 min and allowed to cool before use) to exclude non-complement protein cytotoxic components in the lot of complement being tested. Once HIC has been shown to be nontoxic (i.e., all cytotoxic activity is attributable to formation of the complement membrane attack complex), it is not necessary to include HIC in subsequent assays, as long as the same lot of complement is in use.
27. The endpoint is the most dilute you can make a particular lot of C′ to cause consistent complement-dependent cell death. Avoid using undiluted C′. It is best to use C′ in diluted form as the calcium and magnesium in the VBS diluent enhance C′ fixation. We dilute C′ to at least 1:1.5 (1 part C′ and ½ part VBS).
28. It may be necessary to test multiple lots of AHG to find one that results in optimal reactivity. If identifying an AHG lot for the first time, it is usually easiest to obtain serum with a known titer from a lab that is already performing AHG testing so that you have a starting point to identify an acceptable lot.
29. We usually obtain small samples of many different lots of AHG from a vendor or vendors, and do the initial evaluation and titration testing on the samples. Then, when the optimal lot is identified, a large volume is purchased to ensure a continuous supply to minimize the complex evaluation assays that need to

Table 4
Example of reagent volumes used when determining optimal dilution of premixed AHG and complement

Final dilutions		Volumes (μL)			
AHG	C′	C′	AHG (1:40)	VBS	Total
1:1,600	1:1.5	400	15	185	600
1:800	1:1.5	400	30	170	600
1:400	1:1.5	400	60	140	600
1:200	1:1.5	400	120	80	600
1:1,600	1:2	300	15	285	600
1:800	1:2	300	30	270	600
1:400	1:2	300	60	240	600
1:200	1:2	300	120	180	600

be done. (AHG can last for many years in the freezer with repeat titrations each year or whenever a new lot of C′ is introduced to determine if optimal dilution needs to be adjusted.) Once the large volume is received, aliquots are made and testing is done to determine optimal AHG-C′ dilution.

30. If the endpoint of the lot of complement is at 1:2, then evaluation of a new lot of AHG should be done using complement at both 1:2 and 1:1.5 (i.e., 2:3). Recall that you will use 5 μL of AHG-C′ mix per well and should make enough AHG-C′ mix (at the correct dilutions) for all wells to be tested. Note that the optimal dilution of AHG is usually higher when premixed with C′ in the assay compared to when the AHG and C′ are added separately. For example, our current lot of AHG works best at 1:50 when added separately but is used at 1:800 when mixed with C′.

In our experience, using very small volumes of stock AHG or complement to make AHG-C′ mixes can lead to inaccurate dilutions. Therefore, the minimum volume of AHG or complement that should be used to make dilutions should not be <5 μL. Keep AHG-C′ mixes on ice until ready for use.

Table 4 shows an example of volumes that might be used to make the dilutions for the tray layout in Fig. 3b. To avoid small volumes it is best to start with a stock of diluted AHG. In this case, the AHG is diluted to 1:40.

References

1. Bray RA, Nickerson PW, Kerman RH et al (2004) Evolution of HLA antibody detection: technology emulating biology. Immunol Res 29(1–3):41–54
2. Patel R, Terasaki PI (1969) Significance of the positive crossmatch test in kidney transplantation. N Engl J Med 280(14):735–739
3. Rodey GE (2000) HLA beyond tears—introduction to human histocompatibility, 2nd edn. De Novo, Inc., Durango, CO
4. Hopkins KA (2010) The basic lymphocyte and microcytotoxicity tests: standard and AHG enhancement. In: Hahn AB, Land GA, Strothman RA (eds) ASHI laboratory manual. American Society for Histocompatibility and Immunogenetics, Laurel, NJ
5. Pidwell DJ (2010) Interpretation of crossmatch results. In: Hahn AB, Land GA, Strothman RA (eds) ASHI laboratory manual. American Society for Histocompatibility and Immunogenetics, Laurel, NJ
6. Zachary AA, Klingman L, Thorne N et al (1995) Variations of the lymphocytotoxicity test. An evaluation of sensitivity and specificity. Transplantation 60(5):498–503
7. Fleisher T (2008) Laboratory reference values, in clinical immunology—principles and practice. In: RIch R et al (eds) Mosby Elsevier, Philadelphia, p 1513
8. Ting A, Hasegawa T, Ferrone S et al (1973) Presensitization detected by sensitive crossmatch tests. Transplant Proc 5(1):813–817
9. dos Reis AP, Betuel H, Reisner EG et al (1973) The utilization of antiglobulin reagents in cytotoxicity testing for HL-A. Transplantation 15(1):36–41
10. Fuller TC, Phelan D, Gebel HM et al (1982) Antigenic specificity of antibody reactive in the antiglobulin-augmented lymphocytotoxicity test. Transplantation 34(1):24–29
11. Mariuzza RA, Phillips SE, Poljak RJ (1987) The structural basis of antigen-antibody recognition. Annu Rev Biophys Biophys Chem 16:139–159
12. Akkoc N, Scornik JC (1991) Intramolecular specificity of anti-HLA alloantibodies. Hum Immunol 30(2):91–98
13. Taylor CJ, Chapman JR, Ting A et al (1989) Characterization of lymphocytotoxic antibodies causing a positive crossmatch in renal transplantation. Relationship to primary and regraft outcome. Transplantation 48(6):953–958
14. Cross DE, Greiner R, Whittier FC (1976) Importance of the autocontrol crossmatch in human renal transplantation. Transplantation 21(4):307–311
15. Scornik JC, Bray RA, Pollack MS et al (1997) Multicenter evaluation of the flow cytometry T-cell crossmatch: results from the American society of histocompatibility and immunogenetics-college of American pathologists proficiency testing program. Transplantation 63(10):1440–1445
16. Karpinski M, Rush D, Jeffery J et al (2001) Flow cytometric crossmatching in primary renal transplant recipients with a negative anti-human globulin enhanced cytotoxicity crossmatch. J Am Soc Nephrol 12(12):2807–2814
17. Gebel HM, Bray RA (2000) Sensitization and sensitivity: defining the unsensitized patient. Transplantation 69(7):1370–1374
18. Mahoney RJ, Ault KA, Given SR et al (1990) The flow cytometric crossmatch and early renal transplant loss. Transplantation 49(3):527–535
19. Scornik JC, Clapp W, Patton PR et al (2001) Outcome of kidney transplants in patients known to be flow cytometry crossmatch positive. Transplantation 71(8):1098–1102
20. Kerman RH, Susskind B, Buyse I et al (1999) Flow cytometry-detected IgG is not a contraindication to renal transplantation: IgM may be beneficial to outcome. Transplantation 68(12):1855–1858
21. Gebel HM, Bray RA, Nickerson P (2003) Pre-transplant assessment of donor-reactive. HLA-specific antibodies in renal transplantation: contraindication vs. risk. Am J Transplant 3(12):1488–1500
22. Wen R, Wu V, Dmitrienko S et al (2006) Biomarkers in transplantation: prospective, blinded measurement of predictive value for the flow cytometry crossmatch after negative antiglobulin crossmatch in kidney transplantation. Kidney Int 70(8):1474–1481
23. Christiaans MH, Overhof R, ten Haaft A et al (1996) No advantage of flow cytometry crossmatch over complement-dependent cytotoxicity in immunologically well-documented renal allograft recipients. Transplantation 62(9):1341–1347
24. Zeevi A, Girnita A, Duquesnoy R (2007) HLA antibody analysis: sensitivity, specificity, and clinical significance in solid organ transplantation. Immunol Res 36(1–3):255–264
25. Colombo MB, Haworth SE, Poli F et al (2007) Luminex technology for anti-HLA antibody screening: evaluation of performance and of impact on laboratory routine. Cytometry B Clin Cytom 72(6):465–471
26. Warner P (2009) Nebulous humors: defining alloantibodies in the 21st century. Hum Immunol 70(8):623–626
27. Aubert V, Venetz JP, Pantaleo G et al (2009) Low levels of human leukocyte antigen donor-specific antibodies detected by solid phase assay before transplantation are frequently clinically irrelevant. Hum Immunol 70(8):580–583

28. Poli F, Benazzi E, Innocente A et al (2011) Heart transplantation with donor-specific antibodies directed toward denatured HLA-A*02:01: a case report. Hum Immunol 72(11):1045–1048
29. Opelz G, Claas FH (2009) Which human leukocyte antigen antibodies are really clinically relevant? Hum Immunol 70(8):561–562
30. Okuno T, Kondelis N (1978) Evaluation of dithiothreitol (DTT) for inactivation of IgM antibodies. J Clin Pathol 31(12):1152–1155
31. Wohler JE, Barnum SR (2009) Nylon wool purification alters the activation of T cells. Mol Immunol 46(5):1007–1010
32. Amos DB, Bashir H, Boyle W et al (1969) A simple micro cytotoxicity test. Transplantation 7(3):220–223
33. Rodey G, Bollig B, Oldfather J et al (1987) Extra reactivities detected in flow-cytometry-positive, CDC-negative crossmatches are definable HLA specificities. Transplant Proc 19(1 Pt 1):778–779
34. Quintanilla-Martinez L, Preffer F, Rubin D et al (1994) CD20+ T-cell lymphoma. Neoplastic transformation of a normal T-cell subset. Am J Clin Pathol 102(4):483–489
35. Nagakura S, Nakakuma H, Horikawa K et al (1993) Expression of decay-accelerating factor and CD59 in lymphocyte subsets of healthy individuals and paroxysmal nocturnal hemoglobinuria patients. Am J Hematol 43(1):14–18
36. Cui W, Fan Y, Yang M et al (2004) Expression of CD59 on lymphocyte and the subsets and its potential clinical application for paroxysmal nocturnal hemoglobinuria diagnosis. Clin Lab Haematol 26(2):95–100
37. Pellegrino MA, Belvedere M, Pellegrino AG et al (1978) B peripheral lymphocytes express more HLA antigens than T peripheral lymphocytes. Transplantation 25(2):93–95

Chapter 14

Lymphocyte Crossmatching by Flow Cytometry

Robert A. Bray

Abstract

Flow cytometry is an invaluable tool for studying lymphocyte biology. In transplantation, flow cytometry represents the most sensitive method for demonstrating the binding of HLA antibodies to cellular targets. Referred to as the flow cytometric crossmatch (FCXM), the implementation of this method has revolutionized HLA antibody assessments and facilitated increased allograft survival among highly sensitized recipients. Here we describe the methods for performing the FCXM and discuss its critical aspects, as well as the presentation of data and interpretation of results.

Key words Flow cytometry, Lymphocyte, Crossmatch, Anti-human IgG, HLA, Alloantibody, Transplantation

1 Introduction

The detection of circulating HLA antibodies in the serum of potential allograft recipients is an essential assessment performed prior to and after transplantation [1]. If HLA antibodies are directed against the mismatched antigens of the donor, there may be serious clinical consequences. Depending upon the strength of the antibody and possibly the HLA specificity, the clinical impact may range from benign to severe constituting a contraindication for transplantation. The lymphocyte crossmatch is one tool used to help assess the risk posed by the presence of donor-specific HLA antibodies (DSA). While there have been many methods for performing a lymphocyte crossmatch, currently, one of the most widely used employs flow cytometry. Early crossmatch methods utilized a complement dependent cytotoxicity assay which was adequate for detecting most HLA antibodies that were responsible for hyperacute graft rejection. However, this methodology did not detect low concentrations of antibodies that may have led to accelerated graft rejection and, in some instances, early graft loss. Consequently, new and more sensitive crossmatching methods

Andrea A. Zachary and Mary S. Leffell (eds.), *Transplantation Immunology: Methods and Protocols, Second Edition*, Methods in Molecular Biology, vol. 1034, DOI 10.1007/978-1-62703-493-7_14, © Springer Science+Business Media, LLC 2013

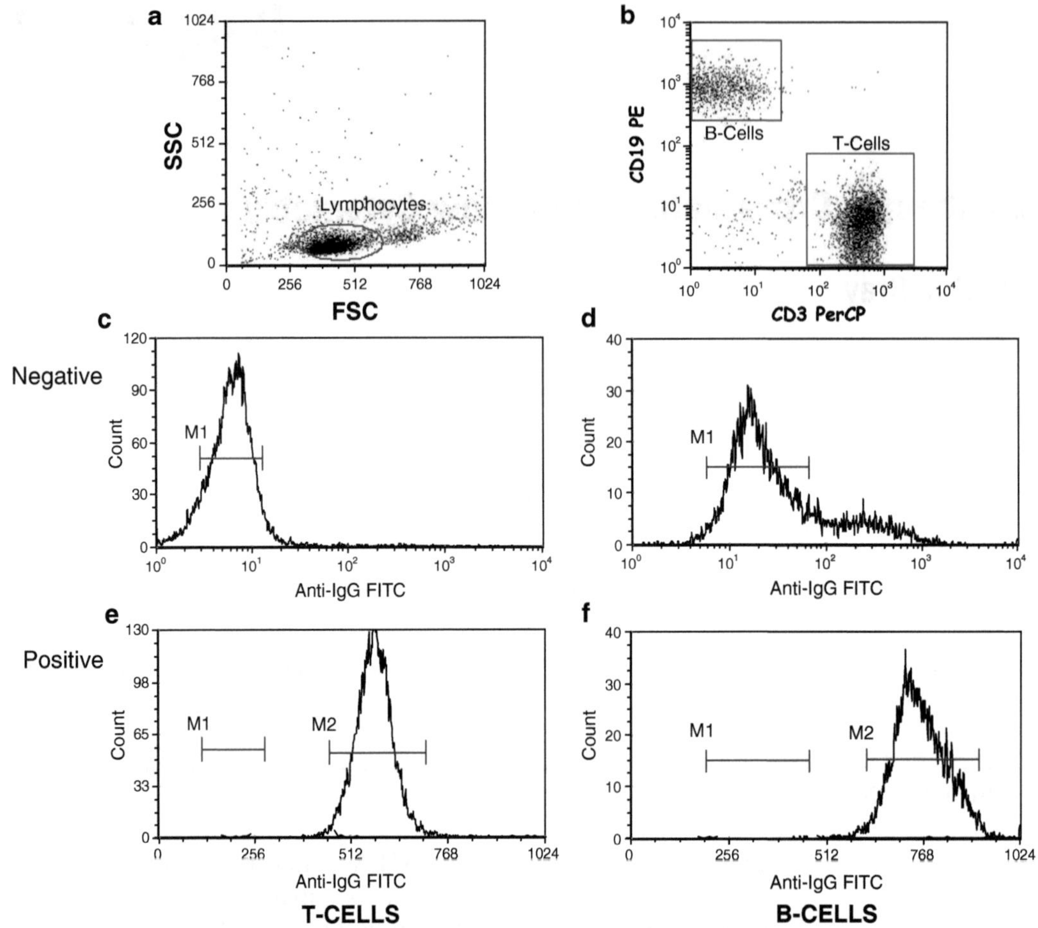

Fig. 1 Illustrates the cytometer acquisition setup for performing the flow cytometric crossmatch. (**a**) Gating of lymphocytes using forward scatter (FSC) versus side scatter (SSC) plot. This is an example of the scatter pattern from a lymph node. (**b**) Gating strategy for identifying T-Cells (CD3 PerCP) and B-Cells (CD19 PE). (**c**, **d**) Examples of fluorescence from anti-human IgG staining with a negative control serum. (**e**, **f**) Examples of fluorescence from anti-human IgG staining with a positive control serum

were developed ultimately leading to the utilization of flow cytometric as a preferred approach [2, 3].

The flow cytometric crossmatch (FCXM) is performed by incubating donor cells with the serum from a potential recipient. If donor-specific HLA antibodies are present, they will be deposited on the surface of the target cell. Assessment of alloantibody binding is performed by the addition of a fluorochrome labeled goat, anti-human immunoglobulin reagent. The level of measured fluorescence is then proportional to the amount of alloantibody bound to the target cell. In order to help differentiate the class of antibody that may be binding to lymphocytes, labeled monoclonal antibodies are used to identify T-cells (CD3) or B cells (CD19) (Fig. 1). This three-color combination allows for the simultaneous

Table 1
Potential reactivity patterns in the flow cytometric crossmatch

T cell	B cell	Interpretation[a]
Negative	Negative	No HLA antibody or very low titer
Negative	Positive	Predominantly Class II antibody
Negative	Wk positive	Weak Class I or II antibody
Positive	Positive	Strong Class I antibody or a combination of Class I and Class II
Positive	Negative	Likely non-HLA reactivity

[a]Assumes that HLA specificity has been confirmed via alternative solid-phase testing methods

detection of alloantibodies reacting with T cells and/or B cells and eliminates confounding background staining due to natural killer (NK) cells or monocytes [4]. Table 1 shows the possible reaction patterns of the flow cytometric crossmatch and their interpretations. Results are then analyzed by comparing the fluorescence value of the patient's serum to the fluorescence value of a control serum (i.e., one lacking HLA antibodies). Depending upon the specificity and strength of reactivity, the transplant may proceed, be cancelled or proceed with the knowledge that the patient may require additional therapeutic intervention(s) prior to or soon after transplantation [5]. The FCXM is usually the last hurdle to be cleared by a patient on their way to a successful transplant [6].

2 Materials

2.1 Specimen Requirements

1. Lymphocytes, purified from peripheral blood, spleen, or lymph nodes, are the preferred target cell population. Mononuclear cells obtained from peripheral blood may be used provided the lymphocyte percentage is >50 %. Pre test cell viability should be >80 %. There should be a sufficient number of lymphocytes to run the test. Minimum concentration of viable lymphocytes is approximately, 1×10^6 cells (1×10^5 cells/tube for five tubes—see below).
2. Cells may be pronase treated prior to testing [7, 8].
3. Serum (1 ml minimum) from patient(s) being evaluated. Pretreatment of serum prior to use in the crossmatch may be useful (*see* **Note 1**). Pretreatment may also include high-speed or ultracentrifugation to remove large immune aggregates (*see* **Note 1**).

2.2 Testing Components

1. Fluoroscein-conjugated goat, anti-human IgG [F(ab)'$_2$, Fc specific] (Jackson Labs. Cat # 109-016-098) (*see* **Note 2**).
2. Anti-human CD3 PerCP (peridinin chlorophyll protein) Becton-Dickinson, Inc. San Jose, CA) (*see* **Note 3**).
3. Anti-human CD19, phycoerythrin-conjugated. Becton-Dickinson, Inc., San Jose, CA (*see* **Note 3**).
4. Flow Wash Buffer (Phosphate buffered saline, 2 % fetal bovine serum and 0.1 % sodium azide, NaN_3).
5. Serum (at least 100 μl minimum) from the patient(s) to be tested (*see* **Note 3**).
6. Quantum™ FITC 5 MESF microspheres (product #555p) and Quick Cal™ v 2.3 data analysis program (Bangs laboratories, Fishers, IN.).

2.3 Equipment and Supplies

1. Eppendorf Pipettes with tips. A pipettor with a range of 20–200 μl is sufficient. Both single channel and multiple channel pipettors may be used.
2. 6 × 50 mm glass tubes (Kimble/Chase Scientific #: 73500-650), 1.5 ml plastic centrifuge tubes (Robbins Scientific, #101-000-00 or similar)

   OR

   96 well, U-bottom, tissue culture treated tray (Costar, #3799).
3. Beckman Airfuge (Ultracentrifuge) with microultracentrifuge tubes and protective caps (Beckman-Coulter, #342630)

   OR

   High-speed centrifuge capable of spinning small tubes and attaining >5,000 × *g*.
4. Centrifuge capable of spinning small tubes and/or 96 well trays.
5. Vacuum aspirator.
6. Flow cytometer.

2.4 Control Serum

1. Negative control (normal human (single donor) or pooled human sera) is thoroughly tested to ensure that it is devoid of HLA antibody and that it has a background fluorescence signal comparable to that of the patients being tested.
2. Positive control (Pooled positive serum), titered for flow cytometry. Positive control serum should be tested to ensure that it contains reactivity to a majority of common HLA phenotypes. Usually this is accomplished by combining samples containing broadly reactive HLA Class I and Class II antibodies.

3 Methods

3.1 Initial Serum/Cell Incubations

1. Place no more than 200,000—250,000 cells in tubes (6×50 or 1.5 ml) or wells of a 96 well tray. An absolute minimum is 100,000. *NOTE*: In using a cell preparation that is not >90 % lymphocytes, count *ALL nucleated cells*, lymphocytes, monocytes and neutrophils, as they all have HLA Class I antigens on their surface. Make sure that your tubes indicate the cell sample—i.e., a label, colored tape, etc. *Mix the cell prep well before adding the cells suspension to the tubes/trays* (*see* **Note 4**).

   Tubes/Wells should be labeled and set up as follows:

Tube #	
Well #	**Primary antibody/serum**
1	Negative control
2	Pooled positive serum
3	Negative control (may be different from or same as tube #1)
4	Cell control (i.e., Flow Wash Buffer Only)
5	Patient serum sample #1[a]
6	Patient serum samples #2 – *n*[a]

[a]For flow cytometric crossmatches, it is recommended that the patient serum be tested in duplicate

2. (a) For 6×50 or 1.5 ml tubes centrifuge cells to a pellet (*see* **Note 5**).

   (b) For 96 well trays, centrifuge for 3 min at 900×*g* in a centrifuge designed for 96 well plate centrifugation.

3. *For tubes*, aspirate supernatant *being careful not to aspirate the cell pellet*. Pellet should be *nearly dry*. Residual fluid volume should be <10 μl.

   For trays, flick trays by quickly turning upside down to force supernatant from the wells. Leaving the tray upside down, blot vigorously onto paper towels (*see* **Note 6**).

3.2 Primary Serum/Cell Incubation

1. Add 25 μl of the appropriate serum (or Wash Buffer for cell control tube) *directly* to the cell pellet in each corresponding tube or well of a tray (*see* **Note 3**). Exercise caution when pipetting and do not to allow the serum to run down the side of the tube or well (*see* **Notes** 7 and **8**).

2. Incubate tubes or trays for ~30 min at 4 °C (in refrigerator or on ice) or room temperature with constant or intermittent mixing. The temperature is *not* a critical aspect of this test but the mixing step is. Alternative incubation times may also be appropriate [9, 10]. However, each laboratory should establish its own protocol and consistently follow such protocol.
3. *For 6×50 tubes*, wash cells with 400 μl of *Cold* Flow Wash Buffer (Add 200 μl, vortex, then add the additional 200 μl).

   For 1.5 ml tubes, wash cells with 1 ml of *Cold* Flow Wash Buffer (Add 500 μl, vortex, then add the additional 500 μl).

   For 96 well trays, wash cells with 150 μl of *Cold* Flow Wash Buffer (Add 75 μl, vortex, then add the additional 75 μl).
4. *For tubes*, centrifuge cells to a pellet—1 min at 700×*g* or comparable.

   For trays, centrifuge for 3 min at 900×*g* in a centrifuge designed for a 96 well plate centrifugation. Place brake on low.
5. Aspirate supernatant (as in **step #3**) or flick trays (**step #3**) and repeat wash as in **steps #6** and 7 two more times for a total of *three washes for tubes* and three more times for a total of *four washes for trays* (*see* **Notes 9** and **10**).

3.3 Addition of Anti-human IgG and Monoclonal Antibodies

1. Following the last wash, including aspiration or flicking, vortex cells to disaggregate the cell pellet. Carefully add 25 μl of pre-titered FITC anti-IgG to each tube (*see* **Notes 11** and **12**). Next, add 20 μl of CD3 PerCP and 20 μl of CD19-PE *OR* add 40 μl of CD3 PerCP/CD19-PE combined to each tube or well. Vortex gently and incubate at 4 °C or room temperature *in the dark*, for 20–30 min (*see* **Note 13**).
2. *For tubes* wash cells 2× with *Cold* wash buffer (400 μl washes for 6×50 tubes and 1 ml washes for 1.5 ml tubes) and centrifuge as in **steps #6** and 7 above.

   For trays wash cells 3× with *cold* wash buffer as in **step #6** and 7 above.
3. *For tubes*, resuspend cell pellet in 200–500 μl of *Cold* wash buffer depending upon the tube used.

   For trays, resuspend cell pellet in 150 μl of *cold* wash buffer (*see* **Note 14**).
4. If using trays and a flow cytometer that does not accommodate 96 well trays, transfer samples to tubes before analyzing on the flow cytometer (*see* **Note 15**).

3.4 Data Acquisition and Analysis

1. Set up cytometer and run daily calibration and compensation controls.

   Since there are several types of commercial cytometers each with their own setup and calibrations procedures, individual cytometer setup and calibrations are not covered in this chapter.

2. After the cytometer is set up and calibrated. Acquire samples based on acquisition template shown in Fig. 1. The parameters for data acquisition are as follows:
   (a) Gate initially on lymphocyte population from forward versus side scatter plot (Fig. 1a).
   (b) Ensure that CD3 positive events and CD20 positive events are present and align within their respective gate (Fig. 1b).
   (c) Ensure that events are being collected in both the CD3 and CD19 histograms (Fig. 1c, d).
   (d) Set acquisition stop gate on CD19 events. Set cell count number to between 1,000 and 2,000 events. This will ensure that a sufficient number of B-cell events will be collected for analysis. There will be sufficient T cell events collected.
   (e) Acquire all data using a high resolution or 1,024 channel scale or the linear values obtained from the log scale on the cytometer.
   (f) Set marker regions around the control populations (Fig. 1c, d). When acquiring patient samples and a sample appears positive, (i.e., not falling within the regions formed by the negative control serum) set a second region marker around the major cell population in the histogram (Fig. 1e, f).
3. Run all patient samples and controls and store appropriately labeled FCS files on computer hard drive for subsequent analysis.
4. Once all samples have been acquired, results can be analyzed using analysis template created with cytometer software or other third party flow cytometry analysis software. Nonetheless, analysis should contain all of the data elements shown in Fig. 1.
5. For data analysis one calculates the change in fluorescence of a patient's sample compared to the negative control. This is referred to as the delta fluorescence value. For positive samples, a significant increase in fluorescence will be observed. For negative samples, either no change in fluorescence or a decreased florescence value may be observed. Delta fluorescence may be represented as a difference in channel values, linear values, a ratio of linear values or by converting to Molecules of Equivalent Soluble Fluorochrome (Figs. 2 and 3). Converting to MESF values provides a true linear representation of the data and is independent of the day-to-day differences in cytometer setup that may occur. MESF values can also be used to "normalize" values between two different instruments either at the same institution or at different institutions/

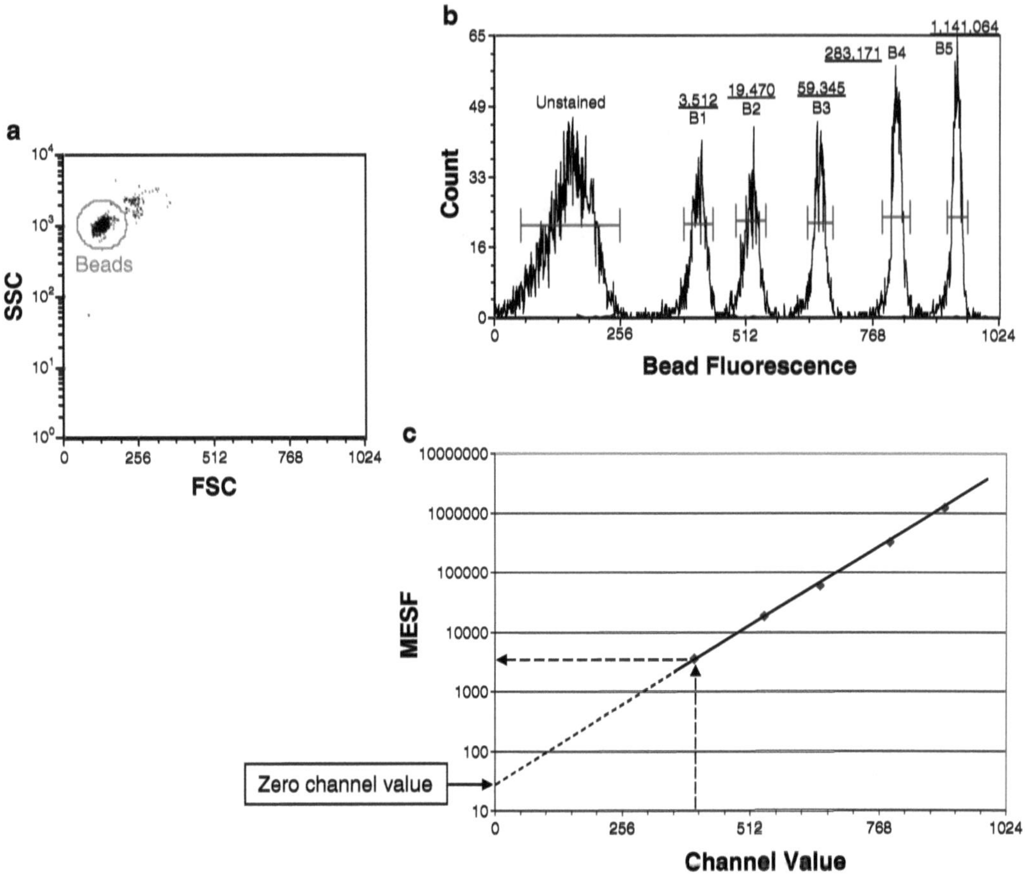

Fig. 2 Illustrates the cytometer display of the Quantum™ MESF beads. (**a**) Gating display using forward light scatter (FSC) versus side scatter (SSC). Note for this plot the SSC parameter is collected with logarithmic amplification while FSC is collected with linear amplification. The result is a tighter bead population for gating and the ability to exclude doublets (e.g., larger cell clusters). (**b**) Histogram of the FL1 fluorescence of the gated MESF beads. Note six distinct bead peaks; one negative bead and five positive peaks of varying fluorescence intensity. The values above each peak are the corresponding MESF (Molecules of Equivalent Soluble Fluorochrome) for each bead. (**c**) Plot showing the linear relationship between channel value and MESF when MESFs are plotted on a log scale. Any channel value can be converted to a corresponding MESF value (*dashed arrows*). The dashed line is the extrapolation of the fluorescence regression line to the "Zero channel value". This value represents the approximate background fluorescence of the instrument. That is, the inherent instrument background fluorescence at the "0" channel

Fig. 3 Illustrates three different approaches for analyzing results from the flow cytometric crossmatch. In each of the three examples, the exact same data is plotted. The difference is the approach for determining the result. The "Neg" peak represents the result from the negative control serum. The "Pos" peak represents the results from a potential patient. The *arrows* indicate the difference in median values between the two peaks. (**a**) Histogram overlay of a Negative and Positive crossmatch result. This data is plotted using linear values (i.e., the actual log number). Calculating the difference between the Negative population and Positive population is performed by assessing the ratio of the positive value to the negative value. In this instance, the positive peak has a median fluorescence value that

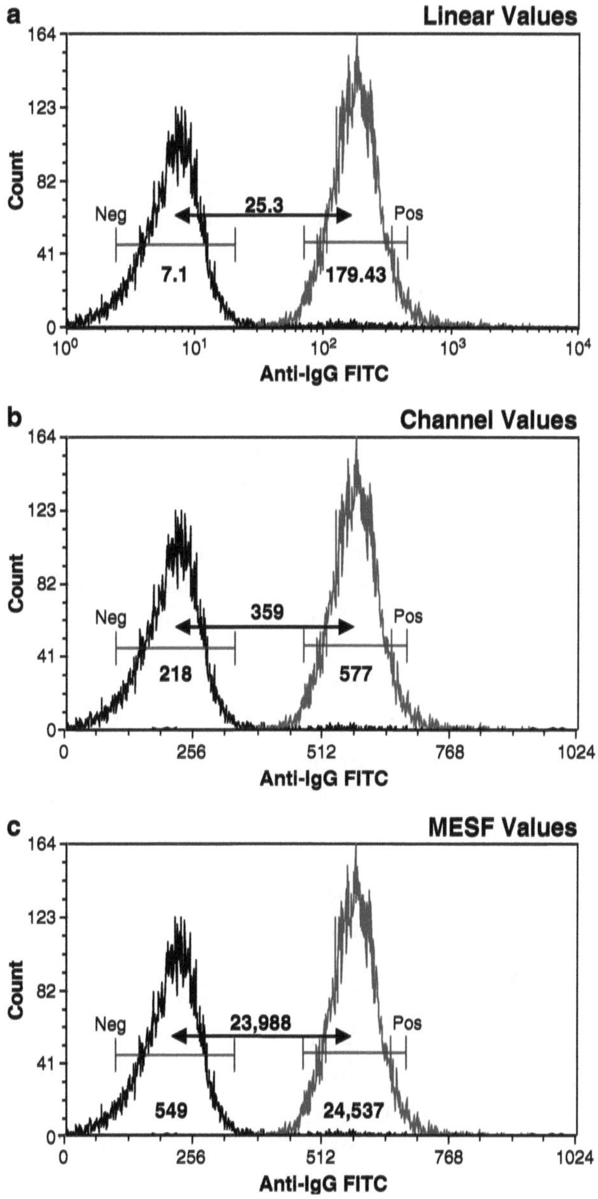

Fig. 3 (continued) is ~25 times greater than the negative control. For such determinations, a ratio of >2 is used to discriminate positive from negative. (**b**) Histogram overlay of the same data but displaying channel values. The median channel value of the negative peak is subtracted from the median channel value of the positive peak. The difference, delta channel shift (delta = +359 channels) is used to discriminate positive from negative. For such determinations, a channel shift of >40 channels (1,024 channel scale) is used as a cutoff. However, each laboratory must define its own range for determining a cutoff value. (**c**) Histogram overlay of the same data but the channel values have been converted in to MESF values (Fig. 2). The MESF value of the Negative control is subtracted from the MESF value of the positive sample. The difference in MESFs (+23,988) is used to discriminate a positive from a negative result. The cutoff value, in MESF, for T and B cells may be different. In general, T-cell values >~2,500 MESF and B-cell values >~4,000 MESF are considered positive. However, each laboratory must define its own MESF cutoff values for these cell populations

locations. This presumes that both centers use the same lot of MESF beads. MESF beads can also serve as an additional quality control material for machine performance. For additional information please see the manufacturer's Web site (http://www.bangslabs.com/).

4 Notes

1. There are important procedures for the pretreatment of serum prior to testing. These procedures may be necessary in order to reduce nonspecific background binding and to remove interfering substances such as IgM, immune complexes, and activated complement components [11, 12]. The use of these procedures is the prerogative of the laboratory director in consultation with his/her clinical team. In addition, high speed or ultracentrifugation of the serum sample may help reduce nonspecific background binding by remove large immune aggregates.
2. After reconstituting the FITC reagent, airfuge (ultracentrifuge or high speed centrifuge) the entire stock to remove aggregates. Dilute with flow wash buffer to the current working dilution and aliquot the pre-titered FITC into 1 ml Sarstedt (product #: 72.694.007 or similar vial) screw-cap microtubes and store at −70 up to 3 months. When ready to use just thaw and mix. Place any unused portion in the −4 refrigerator for storage up to 7 days. Once thawed, store FITC at *4 °C* and *protect from light.*
3. Alternative fluorochromes may be required depending upon the optics of the flow cytometer utilized.
4. Maximum tube volume is 450 μl for 6 × 50 tubes; 1 ml for 1.5 tubes and 200 μl for 96 well trays. The number of tubes/wells will depend upon the number of serum samples to be tested.
5. Generally, 700–900 × *g* for 1 min but the time and speed may vary depending upon the particular centrifuge.
6. Thoroughly vortex cells to disaggregate the cell pellet (tubes or trays) prior to the addition of patient serum.
7. It is recommended that patient serum be added directly to a dry cell pellet. The sensitivity of the assay can be affected by altering this aspect. Generally, when adding patient's serum to cells in liquid suspension, a 2 to 1 (serum volume to cell liquid volume) ratio should be used in order to provide comparable sensitivity to the serum that is added directly to a dry pellet.
8. Vortex the dry pellet prior to adding wash buffer to ensure that cells are completely disaggregated. Failure to completely disaggregate the cell pellet will result in inconsistent results

and potentially high backgrounds. Lack of proper washing can also lead to false negative results due to excess immunoglobulin interfering with the staining of the anti-human IgG.

9. *Be careful* not to cross-contaminate samples with pipette tips when aspirating supernatant. For tubes, be sure to aspirate positive control *last* to decrease the chance of carryover. Rinse tip after aspirating positive control.
10. *Be careful* when flicking trays. Cross-contamination can occur with improper flicking technique.
11. Check titer and proper dilution of *all* reagents prior to use. FITC anti-human IgG must be properly titered prior to use. Titration is performed to establish the optimal signal-to-noise ratio.
12. Although using monoclonal antibodies at the manufacturers recommended concentration is acceptable, some monoclonal antibodies may be titered further prior to use. It is up to each laboratory to determine the working concentration for all monoclonal antibodies.
13. CD3 PerCP and CD19 PE may be combined using equal volumes of the appropriate dilution of each reagent. The combination may be stored in the refrigerator for up to 1 month. *Do not freeze any phycoerythrin-conjugated antibody.*
14. It is important to remember to store the *all* reagents *Cold and fluorescent reagents in the Dark as well!*
15. *Be accurate*: Due to the high sensitivity of flow cytometry, all cell concentrations, serum dilutions, and serum volumes must be *exact* and *accurate*. Small fluctuations in cell numbers and serum volumes or dilution errors will result in erroneous and inconsistent results. The two aspects with the greatest potential for error are (1) inaccurate cell counts and (2) incomplete wash steps. Both of these aspects can lead to false negative results.

References

1. Gebel HM, Bray RA (2010) The evolution and clinical impact of human leukocyte antigen technology. Curr Opin Nephrol Hypertens 19:598–602
2. Garovoy MR, Rheinschmilt MA, Bigos M, Perkins H, Colombe B, Feduska N, Salvatierra O (1983) Flow cytometry analysis: a high technology crossmatch technique facilitating transplantation. Transplant Proc 15:1939
3. Cook DJ, Terasaki PI, Iwaki Y, Terashita GY, Lau M (1987) An approach to reducing early kidney transplant failure by flow cytometry crossmatching. Clin Transplantation 1:253–258
4. Bray RA, Lebeck LK, Gebel HM (1989) The flow cytometric crossmatch: dual color analysis of T and B cell reactivities. Transplantation 48:834–840
5. Gebel HM, Bray RA, Nickerson P (2003) Pretransplant assessment of donor reactive HLA-specific HLA antibodies in renal transplantation: contraindication vs risk. Am J Transplant 3:1488–1500
6. Bray RA, Tarsitani C, Gebel HM, Lee JH (2011) Clinical cytometry and progress in HLA antibody detection. Methods Cell Biol 103:285–310

7. Lobo P, Spencer CE, Stevenson WC et al (1995) The use of Pronase digested lymphocytes to improve the specificity of the flow cytometric crossmatch. Tranplant Int 8:472
8. Vaidya S, Cooper TY, Avandsalehi J, Barnes T, Brooks K, Hymel P, Noor M, Sellers R, Thomas A, Stewart D, Daller J, Fish JC, Gugliuzza KK, Bray RA (2001) Improved flow cytometric detection of HLA alloantibodies using pronase: potential implications in renal transplantation. Transplantation 71(3): 422–428
9. Liwski R, Adams G, Peladeau G, Eckels D, Bray R, Gebel H (2011) An Optimized flow cytometric crossmatch assay expedites pre-transplant immunologic risk assessment. Hum Immunol 72(suppl. 1):s48
10. Liwski R, Pochinco D, Tinckam K, Gebel H, Campbell P, Nickerson P (2012) Canada-wide evaluation of rapid optimized flow crossmatch (rofcxm) protocol. Hum Immunol 73 (suppl. 1):26
11. Zachary AA, Lucas DP, Detrick B, Leffell MS (2009) Naturally occurring interference in Luminex assays for HLA-specific antibodies: characteristics and resolution. Hum Immunol 70(7):496–501
12. Schnaidt M, Weinstock C, Jurisic M et al (2011) HLA antibody specification using single-antigen beads—a technical solution for the prozone effect. Transplantation 92(5):510–515

Chapter 15

Solid Phase Assay Measuring C4d Deposition to Determine Complement Fixation by HLA-Specific Antibodies

John D. Smith and Marlene L. Rose

Abstract

The definition of HLA-specific antibodies in solid organ transplant patients is a necessary tool for recipient selection prior to transplantation and monitoring for rejection post transplant. Solid phase assays can detect both complement fixing and non-complement fixing HLA-specific antibodies. Here we describe a method for determining the presence of complement fixing HLA-specific antibodies using a sensitive solid phase assay.

Key words Complement, HLA antibodies, C4d, Multiplexed bead assays

1 Introduction

Historically, HLA antibodies were detected by the complement-dependent cytotoxicity assay (CDC) with a strong correlation between the presence of CDC donor-specific HLA antibodies (DSA) and poor graft survival after renal, cardiac, and lung transplantation [1–4]. With the advent of solid phase assays, particularly those using Luminex® x-map microspheres, both complement and non-complement fixing antibodies are detected and at much lower levels than seen with CDC assays. Luminex®-based assays have been shown to detect HLA-specific antibodies in 5–10 times more patients than conventional CDC methods [5].

It is clear that transplantation of kidney, heart, or lungs in the presence of preformed CDC detected DSA leads to hyperacute rejection or accelerated antibody-mediated rejection (AMR) in the majority of cases [1–4]. The role of HLA DSA detected by solid phase assays alone is less clear [6, 7]. It is possible that there will be increased rejection and graft loss compared to patients with no HLA-specific antibodies, but hyperacute rejection is unlikely.

Many laboratories no longer use CDC as part of their antibody screening programs relying instead on the more sensitive solid phase bead assays to detect and define the presence of HLA

Andrea A. Zachary and Mary S. Leffell (eds.), *Transplantation Immunology: Methods and Protocols, Second Edition*, Methods in Molecular Biology, vol. 1034, DOI 10.1007/978-1-62703-493-7_15, © Springer Science+Business Media, LLC 2013

antibodies. Whilst this approach will maximize the detection of HLA-specific antibodies, definition of unacceptable HLA antigens in the donor (UDA) when listing patients is challenging as the Luminex® bead assays are at best semiquantitative.

The C4d assay developed using the Luminex® bead assays provides a more functional aspect to antibody definition than other solid phase methods of antibody detection. This type of assay was first developed by Wahrmann et al. [8] in flow cytometry assays utilizing FlowPRA® beads and used for the detection of HLA antibodies in renal transplant patients [9]. We modified the assay for Luminex® beads. Using the C4d fixing Luminex® assay, we compared it to CDC for detection of pre-transplant HLA antibodies in 653 cardiac transplant patients transplanted between 1991 and 2005 [5]. We demonstrated that the assay was considerably more sensitive than CDC. In our study, the C4d assay detected complement fixation by HLA-specific antibodies in 22 patients prior to cardiac transplantation (11 DSA, 11 non-DSA) compared to CDC which detected HLA antibodies in only nine patients. Moreover, it was demonstrated that patients transplanted with C4d fixing HLA DSA had a significantly reduced 1 year graft survival of 20 % compared with 54 % for patients transplanted with DSA which did not fix C4d in the assay, $p = 0.0002$ [5].

The potential uses for this assay are not only for definition of UDA in sensitized patients awaiting transplantation but also for detection of DSA/HLA produced after transplantation. Studies have shown that de novo production of DSA is detrimental for cardiac allograft survival [10]. Defining UDA by C4d fixation prior to transplantation could lead to an expansion of the potential donor pool for sensitized patients compared to UDA defined by the standard IgG binding assay, shorten the time to transplantation whilst still avoiding the risk of hyperacute rejection. The assay has been shown to be useful for post-transplant monitoring of HLA-specific antibodies, in patients transplanted in the absence of pre-transplant DSA. For example, in a recent study [11], 13 of 15 patients who developed late AMR (i.e., years after their transplant) were shown to be producing C4d–fixing DSA at the time AMR was diagnosed.

There are four stages to the assay: (1) HLA-specific antibody binding to antigen, (2) complement fixation, (3) binding of antibody to human C4d, and (4) detection stage. The assay relies upon HLA-specific complement binding antibodies (IgM, IgG1, and IgG3) binding to target antigen causing activation of the complement cascade resulting in fixation of the complement split product C4d to the microsphere. Although the test serum (i.e., patient's serum) may contain complement, in our experience it is necessary to add an exogenous source of complement such as normal human serum to maximize detection of C4d. Here we use a two stage process for the detection of complement deposition, first, a monoclonal antibody raised in mouse targeted to human C4d followed by an antibody to mouse immunoglobulins conjugated to phycoerythrin for detection in the Luminex® analyzer.

2 Materials

2.1 Luminex® X-Map Microspheres

1. LABScreen® Single Antigen HLA Class I—Combi (Catalog No. LS1A04) (One Lambda).
2. LABScreen® Single Antigen HLA Class II Antibody Detection Test—Group 1 (Catalog No. LS2A01) (One Lambda).

2.2 Equipment

1. Luminex® LABScan™ 100/200 flow analyzer (Luminex® Corporation).
2. Millipore filter plates.
3. MultiScreen™ Vacuum Manifold 96-well (Millipore).
4. Vacuum pump with a pressure less than 100 mmHg.
5. Sheath fluid.

2.3 Antibodies and Conjugates

Mouse anti-human C4d (*see* **Note 4**) (Ab Serotec 222-8004).

Normal Human serum (*see* **Notes 2, 3**).

Donkey anti-mouse IgG-PE Conjugate (Jackson Immunoresearch).

3 Methods

Carry out all procedures at room temperature unless otherwise specified.

C4d assay using Labscreen Single antigen kits

1. Cover the unassigned wells of the filter plate with an adhesive plastic cover. Pre-wet the wells to be used with 200 μl of wash buffer. Leave for 5 min after which time aspirate the plate using the vacuum manifold.
2. Centrifuge the beads briefly to remove any liquid from the cap of the tube. Thoroughly vortex the beads for approximately 1 min to evenly resuspend the beads.
3. Incubate 5 μl of LABScreen® beads with 20 μl of test serum and negative/positive controls to the appropriate wells of a 96-well plate in the dark for 30 min at 20–25 °C with gentle shaking (*see* **Note 5**).
4. After incubation add 250 μl 1× wash buffer to each test well. Aspirate the plate using the vacuum manifold. Repeat two times. NOTE: Do not exceed 100 mmHg vacuum pressure. A rapid vacuum will cause loss of beads due to entrapment in the pores of the filter paper. Failure to wash sufficiently to remove all

unbound immunoglobulin may reduce the ability of the conjugate to detect IgG bound the beads and cause false-negative results (*see* **Note 1**).

5. The Normal Human Serum must be taken out to thaw ~15 min prior to use. Centrifuge the serum at 16,000 × *g* for at least 3 min. Add 50 μl of Normal Human serum to each of the wells making sure the pellet at the bottom of the tube is not disturbed. Incubate in the dark for 30 min at 20–25 °C with gentle shaking.
6. After incubation add 250 μl 1× wash buffer to each test well. Aspirate the plate using the vacuum manifold. Repeat four times.
7. Prepare a 1/100 dilution of the mouse anti-human C4d antibody in PBS. Add 50 μl of the antibody to all of the test wells (including control wells) on the plate. Incubate in the dark for 30 min at 20–25 °C with gentle shaking.
8. Repeat wash **step 6**.
9. Immediately prepare a 1/100 dilution of the donkey anti-mouse IgG-PE conjugate with PBS for the appropriate number of test samples. Add 50 μl of the antibody to all of the test wells (including control wells) on the plate. Incubate in the dark for 30 min at 20–25 °C with gentle shaking.
10. Repeat wash **step 6**. Aspirate the plate using the vacuum manifold and add 100 μl PBS to each well and mix gently in the dark for at least 5 min.
11. Load the plate into the Labscan Flow analyzer and proceed with acquisition.
12. Analyze using the HLA Fusion software.

4 Notes

1. There are an increased number of wash steps in this procedure in comparison to the standard antibody binding assays. It is important therefore to ensure that during the wash steps beads do not get trapped in the membrane as this will result in low bead counts in the assay. Do not exceed 100 mmHg vacuum pressure. Modifying the assay to use in 96-well plates with centrifugation wash steps may remove this potential problem.
2. The assay relies on a source of human complement. It is therefore important to ensure that the source used has relatively high levels of complement activity. It is important that the serum is separated within 4 h. It is advisable to test a number of different volunteer samples in the assay for complement activity. When doing so use a positive control serum that has

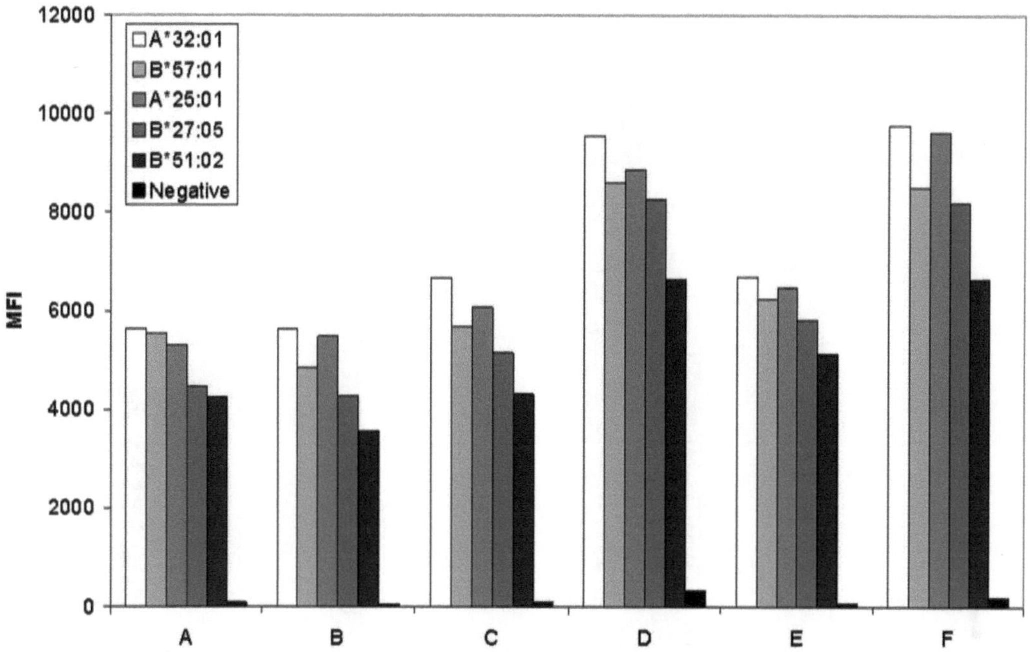

Fig. 1 C4d deposition on Luminex beads. A CDC positive control serum with specificity for Bw4 was incubated with Labscreen Single Antigen class I microbeads. Data from five HLA-coated microbeads and a negative control bead are shown. After serum/bead incubation six different (A–F) normal human serum (NHS) were used as a source of complement. C4d deposition was visualized using monoclonal antibody to C4d as described. The amount of C4d, measured by mean fluorescence intensity (MFI) is shown on the *y*-axis. Individual bars represent the five specific microbeads and the negative control bead (no HLA present). Serum samples (D) and (F) gave stronger signals and would be selected for use in the assay, although all would be suitable

been shown to have a broad range of HLA antibody specificities by CDC (Fig. 1).

3. The serum used for the source of complement should be separated, aliquoted, and frozen within 4 h, although ideally within 1–2 h. The serum should be a single use only and should not be refrozen. The aliquot volume therefore should be selected for a small number of samples so that wastage is minimized. We use aliquots of 500 μl (sufficient for at least eight wells) in our laboratory.
4. There are limited sources of antibodies to human complement component C4d. It is advisable to titrate the antibody to determine optimum concentrations for the assay. The anti-mouse IgG-PE conjugate also needs to be titrated.
5. In every assay both negative and positive controls should be included. The negative control should be a serum screened by single antigen assays and confirmed to be negative for both IgG and IgM antibody binding. The positive control should

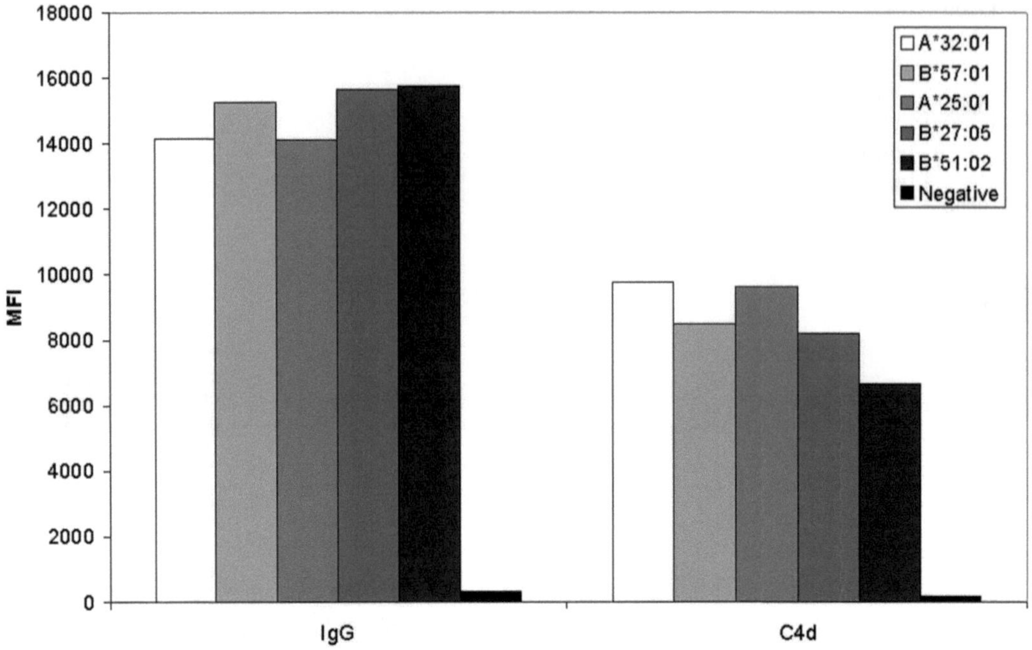

Fig. 2 Comparison of MFI signal intensity of IgG binding assay and C4d deposition on Luminex beads. A CDC positive control serum with specificity for Bw4 was incubated with Labscreen Single Antigen class I microbeads. IgG binding and C4d fixation was measured. MFI values for the C4d fixation were approximately 50 % of the intensity seen with IgG HLA antibody binding

be sera with broad HLA antibody reactivity, in the first instance, confirmed by CDC assays.

6. The MFI values obtained from this assay are reduced in comparison to the standard IgG assay. The MFI levels are generally between 25 and 65 % of those seen with the standard assay (Fig. 2). Care needs to be taken with interpretations. If MFI cut-off values are used in the laboratory it may be necessary to adjust these for the C4d assay.
7. The MFI values for the positive control bead(s) in the commercially available HLA single antigen kits do not perform as for the standard IgG binding assay. The MFI values are greatly reduced and are often below 500. It is therefore imperative that a good positive control serum is used in order to use this to validate the assay.
8. This method can also be used with the Gen-Probe Lifematch single antigen beads. The bead volume is 40 μl incubated with 20 μl of serum. The remaining steps of the assay are identical (Lifecodes LSA class I (Catalog No. 265100), Lifecodes LSA class II (Catalog No. 265200) (Gen-Probe)).

9. It is possible to use reduced bead volumes, such as 2.5 μl, to increase the sensitivity of the assay. This increases the risk of bead loss during the wash steps.
10. It is possible to perform the assay excluding the first wash step after incubation of test serum with beads.

References

1. Patel R, Terasaki PI (1969) Significance of the positive crossmatch test in kidney transplantation. N Engl J Med 280(14):735–739
2. Smith JD, Danskine AJ, Laylor RM, Rose ML, Yacoub MH (1993) The effect of panel reactive antibodies and the donor specific crossmatch on graft survival after heart and heart-lung transplantation. Transpl Immunol 1(1):60–65
3. Williams GM, Hume DM, Hudson RP Jr, Morris PJ, Kano K, Milgrom F (1968) "Hyperacute" renal-homograft rejection in man. N Engl J Med 279(12):611–618
4. McCloskey D, Festenstein H, Banner N et al (1989) The effect of HLA lymphocytotoxic antibody status and crossmatch result on cardiac transplant survival. Transplant Proc 21 (1 Pt 1):804–806
5. Smith JD, Hamour IM, Banner NR, Rose ML (2007) C4d fixing luminex binding antibodies – a new tool for prediction of graft failure after heart transplantation. Am J Transplant 7(122809–15):122809–122815
6. Gupta A, Iveson V, Varagunam M, Bodger S, Sinnott P, Thuraisingham RC (2008) Pretransplant donor-specific antibodies in cytotoxic negative crossmatch kidney transplants: are they relevant? Transplantation 85(8):1200–1204
7. Susal C, Ovens J, Mahmoud K et al (2011) No association of kidney graft loss with human leukocyte antigen antibodies detected exclusively by sensitive Luminex single-antigen testing: a Collaborative Transplant Study report. Transplantation 91(8): 883–887
8. Wahrmann M, Exner M, Haidbauer B et al (2005) [C4d]FlowPRA® screening – a specific assay for selective detection of complement-activating anti-HLA alloantibodies. Hum Immunol 66(5):526–534
9. Wahrmann M, Exner M, Schillinger M et al (2006) Pivotal role of complement-fixing HLA alloantibodies in presensitized kidney allograft recipients. Am J Transplant 6(5 Pt 1):1033–1041
10. Smith JD, Banner NR, Hamour IM et al (2011) De novo donor HLA-specific antibodies after heart transplantation are an independent predictor of poor patient survival. Am J Transplant 11(2):312–319
11. Hodges AM, Lyster H, McDermott A, et al (2012) Late antibody-mediated rejection after heart transplantation following the development of de novo donor-specific human leukocyte antigen antibody. Transplantation (Epub ahead of print)

Chapter 16

C1q Assay for the Detection of Complement Fixing Antibody to HLA Antigens

Ge Chen and Dolly B. Tyan

Abstract

Solid phase Luminex® and flow cytometric single antigen bead assays offer exquisite sensitivity and specificity for HLA antibody detection. Unlike the historical complement-dependent cytotoxicity (CDC) method, these assays do not distinguish complement fixing from non-complement fixing antibody, the former of which are considered the most clinically relevant in the peri-transplant period. This chapter describes a novel solid phase C1q binding assay to distinguish HLA antibodies that can bind the first component of complement (C1q). These antibodies have the capacity to initiate the complement cascade irrespective of whether that actually occurs. The C1q assay detects many more complement fixing antibodies than are observed by the less sensitive and less specific CDC assay.

Key words HLA antibody, Solid phase assay, Single antigen beads, Luminex®, Transplantation, Complement, C1q

1 Introduction

The complement-dependent cytotoxicity (CDC) method has been used for more than 40 years to define clinically relevant HLA antibodies that have a very high correlation with adverse outcome in the transplant setting when they are specific to the donor [1]. The test uses rabbit, not human, complement and is both insensitive and nonspecific. The advent of solid phase immunoassays on the Luminex® platform and flow cytometric bead assays have overcome the sensitivity and specificity drawbacks of the CDC method [2, 3]. These assays detect IgG antibody that can bind to HLA class I (A,B,C) and class II (DR,DQ,DP) antigens present on beads. However, they do not distinguish complement fixing from non-complement fixing antibody. A series of modifications to the solid phase assays have been developed [4–8] to define clinically important antibodies that can bind the complement component, C4d. The C4d assays are functional assays, requiring progression through the early part of the complement cascade, use a variable source of

Andrea A. Zachary and Mary S. Leffell (eds.), *Transplantation Immunology: Methods and Protocols, Second Edition*, Methods in Molecular Biology, vol. 1034, DOI 10.1007/978-1-62703-493-7_16, © Springer Science+Business Media, LLC 2013

human complement and have low sensitivity with maximum mean fluorescence intensity (MFI) on the beads of ~3,500 [5].

The C1q assay [9], developed on Luminex® single antigen beads, measures the binding of C1q to the antibody and detects the array of antibodies capable of binding complement and initiating the classical pathway, irrespective of whether the cascade is actually activated. It does not require complement activation and is not affected by complement regulatory factors, except perhaps by C1INH [10]. The method has undergone incremental developmental modifications including two different two-step methods using autologous serum as the source of human C1q (hC1q) or spiking with purified hC1q and detecting bound C1q with purified custom labeled sheep anti-human hC1q (*see* **Notes 1** and **2**). The current C1q assay is a one-step assay (*see* **Note 3**) in which the beads are incubated with patient serum and a standard amount of purified, directly PE-labeled hC1q, simultaneously. The assay is highly sensitive, with maximum MFI values on the SAB of greater than 30,000. The assay also detects IgM. While this could be considered a potential drawback, the definition of IgM+ DSA has been shown to be clinically relevant [9]. Likely because of its ability to detect both IgG and IgM that is DSA, the C1q assay is always positive when the CDC is positive. Remarkably, it detects 513 % more antibodies capable of fixing complement than CDC when compared with the universe of IgG positive antibodies detected by IgG [9]. The C1q assay is highly correlated with clinical outcome in kidney and heart transplant recipients [11–13].

2 Materials

2.1 Reagents

1. LABScreen Class I Single Antigen Bead Mix (OneLambda LS1A04, Canoga Park, CA). Store at 4 °C.
2. LABScreen Class II Single Antigen Bead Mix (OneLambda LS2A01, Canoga Park, CA). Store at 4 °C.
3. 10× Wash Buffer (LABScreen, OneLambda, Canoga Park, CA). Store at 4 °C. If crystals are present, dissolve in a 37 °C water bath before use.
4. 1× Wash Buffer (sufficient for 48 wells): 5 mL 10× Wash buffer, 45 mL double-distilled water (Mix well).
5. Bio-C1q: Biotin-labeled human complement component C1q (One Lambda, Canoga Park, CA). Store at −70 °C.
6. SA-PE: Phycoerythrin-conjugated streptavidin (OneLambda LT-SAPE, Canoga Park, CA). Lyophilized. Store at 4 °C. DO NOT FREEZE.
7. HEPES Buffer: 10 mM HEPES, 0.3 M NaCl, pH 7.2. Store at room temperature.

8. Deionized H_2O.
9. 20 % bleach in deionized H_2O.
10. LiquiChip Calibration Bead Kit containing Cal1 and Cal2 beads (Qiagen, Valencia, CA).
11. LiquiChip Control Bead Kit containing Con1 and Con2 beads (Qiagen, Valencia, CA).
12. Absorption Beads: Polystyrene particles 0.4–0.6 μm diameter, in solution (Spherotech, Lake Forest, IL).

2.2 Equipment and Supplies

1. LABScan 100 or 200 flow analyzer (also known as LiquiChip or Luminex® instrument).
2. Luminex® XY platform.
3. Eppendorf 5810R/Sorvall Legend Centrifuge with holders for 96-well microplates.
4. Vortex Genie 2 mixer.
5. IKA MS3 digital microplate shaker.
6. Barnstead/LabLine horizontal tray shaker (Model 4625).
7. Eppendorf Centrifuge 5424.
8. Electronic pipettes and pipette tips.
9. Greiner Bio-One V-Bottom 96-well microplates (VWR 651201).
10. Reagent boats (Art Robbins Instruments, Sunnyvale, CA).
11. 0.2 mL PCR strip vials.
12. Bullet tubes: 0.6 mL microcentrifuge tubes.
13. Fusion analysis program (One Lambda, Canoga Park, CA).

3 Methods

3.1 Serum Preparation

Keep sera on ice or at 4°C at all times unless otherwise indicated.

1. (Samples must be frozen before testing). Thaw serum on ice.
2. Centrifuge serum at 21,130 rcf for 10 min in the Eppendorf 5424 centrifuge prior to test.
3. Transfer serum to a clean, labeled tube avoiding any sediment at the bottom.
4. In a bullet tube, mix Spherotech adsorption beads with serum at 1:10 ratio, i.e., one part beads plus ten parts serum, e.g., 3 μL of beads + 30 μL of patient serum per test (*see* **Note 4**).
5. Incubate 10 min at room temperature with gentle shaking on Vortex Genie 2 (speed 6).
6. Pellet beads by spinning for 10 min in an Eppendorf 5424 centrifuge at maximum speed.

7. Transfer the serum into a clean, labeled bullet tube containing 3 μL Spherotech beads.
8. Repeat **steps 5** and **6**.
9. Transfer the absorbed serum into a clean, labeled bullet tube.
10. Arrange tubes according to the plate plan.

3.2 Testing

1. Remove single antigen beads from refrigerator and verify bead lot numbers (*see* **Note 5**).
2. Vortex bead mixture vigorously.
3. Use a multi-dispense pipette to add 2.5 μL of appropriate beads to the bottom of each test well.
4. Use a Rainin 5–50 μL multichannel pipette to dispense 10 μL of each serum sample into the corresponding test well. *Be sure that tips are equally filled for each serum sample, and no air bubbles are present. Verify that all 10 μL have been dispensed into the test wells* (*see* **Note 6**).
5. Vortex the plate on the IKA shaker 30 sec at 750 RPM (*see* **Note 7**).
6. Add 10 μL Bio-C1q to each test well using the same Rainin multichannel pipette.
7. Vortex the plate on an IKA shaker 30 sec at 750 RPM.
8. Cover plate with aluminum foil to keep it dark.
9. Place the covered plate on the Barnstead/Lab line tray shaker.
10. Incubate the plate in the dark at room temperature, shaking at speed 2.5, for 30 min.
11. Make the SAPE dilution 2 min before end of the first incubation. SAPE is diluted according to lot specification of Bio-C1q and SAPE. Dilution factor varies with each lot. 10 μL of diluted SAPE is needed for each test well. Add the HEPES buffer first to the dilution tube. Add the correct amount of SAPE to the HEPES buffer with 1–10 μL Rainin pipette at speed 3. Rinse the pipette tip once (*see* **Note 8**).
12. When the incubation is finished, use the same Rainin pipette to add 10 μL diluted SAPE to each test well.
13. Vortex the plate on an IKA shaker for 30 sec at 750 RPM.
14. Cover plate with aluminum foil to keep it dark.
15. Place the covered plate on the Barnstead/Lab line tray shaker.
16. Incubate the plate in the dark at room temperature, shaking at speed 2.5 for 20 min.
17. During the incubation, make 1× wash buffer from 10× stock solution, as per instructions in Subheading 2.1 (**step 4**). 500 μL per test well is required.
18. At the end of the incubation, add 100 μL 1× wash buffer to each well.
19. Vortex the plate on an IKA shaker for 30 sec at 750 RPM.

20. Add another 100 μL of 1× wash buffer.
21. Cover and centrifuge the plate at 1,500×*g* in Eppendorf 5810R centrifuge for 3 min.
22. Immediately flick the plate **hard** to remove the liquid and blot upside down twice by banging the tray on a stack of paper towels *BEFORE TURNING TRAY RIGHT SIDE UP* (*see* **Note 9**).
23. Resuspend the dry pellet on the IKA shaker at 1,300 RPM for 30 sec.
24. Repeat wash **steps 18–22** once more, for a total of two washes.
25. Add 60 μL 1× wash buffer to each test well.
26. Vortex the plate on an IKA shaker for 30 sec at 750 RPM.
27. Acquire sample data using the LABScan 100 Flow Analyzer (Luminex® instrument) (*see* **Notes 10** and **11**).

3.3 Analysis and Interpretation

1. Open HLA Fusion software.
2. Log in.
3. Click *Analyze Data* and *Labscreen.*
4. Select the run from Z:\HLAVNet\LABSCREEN_OUTPUT\OUTPUT.
5. Check mark *ABNeg sample* as control.
6. Click on *Import.* The run will appear in the "Navigator" screen (*see* **Note 12**).
7. Select *Baseline* in the lower left corner of the screen.
8. Arrange the baseline MFI values from highest to lowest and reading from the lowest up, find the first increment of 300 MFI or greater. Record the MFI value of the lower MFI bead where that break occurs.
9. Click on *Graph Raw* in upper right corner of screen.
10. On the graph in Fusion, drag all cutoff lines to the MFI value that you have just recorded (i.e., all MFIs above this cutpoint are Positive and have a score of eight and all MFIs below this cutpoint are negative and have a score of one). Scores are automatically assigned by Fusion after the lines have been moved.
11. Add 1,000 MFI to the MFI value of the highest negative bead (i.e., highest MFI value with a score of one).
12. *Positive* calls start at this value or higher (sum of highest negative MFI plus 1,000).
13. Any reaction with a score of eight but below the Positive antibody threshold is called *Possible.*
14. Double-click specificities to add them to the "Final Assignment" box.
15. Click *Save.*
16. Report.

4 Notes

1. The C1q method was modified by adding a standard (physiologic) amount of exogenous purified hC1q to the patient serum prior to incubation with the beads when it became obvious that patients with protein losing enteropathy did not have sufficient native C1q for the assay to work.
2. The C1q method is equally applicable to any solid platform including the flow cytometer.
3. Because the procedure is a one-step procedure, dithiothreitol (DTT) cannot be used to reduce IgM antibody. The C1q molecule is a six part structure which is held together by disulfide bonds. Thus, reducing the disulfide bonds for IgM also destroys the C1q. Reduction of IgM from the serum by heat treatment (63 °C × 13 min) can remove high background but the effect on the patient-specific antibody is currently unknown. Removal of IgM is best achieved by adsorption with beads specific for IgM (i.e., coated with anti-IgM antibody) which are currently custom reagents.
4. Absorption is CRITICAL to achieving valid test results. It removes sporadic blocking factors of unknown origin which maximize the signal to noise ratio and results in valid controls. In the absence of absorption, the positive control (bead #2) can be very low (~300 MFI) making the test invalid. In some cases, absorption with the usual absorption beads is inadequate to remove high background on the negative control (bead #1). In rare instances, the negative control value can be >20,000 MFI. This can be due to IgM which must be removed to obtain a valid test.
5. The thaw date must be entered on the Bio-C1q bottle label. The expiration date is 3 months from the thaw date and must not exceed original kit expiration date.
6. Because the volumes of beads and serum are so small per test well, it is essential to assure that the serum is fully coating the beads and not dispersed in bubbles around the circumference of the well. This step is CRITICAL.
7. The vortexing is critical to the reproducibility of the assay. It is important to use a validated shaker at the programmed speed to have consistency between technologists and between runs.
8. SAPE is not stored after dilution. Make only as much as you need. The first time this step is performed, it is likely to take more than 2 min. It is important to have all details regarding the required dilution factor ready.
9. The flicking and blotting steps are CRITICAL to the success of the assay. The beads are well embedded in the V-bottom

wells. As soon as the centrifugation is over, it is important to flick the liquid off hard into the sink and bang the wells (upside down) on a pad of paper towels to get off ALL the liquid.

10. Collect a minimum of 100 of each bead to assure validity of results.
11. Currently the LabXpress robot (One Lambda, Canoga Park, CA) is not programmed for testing by C1q. It cannot be used for methods using less than 5 μL of beads.
12. Before the run is analyzed, check the negative and positive controls to make sure they fall within acceptable limits (predetermined by local validation). In general, the negative control (Bead #1 on the SAB) should be less than 500 MFI and the positive control (Bead #2 on the SAB) should be more than 3,000 MFI. The positive control bead was not designed for the C1q assay and is a bead coated with IgG. However, achieving values over 3,000 MFI should be routine and many go up to 12,000 MFI.

References

1. Patel R, Terasaki PI (1969) Significance of positive crossmatch test in kidney transplantation. N Engl J Med 280:735–739
2. Pei R, Lee JH, Chen T et al (1999) Flow cytometric detection of HLA antibodies using a spectrum of microbeads. Hum Immunol 60:1293–1302
3. Pei R, Lee JH, Shih NJ et al (2003) Single human leukocyte antigen flow cytometry beads for accurate identification of human leukocyte antigen antibody specificities. Transplantation 75:43–49
4. Bartel G, Wahrmann M, Exner M et al (2008) In vitro detection of C4d-fixing HLA alloantibodies: associations with capillary C4d deposition in kidney allografts. Am J Transplant 8:41–49
5. Smith JD, Hamour IM, Banner NR et al (2007) C4d fixing, luminex binding antibodies - a new tool for prediction of graft failure after heart transplantation. Am J Transplant 7:2809–2815
6. Wahrmann M, Bartel G, Exner M et al (2009) Clinical relevance of preformed C4d-fixing and non-C4d-fixing HLA single antigen reactivity in renal allograft recipients. Transpl Int 22:982–989
7. Wahrmann M, Exner M, Haidbauer B et al (2005) [C4d]FlowPRA screening – a specific assay for selective detection of complement-activating anti-HLA alloantibodies. Hum Immunol 66:526–534
8. Wahrmann M, Exner M, Regele H et al (2003) Flow cytometry based detection of HLA alloantibody mediated classical complement activation. J Immunol Methods 275:149–160
9. Chen G, Sequeira F, Tyan DB (2011) Novel C1q assay reveals a clinically relevant subset of human leukocyte antigen antibodies independent of immunoglobulin G strength on single antigen beads. Hum Immunol 72:849–858
10. Heeger PS (2010) A complementary approach to treating antibody-mediated transplant rejection. Kidney Int 78:125–127
11. Chin C, Chen G, Sequeria F et al (2011) Clinical usefulness of a novel C1q assay to detect immunoglobulin G antibodies capable of fixing complement in sensitized pediatric heart transplant patients. J Heart Lung Transplant 30:158–163
12. Sutherland SM, Chen G, Sequeira FA et al (2012) Complement-fixing donor-specific antibodies identified by a novel C1q assay are associated with allograft loss. Pediatr Transplant 16:12–17
13. Yabu JM, Higgins JP, Chen G et al (2011) C1q-fixing human leukocyte antigen antibodies are specific for predicting transplant glomerulopathy and late graft failure after kidney transplantation. Transplantation 91:342–347

Chapter 17

Tetramer Staining for the Detection of HLA-Specific B cells

Donna P. Lucas, Mary S. Leffell, and Andrea A. Zachary

Abstract

HLA-specific B cells can be identified, quantified, and isolated after staining with HLA tetramers. Quantification of these B cells can in turn identify individuals who are sensitized to HLA antigens and the isolation of these cells facilitates a variety of experimental investigations.

Key words HLA tetramers, B lymphocytes, HLA specific B Lymphocytes, HLA sensitization, HLA antibodies

1 Introduction

The detrimental effects of antibodies specific for donor HLA are well documented and are a major barrier to outcome and access in transplantation. The development of solid phase immunoassays for the detection and characterization of HLA-specific alloantibodies has led to increased insight into the role of antibodies in transplantation and has strengthened our understanding of the efficacy of treatment modalities to overcome incompatibility [1, 2]. The ability to examine the mechanisms and regulatory processes involved in the humoral response has not kept pace however. Staining with HLA-tetramers provides the tool for identifying, isolating and enumerating HLA-specific B cells [3].

Conformational epitopes on intact antigens are the ligands for the surface immunoglobulin antigen receptors of B lymphocytes [4]. HLA-specific B cells bind the HLA molecule that has the same specificity to the immunoglobulins that it secretes. Direct measurement of frequencies of antigen-specific B cells is possible using HLA tetramers which are complexes of four peptide-loaded HLA molecules that are conjugated with a fluorescent protein [5]. The antigen-specific B lymphocytes may then be enumerated by flow cytometry which allows rapid and sensitive quantitation of a patient's B cell response to the given MHC antigen [6].

Andrea A. Zachary and Mary S. Leffell (eds.), *Transplantation Immunology: Methods and Protocols, Second Edition*, Methods in Molecular Biology, vol. 1034, DOI 10.1007/978-1-62703-493-7_17, © Springer Science+Business Media, LLC 2013

2 Materials

2.1 Materials and Equipment

1. 20–40 ml anti-coagulated peripheral blood on recipient (*see* **Note 1**).
2. 50 ml polypropylene centrifuge tubes.
3. 12×75 mm round bottom polystyrene tubes.
4. Adjustable micropipettes and tips to deliver 1–10 and 10–100 μl.
5. Serological pipette to deliver 10 ml.
6. Centrifuge with swinging bucket rotor and adjustable speed.
7. Rotator or mixer that allows both tilting and rotation.
8. Magnetic bead/particle collector (*see* **Note 2**).
9. 4 °C Refrigerator.
10. Flow cytometer capable of detecting three colors.

2.2 Reagents

1. Phosphate Buffered Saline (PBS): pH 7.4, without Ca^{2+} or Mg^{2+}: 9.0 g/l NaCl, 144 mg/l KH_2PO_4, 795 mg/l Na_2HPO_4 (anhydrous).
2. Ficoll-Hypaque: density of 1.077 g/ml.
3. Isolation buffer: Phosphate Buffered Saline (PBS) pH 7.4, without Ca^{2+} or Mg^{2+} with 1 % (wt/vol) BSA and 2 mM EDTA. Alternatively EDTA can be replaced by 0.6 % sodium citrate and BSA can be replaced by 2 % fetal bovine serum (FBS).
4. Dynabeads® Untouched™ Human B cell kit containing antibody mix to non-B cells and MyOne™ SA Dynabeads® (Life Technologies™, Grand Island, NY).
5. Trypan Blue Stain: 0.4 % (wt/vol) Trypan Blue in PBS.
6. HLA tetramers conjugated with phycoerythrin for identifying HLA-specific cells (*see* **Note 3**).
7. Mouse anti-human CD45 monoclonal antibody conjugated with fluorescein isothiocyanate for identifying leukocytes (CD45-FITC).
8. Mouse anti-human CD19 monoclonal antibody conjugated with allophycocyanin for identifying B cells (CD19-APC) (*see* **Note 4**).

3 Methods

3.1 Isolation of Peripheral Blood Mononuclear Cells (PBMC)

1. Transfer 20 ml of anti-coagulated peripheral blood into each of two labeled 50 ml centrifuge tubes.
2. Dilute with PBS to a total volume of 35 ml.
3. Underlay diluted blood with 10 ml Ficoll-Hypaque being careful not to mix the blood–Ficoll interface.

4. Centrifuge for 20–30 min at 1,650 × *g*.
5. Carefully aspirate the mononuclear cell layer at the interface from each centrifuge tube and transfer into a clean labeled tube and bring the volume to 50 ml with PBS.
6. Pellet the cells by centrifuging for 10 min at 500 × *g*.
7. Decant the supernatant and resuspend the pellet in 50 ml of PBS.
8. Centrifuge for 10 min at 500 × *g*.
9. Resuspend the cell pellets and pool in 2–4 ml of Isolation buffer.
10. Adjust the cell count to 10×10^6 cells/ml.

3.2 B Cell Enrichment with Untouched Human B Cell Kit

1. Resuspend the Dynabeads® by mixing on a Vortex mixer for 30 s and transfer 100 μl of the suspension for every 1×10^7 PBMC to a 12 × 75 mm round bottom tube.
2. Add 1 ml of Isolation Buffer to the tube and mix.
3. Place the tube on the magnet for 1–3 min depending on the magnet's strength and discard the supernatant.
4. Remove the tube from the magnet and resuspend the Dynabeads® in the same volume of cold Isolation Buffer as for the initial volume of beads used in **step 1**. Set aside.
5. Add up to 5×10^7 PBMCs at a concentration of 1×10^8 cells/ml in Isolation Buffer to a labeled 12 × 75 mm round bottom tube.
6. Add 100 μl of the antibody mix provided in the kit for every 5×10^7 cells.
7. Mix well and incubate for 20 min at 2–8 °C.
8. Wash the cells by filling the tube with Isolation Buffer. Mix well and centrifuge at 350 × *g* for 8 min. Discard the supernatant.
9. Resuspend the cells in Isolation Buffer to a concentration of 10^8 cells/ml.
10. Add the prewashed Dynabeads®.
11. Incubate for 15 min at 18–25 °C on a mixer or rotator.
12. Resuspend the bead-bound cells by vigorously pipetting ≥10 times using a pipette with a narrow tip opening.
13. Add 3 ml of Isolation buffer and place the tube on the magnet for 2 min.
14. Transfer the supernatant, containing the untouched B cells, to a new labeled tube.
15. Add 4 ml of Isolation Buffer to the tube containing the beaded cells from **step 13**.
16. Repeat **steps 12–13** to recover remaining B cells.
17. Combine all supernatants containing untouched B cells.

18. Pellet the cells by centrifugation at 350 × *g* for 8 min.
19. Resuspend the cell pellet in 1 ml Isolation Buffer.
20. Count the enriched B cells and determine viability by staining with Trypan blue.

3.3 Tetramer Staining

1. Place 2–5 × 10^5 B cells in each 12 × 75 mm tube, add 1.0 ml of Wash Buffer and mix. Centrifuge to pellet (750 × *g* for 5 min).
2. Decant the supernatant and blot the tube on absorbent pad until the pellet is nearly dry.
3. Add 10 μl of appropriate tetramer suspension to dry cell pellets and resuspend the pellet. Incubate for 15 min at room temperature (20–25 °C) in the dark.
4. Add 10 μl of CD19-APC monoclonal antibody and additionally 10 μl of CD45-FITC to tubes if cell population contains contaminating erythrocytes or granulocytes.
5. Mix and Incubate in the dark for 30 min at 2–8 °C.
6. Wash cells with 3 ml of cold Isolation buffer. Centrifuge to pellet (750 × *g* for 10 min).
7. Resuspend cells in 500 μl of cold Isolation buffer. Cells are ready for acquisition on the flow cytometer (*see* **Note 5**).

3.4 Flow Cytometric Analysis

The flow cytometer instrument must be set up correctly before use. The manufacturer's daily start-up and shutdown procedures must be followed and a daily calibration using commercial standard reagents performed. In addition, optimization (*see* **Note 6**) and color compensation must be performed (*see* **Note** 7). An example of the progressive gating from the lymphocyte population to the tetramer binding, HLA specific B lymphocytes is shown in Fig. 1.

1. Acquire and record list mode data on 10,000 B cells events as follows:
   (a) Using the cytometer acquisition and analysis software create a forward scatter (FSC) versus side scatter (SSC) dot or density plot.
   (b) Draw a gate around the lymphocyte population and use this gate to create a four decade log CD19 (APC) versus CD45 (FITC) plot. Draw a rectangular gate around the double positive population and use this gate to identify the B cells.
   (c) Use the CD45+/CD19+ gate to create a plot displaying CD19-APC (FL4) versus PE conjugated HLA Tetramer and draw a gate around the tetramer positive B cells.
   (d) The data are presented as the percent tetramer-positive cells of CD19-positive cells.

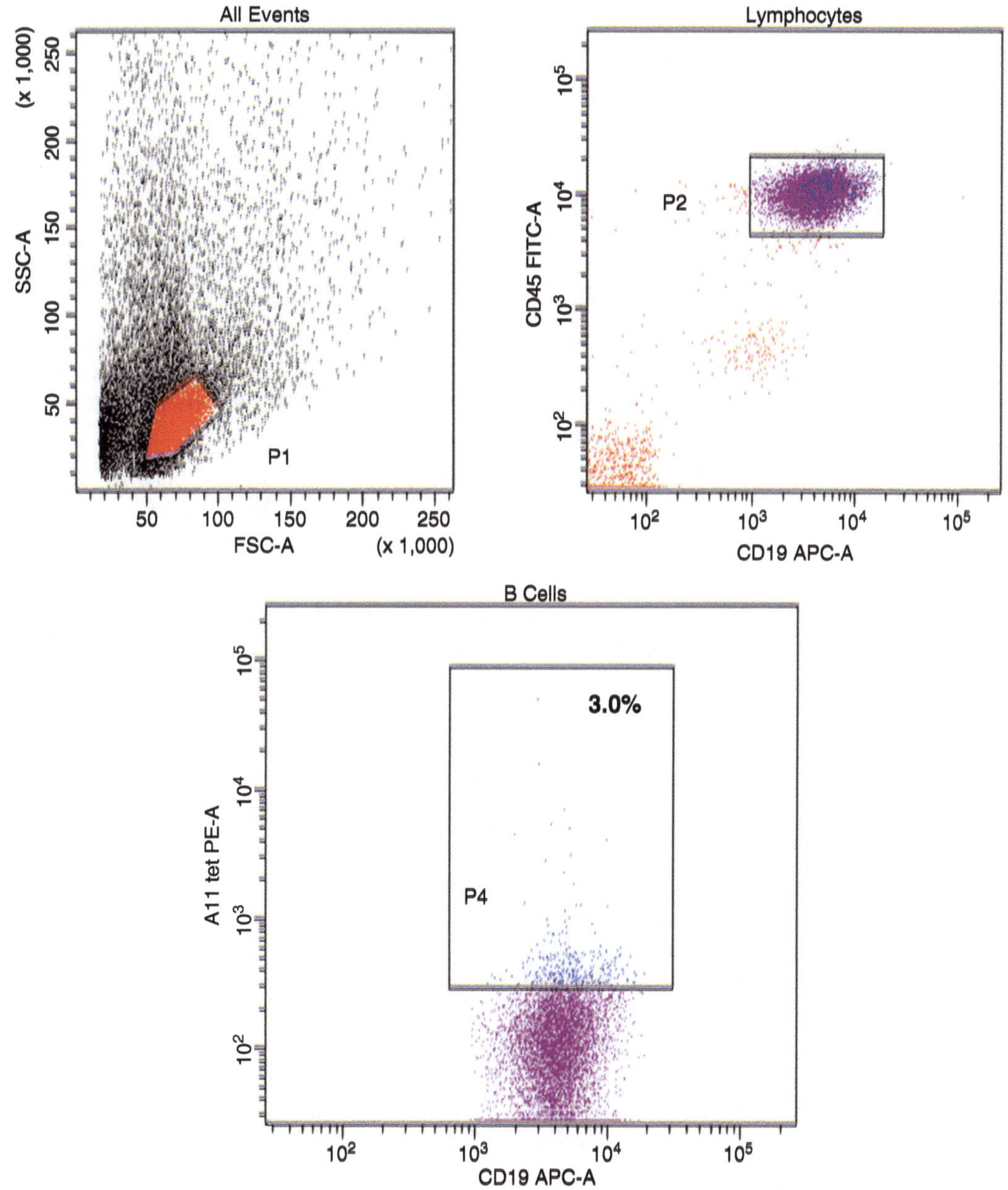

Fig. 1 Gating strategy for tetramer positive B cells. The percentage of HLA-A11 tetramer positive B lymphocytes is determined with sequential gates. The lymphocyte population is defined by the P1 gate which is based on forward and side scatter (FSC and SSC, respectively). The P2 gate is set around CD19+ B lymphocytes, and the P4 gate is then set on CD19+ Tetramer+ B lymphocytes

4 Notes

1. Common anticoagulants such as ethylenediaminetetracetic acid (EDTA), acid citrate dextrose (ACD), and Sodium heparin are suitable for the collection of blood used to obtain lymphocytes for flow cytometric analysis, but ACD is better at

maintaining cell viability. Blood should be maintained at room temperature prior to staining and analysis.

2. Magnetic cell separators are available from several companies such as Stemcell™ Technologies and Life Technologies™. The magnet chosen needs to hold a 5 ml 12×75 mm tube and contain a strong rare earth magnet capable of isolating 1 μm beads.
3. We use HIV peptides and all patients tested are HIV negative, but we have shown that the binding of tetramer by B cells was not affected by the HLA-bound peptide [3].
4. Different fluorochrome combinations can be used for the tetramers and monoclonal antibodies being mindful of the excitation and emission spectra of the different fluorochromes as well as the instrument configuration.
5. Keep cells in the dark until ready for analysis. Perform analysis within an hour of the end of the assay. Alternatively a cell fixing reagent such as *para*-formaldehyde can be used to preserve the cells for up to 24 h.
6. The flow cytometer must be set up before acquisition in order to optimally record the amount of tetramer binding to cells. Adjust the FSC amperage gain and SSC voltage to display the lymphocytes on a FSC versus SSC plot. Adjust the FSC threshold to exclude the collection of data on unwanted small particulate matter and cellular debris.
7. Prior to sample acquisition compensation should be performed to optimize settings and minimize detection of overlapping emission spectra of fluorophores. This can be performed with lymphocytes or alternatively with beads such as CompBeads Plus (BD Biosciences, Mountain View, CA) according to the manufacturer's instructions.

References

1. Leffell M, Zachary A (2012) Antiallograft antibodies: relevance, detection, and monitoring. Curr Opin Organ Transplant 15:2–7
2. Zachary A, Vega R, Lucas D et al (2010) HLA antibody detection and characterization by solid phase immunoassays – methods and pitfalls. In: Christiansen F, Tait DB (eds) Methods in molecular biology™. Springer, New York, pp 289–308
3. Zachary A, Kopchaliiska D, Montgomery R et al (2007) HLA-specific B cells: method for their detection, quantification, and isolation using HLA tetramers. Transplantation 83: 982–988
4. Bjorkman P, Saper M, Samraoui B et al (1987) The foreign antigen binding site and T cell recognition regions of class I histocompatibility antigens. Nature 329:512–518
5. Altman J, Moss P, Goulder P et al (1996) Phenotypic analysis of antigen-specific T lymphocytes. Science 274:94–96
6. Zachary A, Kopchaliiska D, Montgomery R et al (2007) HLA-specific B cells: application to transplantation. Transplantation 83:988–994

Chapter 18

A Flow Cytometric Crossmatch Test Using Endothelial Precursor Cells Isolated from Peripheral Blood

Annette M. Jackson, Donna P. Lucas, and Jessica L. Badders

Abstract

Flow cytometric crossmatch tests provide a donor-specific, cell based method for the detection of alloreactive antibodies in the sera of transplant patients. Conventional crossmatch tests used in solid organ transplantation utilize lymphocytes as target cells to detect the presence of alloreactive HLA antibodies. Isolation of endothelial precursor cells (EPCs) from peripheral blood now allows testing for antibodies reactive with non-HLA endothelial cell antigens.

Key words Endothelial cell, Non-HLA antibodies, Transplantation, Flow cytometric crossmatch, Alloantibodies

1 Introduction

Humoral sensitization to ABO and HLA alloantigens remains the major immunological barrier to successful transplantation; however, growing evidence also suggests a role for non-HLA antibodies in allograft rejection [1–5]. Anti-endothelial cell antibodies (AECAs) have been implicated in hyperacute, acute, and chronic rejections of kidney allograft. Moreover, decreased long-term graft survival in sensitized recipients transplanted with kidneys from HLA identical siblings suggests that antigenic targets in addition to HLA and ABO are involved in the alloimmune response [6].

Many non-HLA antigens implicated in allograft survival are expressed on endothelial cells, which serve as a barrier between the recipient's immune system and the transplanted allograft. Potential targets of AECAs that have been associated with rejection in transplanted allografts include antibodies specific for angiotensin II type 1 receptor 1 (AT_1R), vimentin, the glomerular basement membrane protein agrin, and the major histocompatibility complex class I chain-related gene A (MICA) [7–11]. Approaches combining proteomics and genomics are uncovering additional tissue specific

Andrea A. Zachary and Mary S. Leffell (eds.), *Transplantation Immunology: Methods and Protocols, Second Edition*, Methods in Molecular Biology, vol. 1034, DOI 10.1007/978-1-62703-493-7_18, © Springer Science+Business Media, LLC 2013

non-HLA antigens capable of initiating de novo humoral responses in transplant recipient [12, 13].

Recently developed reagents allow for the isolation of EPCs from the peripheral blood of potential allograft donors using anti-Tie2 magnetic nanoparticles and positive selection [9, 10]. Tie2 is an endothelial cell specific tyrosine kinase expressed on the surface of endothelial cells and EPCs. Once isolated, EPCs can be used as target cells in a flow cytometric crossmatch assay (ECXM) to detect donor-specific anti-endothelial cell reactive antibodies (AECAs) in the sera of transplant recipients [14].

In a multicenter clinical trial, 24 % of patients (35/147) tested positive for donor-reactive EPC antibodies and had significantly higher incidences of early rejection ($p = 0.00005$) compared to patients for whom no AECAs were detected [15].

A single center analysis of 60 sequential renal transplants found that 14 recipients, or 23 %, tested positive for donor-specific IgG AECAs. These patients had a significantly higher frequency of rejections (5, 36 %) during the first 3 months post-transplant compared to patients without donor-specific AECAs (8, 17 %; $p < 0.025$) [16]. Mean serum creatinine levels within this early post-transplant period were also significantly higher in patients testing positive in an IgG ECXM compared to those that tested negative (1.5 mg/dl versus 1.2 mg/dl, $p = 0.014$). A higher percentage of patients (42 %, 13/42) tested positive for IgM AECAs but no correlation was found between IgM AECAs and increased incidences of rejection or increased SCr values during the early post-transplant period (<100 days). The absence of donor-specific HLA-antibodies in these patients was determined by flow cytometric crossmatch tests using donor lymphocytes and multianalyte bead immunoassays.

2 Materials and Equipment

2.1 Specimens

1. Four, 10 milliliter (ml) tubes of peripheral blood collected in acid citrate dextrose (ACD) and processed within 24–48 h (*see* **Note 1**).
2. Test serum depleted of immunoglobulin isotype IgM (*see* **Note 2** and Subheading 3.2).

2.2 Reagents Included in XM-ONE® Kit (Absorber, Stockholm Sweden)

1. Cell Preparation Tube™ (CPT) vacutainer tubes containing sodium citrate and cell isolation gel (store at 18–22 °C).
2. Anti-human Tie2 magnetic nanoparticles (store at 2–8 °C).
3. Rabbit anti-human IgG FITC-conjugated antibodies (store at 2–8 °C).
4. Rabbit anti-human IgM FITC-conjugated antibodies (store at 2–8 °C)—*NOT USED at our center.*

2.3 Additional Reagents (All Stored at 2–8 °C Unless Indicated)

1. 1× phosphate buffered saline (PBS) with 5 % heat inactivated fetal calf serum (FCS).
2. Trypan blue, cell viability dye.
3. Flow Wash Buffer: 1× PBS, 1 % bovine serum albumin (BSA), 0.1 % sodium azide (NaN_3).
4. Fluorochrome-conjugated antibodies:

   CD34-allophycocyanin (APC), clone 581.

   HLA class I-fluorescein (FITC), clone G46-2.6.

   HLA class II-FITC, clone Tu39.
5. Negative control serum (NAB), pooled AB serum. Each lot is screened for HLA-specific antibodies using solid phase immunoassays and must yield negative ECXM tests with all EPC donors. Individual test aliquots stored at −20 °C.
6. Positive control serum (POS), pooled sera containing HLA class I and class II antibodies from highly sensitized patients. Individual test aliquots stored at −20 °C.
7. Optional EPC isolation method: Ficoll-Hypaque, specific gravity of 1.076. Bring to room temperature (18–22 °C) before using.
8. Calibration beads for flow cytometer.

2.4 Equipment

1. Centrifuge with swinging buckets, adjustable speed.
2. Beckman Airfuge.
3. Vortex mixer.
4. 63 °C water bath.
5. Hematology mixer.
6. Light microscope and hemocytometer for cell counting.
7. 4 °C Refrigerator and −20 °C freezer.
8. Vacuum aspiration system (optional).

2.5 Additional Supplies

1. Adjustable micropipettes to deliver 1–10, 10–100, and 500 microliters (μl).
2. Pipette tips.
3. 10 ml pipettes.
4. 50 ml polypropylene tubes.
5. Electronic pipetting aide.
6. Interval timer.
7. Indelible marking pen.
8. Test tube rack.
9. 0.5 ml microcentrifuge tubes.

10. 12 × 75 mm polypropylene tubes with caps for EPC isolation.
11. Parafilm.
12. Cell isolation magnet (Dynal or Stem Cell Technologies).
13. 12 × 75 mm polystyrene tubes for acquisition on flow cytometer.
14. 8 × 20 mm Beckman Ultra-clear centrifuge tubes for serum.
15. Absorbent towels for blotting tubes following wash steps.

3 Methods

3.1 EPC Isolation

1. Isolate peripheral blood mononuclear cells (PBMCs) from freshly drawn blood using either of the following methods (*see* **Note 3**).
   (a) Transfer blood collected in ACD tubes into CPT tubes and centrifuge (1,650 × *g*, 30 min).
   (b) Perform density gradient separation by underlayering 10 ml Ficoll-Hypaque solution beneath 30 ml ACD blood that has been diluted 1:2 in 1× PBS and centrifuge (1,650 × *g*, 30 min).
2. Transfer mononuclear cell layers from CPT tubes or from Ficoll-Hypaque gradient into two 50 ml conical tubes. Wash PBMCs in 1× PBS with 5 % FCS (total volume of 50 ml/tube) and centrifuge 500 × *g* for 10 min. Do not use media containing Mg^{2+} or Ca^{2+} (*see* **Note 4**).
3. Repeat **step 2** once for a total of two washes.
4. Decant the supernatant from the last wash, add 0.5 ml of 1× PBS with 5 % FCS, and transfer cells into a labeled 5 ml polypropylene tube.
5. Briefly centrifuge (10 s) the Tie2 nanoparticle vial to remove beads from cap. Add 0.5 ml of 1× PBS with 5 % FCS using a micropipette and resuspend nanoparticles by pipetting up and down. Add Tie2 nanoparticles to the cell tube, cap tube, and place parafilm around cap to prevent leakage. Place tube on rotator 4 °C for 30 min.
6. Following Tie2 nanoparticle incubation, increase the volume of cells to 3 ml with 1× PBS with 5 % FCS. Place cell tube on magnet for 10 min at 18–22 °C. Remove supernatant containing PBMCs. Wash Tie2+ cells by adding 3 ml of 1× PBS with 5 % FCS, gently resuspend cells, reapply magnet for 10 min. Remove supernatant and discard (*see* **Note 5**). Resuspend Tie2+ cells in 1 ml of 1× PBS with 5 % FCS.
7. Make a 1:20 dilution of cells in trypan blue viability dye and count using a hemocytometer (*see* **Note 6**). Cell viability should be equal to or exceed 80 %.

Table 1
Preparation of control and sample tubes for flow cytometric crossmatch analysis

Tube	Incubation #1	Incubation #2	Purpose
1: Negative control	50 μl NAB serum	10 μl anti IgG-FITC	To assess nonspecific binding of human IgG to EPC cells
2: Positive control	50 μl Pos Ctrl serum		To show that test is working and evaluate antigen expression on EPCs
3: No serum	50 μl Wash buffer		To assess nonspecific binding of anti-human IgG antibodies to EPC cells and detect donor-autoreactive antibody bound to donor EPCs
4: Patient #1	50 μl: Test serum #1		To assess presence of donor-specific EPC reactive antibody in recipient's serum
N: Patient #*N*	50 μl: Test serum #*N*		To assess presence of donor-specific EPC reactive antibody in recipient's serum
HLA class I	50 μl Wash buffer	10 μl CD34-APC 10 μl HLA I-FITC	To assess quality of Tie2 bead enrichment and the expression of HLA class I on EPCs
HLA class II	50 μl Wash buffer	10 μl CD34-APC 10 μl HLA II-FITC	To assess the quality of Tie2 bead enrichment and the expression of HLA class II on EPCs

8. Place 5×10^5 cells in each 12×75 mm tube (labeled according to Tubes column of Table 1). Add 1.0 ml of Flow Wash Buffer to each tube and centrifuge to pellet ($500 \times g$ for 5 min).
9. Remove all residual Flow Wash Buffer by blotting with an absorbent towel or using a vacuum aspirator. If vacuum aspirator is used, care must be taken not to aspirate the cell pellets. Do not let the cells dry out; immediately add prepared serum (*see* Subheading 3.2) or wash buffer (*see* Table 1) to the cell pellet.

3.2 Serum Preparation and Incubation

1. Transfer 100 μl of each test serum and NAB into labeled 0.5 ml microcentrifuge tubes and heat inactivate at 63 °C for *exactly* 10 min. Transfer sera to ultracentrifuge tubes and centrifuge for 15 min at $100{,}000 \times g$ (30 psi, 95,000 rpm) in Beckman airfuge (*see* **Note 7**).
2. Add 50 μl of the appropriate serum to the corresponding labeled tubes (*see* Table 1). Vortex each tube briefly to ensure proper mixing of cells and serum. Sera are listed under "Incubation 1" in Table 1. If no serum is added, add 50 μl of Flow Wash Buffer to prevent the cells from drying out.
3. Incubate for 30 min at 18–22 °C
4. Wash cells with 1 ml of *cold* Flow Wash Buffer and centrifuge to pellet ($500 \times g$ for 5 min) (*see* **Note 8**).
5. Decant off the Flow Wash Buffer and vortex tubes to break up the cell pellet. Repeat **step 4** twice for a total of three washes,

making sure to remove all residual Flow Wash Buffer on the last wash. If using aspirator, rinse with distilled water to clean the aspirator between samples to prevent cross-contamination.

3.3 Fluorochrome-Conjugated Antibody Incubation

1. Add the appropriate antibodies, as indicated in the column marked "Incubation 2" in Table 1, to the cells and vortex to mix.
2. Incubate antibodies with cells for 30 min at 2–8 °C and protect from light.
3. Following the incubation, wash cells three times with 1 ml of cold Flow Wash Buffer and centrifuge to pellet (500 × *g* for 5 min).
4. After final wash, resuspend cells in 250 μl of cold Flow Wash Buffer and acquire on calibrated flow cytometer.

3.4 Acquisition and Analysis

1. BD™ Cytometer Setup & Tracking beads (CS&T) are used to calibrate digital flow cytometers at the start of each experiment to increase reproducibility and track flow cytometer performance. CS&T beads contain a mixture of fluorochromes of different fluorescent intensities (dim, mid, and bright). CS&T beads update cytometer settings to achieve the same signal intensity for each fluorochrome, thereby standardizing performance and reducing inter-experiment instrument variability. These data are also automatically entered into Levey–Jennings plots, which allow tracking of cytometer performance and monitoring for potential problems.
2. The emission spectra for FITC and APC, fluorochromes used in this procedure, do not overlap and do not require compensation. If alternate fluorochromes are used fluorescence compensation controls may be required.
3. The EPCs (population P1) can be differentiated from lymphocytes (population P2) by their increased size and granularity using forward and side scatter parameters (Fig. 1).
4. To assess the purity and quality of each EPC isolation and assist in EPC gating, monoclonal antibodies specific for CD34 (a stem cell marker), HLA class I (A, B, Cw) and HLA class II (DR, DQ, DP) are used (*see* Table 1 and Fig. 2.). Set endothelial precursor cell gate (P1) to encompass cells staining positive for both CD34 and HLA class II.
5. Acquire 5,000 EPCs per tube and display on either a 1024 channel scale or a logarithmic scale.
6. All controls must demonstrate appropriate reactivity as follows:

   NAB Control: Median fluorescent values with NAB vary greatly between different EPC donors; however, values for NAB should be lower than the positive control and higher that of the "no serum" tube. Our current NAB produces median fluorescent values that are approximately twice that of the "no serum" tube with all donors tested.

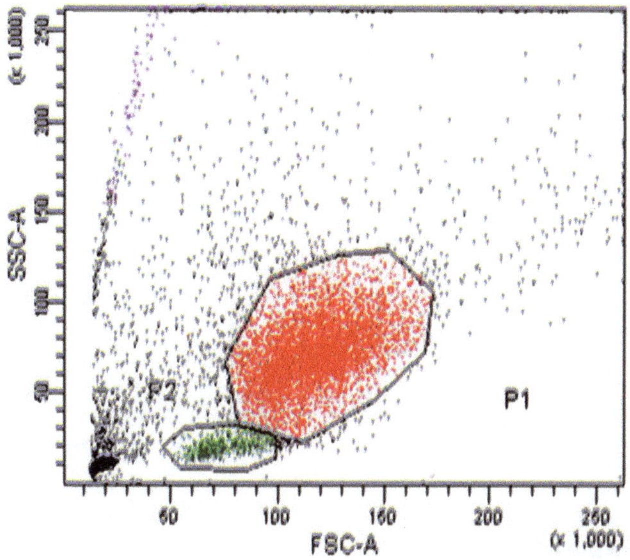

Fig. 1 Forward and side scatter plot of EPCs and lymphocytes following Tie2 positive selection

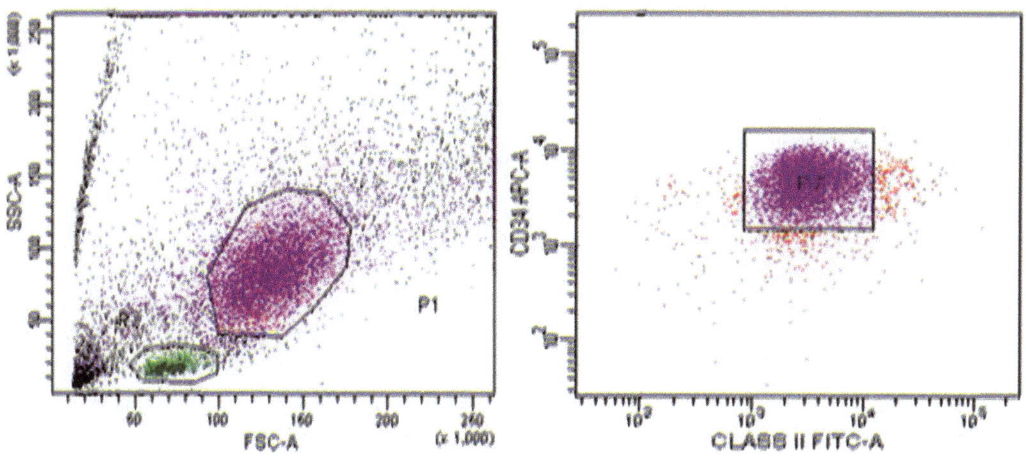

Fig. 2 Verification of EPC gate (P1) via surface expression of stem cell marker CD34 and HLA-class II

Positive Control: The ratio of positive control serum to NAB must be greater than or equal to 1.5. The ratio for our positive serum is consistently ≥2.0. The histogram peak should be sharp, not broad. Broad or double peaks, when using positive control serum that contains both HLA class I and class II antibody, may occur when a dual population of $CD34^{+}$ HLA-class II^{+} and $CD34^{-}$ HLA-class II^{-} cells exist in the EPC population (*see* **Note 1** and Fig. 3).

No Serum: Median fluorescent values must be lower than the NAB tube. Values higher than the NAB control indicate the presence of donor-autoreactive IgG bound to the EPCs at the time of isolation.

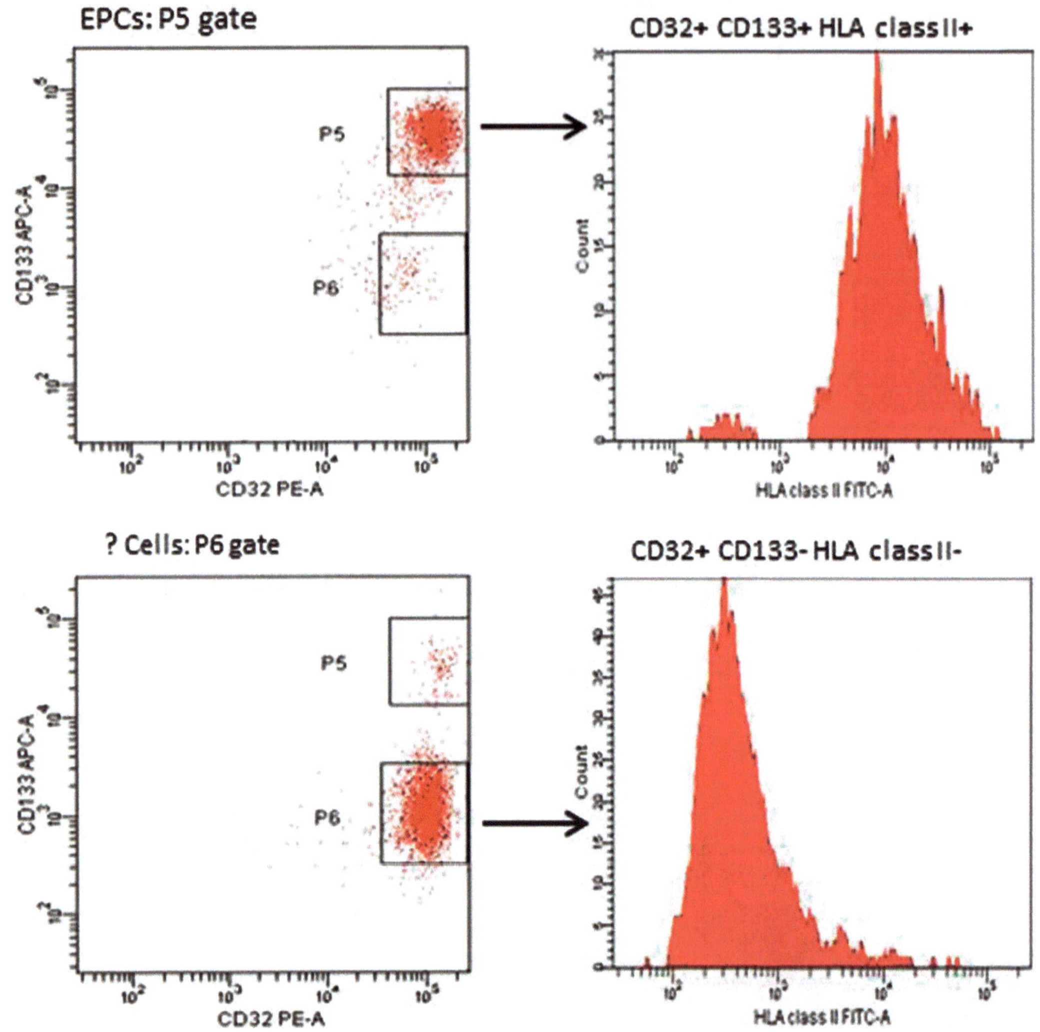

Fig. 3 Dual population of Tie2+ cells isolated from blood >48 h old: loss of CD133 corresponds with loss of HLA class II

7. Determination of a positive ECXM, using channel shifts or ratio to NAB, must be established by each laboratory according to clinical relevance (*see* **Note 9**).

4 Notes

1. Our correlation between a positive ECXM test and early allograft rejection was established using donor blood <48 h from the time of phlebotomy. We have observed decreased surface expression of stem cell marker CD133, CD34, and HLA-class II on EPCs isolated from blood >48 h from time of phlebotomy (Fig. 3). The clinically relevant antigenic targets

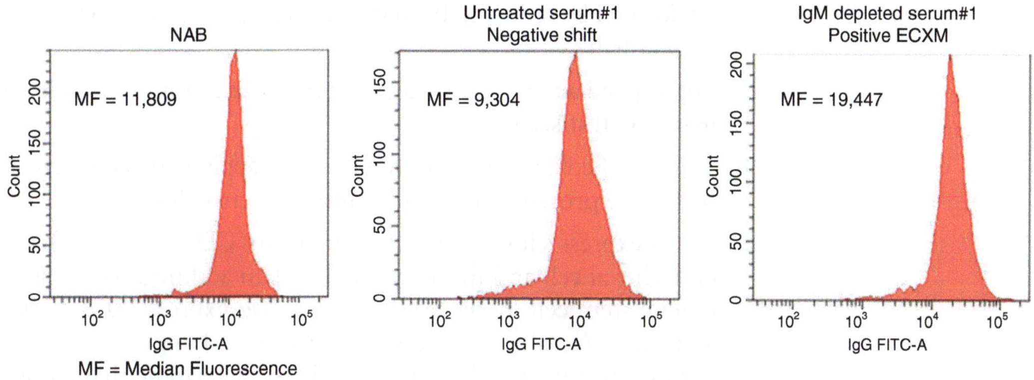

Fig. 4 Serum treated to remove IgM increased ECXM reactivity from negative to positive

expressed on EPCs are not yet known and may also have decreased expression in older blood samples. Therefore, we have strict criteria for testing blood within 48 h of phlebotomy and including stem cell phenotype markers (CD133 or CD34) and HLA class II to assess the purity and quality of the EPCs used in each ECXM.

2. Excess IgM in test serum appears to block the binding or detection of IgG specific for antigens on the EPC surface. This IgM blocking results in an IgG median fluorescence value for the test serum that is below that of the NAB (IgG negative shift) [15]. Further testing in our laboratory has shown that treating sera to remove IgM via hypotonic dialysis and heat inactivation eliminated the IgG negative shift phenomenon (Fig. 4) [15, 17].
3. Density gradient medium contained in the CPT tubes contains Ficoll-Hypaque that is toxic to cells; wash cells immediately after density gradient separation.
4. Manufacturers of magnetic-bead cell isolation kits recommend using wash buffers that contain a protein source (BSA or heat inactivated fetal calf serum) but do not contain Mg^{2+} or Ca^{2+} cations. In addition, sufficient wash buffer volume is needed during the first cell wash to dilute density gradient medium and allow for efficient cell pelleting and cell recovery.
5. Lymphocytes, contained in the supernatant, can be frozen or used immediately for other testing purposes.
6. The number of EPCs isolated from 40 ml of ACD blood (processed within 48 h of collection) varies between donors; however, our mean and standard deviation for EPC yields are $7.7 \times 10^6 \pm 3.1$ compared to a PBMC yield of $49.2 \times 10^6 \pm 19.5$. Purity of the EPC population is greatly enhanced by the wash step performed on the magnet at the time of cell isolation. For consistent test results it is important to keep the cell-to-serum ratio constant. If the EPC yield is low, the test can be

performed by reducing both the cell number and serum volume by one-half.

7. High speed airfuge centrifugation removes immune complexes from the test serum.
8. The use of cold wash buffer reduces the capping and endocytosis of surface proteins induced by antibody cross-linking.
9. EPCs express cluster of differentiation (CD) markers of the endothelial cell and monocyte lineages in addition to hematopoietic stem cell markers [14]. EPCs also express HLA class I and class II, albeit at lower levels than lymphocytes (our unpublished data and [18]). In order to determine that a positive ECXM test is due to donor-specific AECAs and not HLA antibodies, the level of donor-specific HLA antibodies must fall well below that expected to yield a positive lymphocyte flow cytometric crossmatch test.

References

1. Sumitran-Karuppan S, Tyden G, Reinholt F et al (1997) Hyperacute rejections of two consecutive renal allografts and early loss of the third transplant caused by non-HLA antibodies specific for endothelial cells. Transpl Immunol 5:321–327
2. Perrey C, Brenchley PE, Johnson RW et al (1998) An association between antibodies specific for endothelial cells and renal transplant failure. Transpl Immunol 6:101–106
3. Mizutani K, Terasaki P, Bignon JD et al (2006) Association of kidney transplant failure and antibodies against MICA. Hum Immunol 67:683–691
4. Amico P, Honger G, Bielmann D et al (2008) Incidence and prediction of early antibody-mediated rejection due to non-human leukocyte antigen-antibodies. Transplantation 85:1557–1563
5. Sun Q, Liu Z, Chen J et al (2008) Circulating anti-endothelial cell antibodies are associated with poor outcome in renal allograft recipients with acute rejection. Clin J Am Soc Nephrol 3:1479–1486
6. Opelz G (2005) Non-HLA transplantation immunity revealed by lymphocytotoxic antibodies. Lancet 365:1570–1576
7. Jurcevic S, Ainsworth ME, Pomerance A et al (2001) Antivimentin antibodies are an independent predictor of transplant-associated coronary artery disease after cardiac transplantation. Transplantation 71:886–892
8. Sumitran-Holgersson S, Wilczek HE, Holgersson J et al (2002) Identification of the nonclassical HLA molecules, mica, as targets for humoral immunity associated with irreversible rejection of kidney allografts. Transplantation 74:268–277
9. Joosten SA, Sijpkens YW, van Ham V et al (2005) Antibody response against the glomerular basement membrane protein agrin in patients with transplant glomerulopathy. Am J Transplant 5:383–393
10. Zwirner NW, Marcos CY, Mirbaha F et al (2000) Identification of MICA as a new polymorphic alloantigen recognized by antibodies in sera of organ transplant recipients. Hum Immunol 61:917–924
11. Dragun D, Muller DN, Brasen JH et al (2005) Angiotensin II type 1-receptor activating antibodies in renal-allograft rejection. N Engl J Med 352:558–569
12. Li L, Wadia P, Chen R et al (2009) Identifying compartment-specific non-HLA targets after renal transplantation by integrating transcriptome and "antibodyome" measures. Proc Natl Acad Sci 106:4148–4153
13. Dinavahi R, George A, Tretin A et al (2011) Antibodies reactive to non-HLA antigens in transplant glomerulopathy. J Am Soc Nephrol 22:1168–1178
14. Vermehren D, Sumitran-Holgersson S (2002) Isolation of precursor endothelial cells from peripheral blood for donor-specific cross-matching before organ transplantation. Transplantation 74:1479–1486
15. Breimer ME, Rydberg L, Jackson AM et al (2009) Multicenter evaluation of a novel endothelial cell crossmatch test in kidney transplantation. Transplantation 87:549–556

16. Jackson AM, Lucas DP, Melancon JK et al (2011) Clinical relevance and IgG subclass determination of non-HLA antibodies identified using endothelial cell precursors isolated from donor blood. Transplantation 92:54–60
17. Zachary AA, Lucas DP, Detrick B et al (2009) Naturally occurring interference in Luminex assays for HLA-specific antibodies: characteristics and resolution. Hum Immunol 70:496–501
18. Alheim M, Johansson SM, Hauzenberger D et al (2010) A flow cytometric crossmatch test for simultaneous detection of antibodies against donor lymphocytes and endothelial precursor cells. Tissue Antigens 75:269–277

Chapter 19

The Detection of Antibodies to the Angiotensin II-Type 1 Receptor in Transplantation

Duska Dragun

Abstract

The detection of auto-antibodies detection is a major aspect of patient's immunomonitoring. Antibodies directed against the heart and kidney Angiotensin II type 1 receptor (AT_1R) play a major role in antibody mediated rejection after heart and kidney transplantation and in obliterative vasculopathy of autoimmune diseases. Here, a sandwich enzyme-linked immunosorbent assay (ELISA) is the reliable tool for the detection of auto-antibodies targeting AT_1R.

Key words Auto-antibodies, Angiotensin II type 1 receptor, ELISA, Immunoassay

1 Introduction

AT_1R-antibodies (AT_1R-Abs) are causative in the pathogenesis of antibody-mediated rejection with severe vasculopathy [1, 2]. Detection of the auto-antibodies initially relied on a bioassay that measured the chronotropic response to AT_1R-IgG mediated stimulation of cultured neonatal cardiomyocytes and its response to receptor-specific antagonists. Dose–response relationship between AT_1R-Ab concentrations and the chronotropic response is linear [3]. The time and labor consuming setting of the bioassay in rat neonatal cardiomyocytes precluded larger studies and emerged the development of an alternative assay feasible for clinical routine. Auto-antibodies can be determined by means of enzyme immunoassay. This immunoassay is based on enzyme-labelling of one reactant, e.g., the secondary antibody. Solid-phase systems such as plates coated with antigen are advantageous, because removal thereof will not give rise to denaturation of proteins. A sandwich ELISA for detection of AT_1R-Abs in serum has been established and validated (CellTrend GmbH, Luckenwalde, Germany) for transplant recipients and patients with autoimmune diseases [4, 5]. Briefly, the membrane extract of native AT_1R is bound to 96-well plates and incubated with patient's serum. After washing

Andrea A. Zachary and Mary S. Leffell (eds.), *Transplantation Immunology: Methods and Protocols, Second Edition*, Methods in Molecular Biology, vol. 1034, DOI 10.1007/978-1-62703-493-7_19, © Springer Science+Business Media, LLC 2013

steps, the plate is incubated with fluorescent-labelled anti-human secondary antibodies. The ELISA currently has 100 % specificity and 88 % sensitivity as compared to cardiomyocyte bioassay. Interassay variability is 12 % [5].

2 Materials

Prepare all solutions using deionized or distilled water. Bring all reagents to room temperature before use. If crystals have formed, mix gently until the crystals have completely dissolved. Diligently follow all waste disposal regulations when disposing waste materials.

2.1 Sample Collection and Storage

Collect serum or plasma according to standard procedure.

2.2 Preparation of Reagents and Samples

1. The microplate strips have been pre-coated with Angiotensin II type 1 receptor and are ready to use (*see* **Note 1**).
2. Dilute the wash buffer (Buf Wash) 1:10 (*see* **Note 2**).
3. Dilute the horseradish peroxidase (HRP) conjugate with diluent (Dil Conj) 1:100 (*see* **Note 3**).
4. Dilute the human serum or plasma samples with diluent (Dil spe) 1:100 (*see* **Note 4**).

3 Methods

3.1 Assay Procedure

1. Pipette 100 μl of diluted samples, standards, controls, or diluent Dil spe (as blank) into the wells.
2. Seal wells with adhesive strip and incubate for 2 h at 2–8 °C.
3. Aspirate fluid from wells and wash three times with 300 μl wash buffer, prepared as described previously (*see* **Note 5**).
4. Dispense 100 μl of diluted HRP conjugate in each well.
5. Seal the wells with adhesive strip and incubate 1 h at room temperature (*see* **Note 6**).
6. Repeat the wash as in **step 3** (*see* **Note 5**).
7. Dispense 100 μl of TMB (3,3′5,5″-tetramethylbenzidine) substrate (Subs TMB) solution in each well.
8. Incubate for 20 min at room temperature in the dark.
9. Add 100 μl of stop solution (Soln Stop) to each well.
10. Determine the absorbance at 450 nm (*see* **Note 7**).

3.2 Calculation of Results

1. Create a standard curve using computer software capable of generating a curve fit (four parameters fit; *x*-axis: linear, anti-AT_1R-Ab standard points (*see* **Note 8**, 2.5, 5, 10, 20, 40 U/ml);

y-axis: linear, absorbance). The sample concentrations can be calculated from the standard curve.

2. Samples >17 U/ml are positive, samples 10–17 U/ml are at risk. Samples <10 U/ml are negative (*see* **Note 9**).

4 Notes

1. Excess strips can be removed and resealed in the bag with the desiccant. Store at 2–8 °C.
2. The diluted solution is stable for 30 days at 2–8 °C.
3. The required amount of conjugate solution should be prepared freshly.
4. The undiluted samples can be stored at room temperature up to 48 h, at 2–8 °C up to 4 days and long term at −20 °C.
5. After the last wash, invert the plate and tap on a clean paper towel.
6. The plate has to be incubated under shaking.
7. The absorbance has to be determined within 30 min. A reference wavelength of 620 nm/690 nm is recommended.
8. The standards (Cal 1-5) are ready to use.
9. A run is considered valid if the positive control (Control +) is in the expected range (see label) and the negative control (Control –) is less than the cutoff. Samples over the standard curve can be assayed again using a higher dilution factor. In that case the concentration read must be multiplied by the additional dilution factor.

Acknowledgments

We acknowledge Dr. Harald Heidecke, Dr. Kai Schulze-Förster (CellTrend GmbH, Luckenwalde), and Dr. Aurélie Philippe for their methodological inputs.

References

1. Hiemann N, Meyer R, Wellnhofer E et al (2012) Non-HLA antibodies targeting vascular receptors enhance alloimmune response and microvasculopathy after heart transplantation. Transplantation 94:919–924
2. Dragun D, Muller DN, Brasen JH et al (2005) Angiotensin II type 1-receptor activating antibodies in renal-allograft rejection. N Engl J Med 352:558–569
3. Wallukat G, Homuth V, Fischer T et al (1999) Patients with preeclampsia develop agonistic autoantibodies against the angiotensin AT1 receptor. J Clin Invest 103:945–952
4. Reinsmoen NL, Lai CH, Heidecke H et al (2010) Anti-angiotensin type 1 receptor antibodies associated with antibody mediated rejection in donor HLA antibody negative patients. Transplantation 90:1473–1477
5. Riemekasten G, Philippe A, Nather M et al (2011) Involvement of functional autoantibodies against vascular receptors in systemic sclerosis. Ann Rheum Dis 70:530–536

Chapter 20

Detection of Antibodies to Self-Antigens (K-alpha 1 Tubulin, Collagen I, II, IV, and V, Myosin, and Vimentin) by Enzyme-Linked Immunosorbent Assay (ELISA)

Nayan J. Sarma, Venkataswarup Tiriveedhi, and T. Mohanakumar

Abstract

The enzyme-linked immunosorbent assay (ELISA) is a widely used technique for detecting antibodies (Abs) and is employed in clinical laboratories to identify Abs against various self-antigens–autoAb development and quantitation. This method relies on specific antigen–Ab interactions where one of the components is immobilized on a solid surface. Using this method, the concentrations of antigens or Ab present in the serum can be quantified with high specificity and accuracy. Here, we describe the detection of autoAbs to various self-antigens with different tissue restriction patterns which includes collagens, k-α1 tubulin, vimentin, and myosin. We also discuss their relevance in monitoring for rejection following solid organ transplantation.

Key words ELISA, Self-antigen, Auto-antibodies, Collagen, K-α1 tubulin, Myosin, Vimentin

1 Introduction

The methods for the enzyme-linked immunosorbent assay (ELISA) were first demonstrated in early 1970s and have been widely used for quantitative detection of antibodies (Abs) or antigens present in liquid samples such as serum [1]. In this method a solution of the antigens is added to a solid surface such as a 96-well plastic plate. The protein antigens adhere to the surface as a result of electrostatic interactions or passive adsorption. The unbound fraction of the antigen is washed off and a nonspecific protein solution (bovine serum albumin or casein) is applied to the surface to block the areas uncoated by the antigen. Next a primary Ab is added which is specific for the coated antigen. The primary Ab could be a purified Ab or Abs present in serum samples that are to be tested for reactivity towards the antigen of interest. The primary Ab binds to the antigen immobilized on the plastic surface and the unbound

Andrea A. Zachary and Mary S. Leffell (eds.), *Transplantation Immunology: Methods and Protocols, Second Edition*, Methods in Molecular Biology, vol. 1034, DOI 10.1007/978-1-62703-493-7_20, © Springer Science+Business Media, LLC 2013

fraction in the solution is washed off. Following this, a secondary Ab specific for the primary Ab is added to the wells and incubated. The secondary Ab is often conjugated with an enzyme such as horse radish peroxidase (HRP). The unbound fraction of the secondary Ab in the solution is then washed off and a substrate for the conjugated enzyme is added. The enzyme–substrate reaction results in a color change and the intensity of the color is proportional to the amount of the antigen–Ab interaction. Quantification of the color intensity is done in an ELISA plate reader by measuring the absorbance at specified wavelengths of light and further normalizing to the controls or to the standards. This method is widely accepted in clinical diagnosis for detection of autoAbs.

Organ transplantation is the treatment of choice for many diseases resulting in end stage organ failure. However, long-term function of the organs following transplantation has been limited and continued to be a challenge. In many cases chronic rejection following transplantation and loss of function of the transplanted organ is the most important issue facing clinical transplantation. This often leads to retransplantation with markedly reduced allograft function following retransplantation. This also puts a great burden towards finding suitable organ donors with compatibility. Several recent studies have suggested an important role for development of Abs to self-antigens (autoimmunity) in the pathogenesis of allograft rejection [2–4]. Studies from our laboratories following human lung transplantation have shown significant correlation between de novo development of Abs to self-antigens, K-α1 tubulin (K-α1T) and collagen V (ColV), and development of chronic rejection clinically diagnosed as bronchiolitis obliterans syndrome (BOS) [5–7]. We have also demonstrated development of Abs to collagens following human liver transplantation suggesting an important role for autoimmunity in the pathogenesis of hepatitis C virus mediated liver fibrosis [8, 9]. Several studies have shown cardiac myosin, a self-antigen, is associated with the pathogenesis of cardiac allograft vasculopathy (CAV), a correlate of chronic rejection following human heart transplantation [10, 11]. It has been shown that Abs against vimentin, a cytoskeleton protein, also pose an independent risk factor for coronary atherosclerosis following cardiac transplantation and possibly contributing to the pathogenesis of transplant associated CAV [11, 12]. Studies from our laboratory have demonstrated that CAV patients developed Abs to self-antigens including myosin, vimentin, collagens, and K-α1T [13, 14]. In our studies, we have employed an ELISA method to detect de novo development of Abs present in the serum following solid organ transplantation to the various self-antigens discussed above.

2 Materials

1. Prepare all solutions using ultrapure deionized water with a sensitivity of 18 MΩ cm at room temperature (25 °C).
2. Use only molecular biology grade reagents to prepare the solutions.
3. Prepare the solutions at room temperature.
4. Aliquot and store Abs at 4 °C.
5. Follow approved institutional research board guidelines to collect serum samples from human subjects.
6. Aliquot and store serum samples at −20 °C.
7. Store aliquots of the antigens at −80 °C. It is important that serum and antigens are not repeatedly freeze-thawed and ideally samples should be used immediately following thawing.

2.1 Antigens for Coating 96-Well Plates

1. Antigens:
   (a) K-α1T and vimentin (recombinant protein prepared in our laboratory by affinity purification stored at −80 °C).
   (b) Col I (Cell Sciences, CRC 158A), Col II (Meridian, A22314H), Col III (Sigma, C4407), Col IV (Meridian, A33125H), ColV (Sigma, C3657).
   (c) Myosin (Sigma, M0531).
2. Dissolve the antigens in Phosphate Buffered Saline (PBS) to obtain a final dilution of 1 μg/ml.

2.2 Blocking and Loading Serum Samples

1. Blocking buffer: 1 % bovine serum albumin (BSA) in PBS. Add 1 g of BSA to 100 ml PBS.
2. Serum samples obtained from patients and normal individuals.
3. Commercially available Abs for the standards: K-α1T (Santa Cruz, SC-12462), Col I (Abcam, ab34710), Col II (AbD Serotech, 132001), Col III (Santa Cruz, SC-28888), Col IV (Calbiochem, CP20), Col V (Abcam# ab7046), Vimentin (BD Pharmingen, 550513), and Myosin (abcam, ab15).
4. PBS without Tween-20 as wash buffer.
5. Plastic ware: 96-well plates (Corning, NY), pipettes and tips.
6. Incubator at 37 °C.

2.3 Secondary Ab Incubation and Detection

1. Secondary Ab: Anti-human IgG HRP (Jackson laboratories Cat 109-035-064) for test serum.
2. Standards: Goat anti-Rabbit HRP (for anti-K-α1T, Col I and V); mouse anti-Goat HRP (for anti-Col II); Goat anti-Mouse HRP (for Col IV); and Goat anti-Mouse HRP (for anti-Vimentin and anti-Myosin).

3. Wash buffer: 1× PBS with 0.05 % Tween-20. Prepare 10 % Tween-20 stock solution and add 500 µl in 100 ml PBS.
4. TMB (3,3′,5,5″-tetramethylbenzidine) substrate (Millipore ES022).
5. Stop solution: 2 N Hydrochloric acid (HCl). Add 10 ml of 11 N HCl stock into 40 ml water to prepare 50 ml stop solution.
6. ELISA plate washer: (ELx50, Bio Instruments, VT). It is important to use distilled water and NOT filtered water for washing the plates.

2.4 Data Analysis

1. ELISA plate reader (Epoch™, Bioteck Instruments, VT) using the program Gen 5 1.09™ (Bioteck Instruments, VT) provided by the manufacturer. The optical density of the solution in the individual wells of the plate is measured based on spectral absorbance at 450 nm.
2. Software, Gen 5 1.09™, used for data acquisition and concentration calculation.

3 Methods

Carry out the procedures at room temperature (23–25 °C) unless otherwise mentioned.

3.1 Coating Plates

1. Dispense 100 µl of the antigen solution in PBS (see Subheading 2) to each well of a 96 well plate.
2. Incubate the plates overnight at 4 °C. The plates can be stored at 4 °C for up to 2 weeks. It is important NOT to let the plates dry by avoiding prolonged stay outside at room temperature such as under the hood. Put the plates quickly at 4 °C. Wrap plates in aluminum foil to prevent drying.

3.2 Blocking and Loading Serum Samples

1. Prepare a plate map with all the samples, standards, negative controls and the blanks in triplicate.
2. Decant the 96 well plates to discard the uncoated antigen in the solution.
3. To each well add 200 µl of blocking buffer and incubate for 1–2 h at 37 °C.
4. Thaw the serum samples and spin for 5 min at 10,000 × *g*.
5. Prepare the following dilution of the serum samples in blocking buffer. Prepare the serum samples through serial dilutions starting from higher concentrations to lower. Avoid air bubbles while preparing the serum samples.

K-α1T—1:1,250.

Col I—1:250.

Col II and IV—1:500.

Col III—1:100.

Col V—1:1,000.

Vimentin and Myosin—1:750.

6. Prepare the standards by serially diluting the commercially available Abs with known concentration starting from 1:2,000 to 1:32.
7. Wash the 96 well plates with 200 μl of PBS four times. Add PBS to the wells and decant by inverting on a blotting paper or use a plate washer. Do not let the plates dry between washes.
8. Load 100 μl of the standards or serum samples to each well according to the plate map.
9. Incubate the plates for 2 h at room temperature (25 °C) or overnight at 4 °C.

3.3 Secondary Ab Incubation and Detection

1. Wash the 96 well plates with 200 μl of wash buffer (PBS + Tween-20) four times. Add PBS to the wells and decant by inverting on a blotting paper or use a plate washer.
2. Prepare 1: 10,000 dilution of the anti-human IgG HRP secondary Ab in the blocking buffer. Add 100 μl to each well. It is important NOT to expose the solutions and the plates to bright light at this stage. Prepare appropriate secondary Abs for the standards.
3. Wrap the plates in aluminum foil and incubate for 1 h at room temperature.
4. Wash the plates with 200 μl of wash buffer (PBS + Tween-20) four times.
5. Wash the plates with 200 μl of PBS four times. When processing multiple plates, proceed to each of the next steps one plate at the time.
6. Add 100 μl of freshly thawed TMB substrate and incubate the plates for 1 min in dark. The color will change to blue.
7. Stop reaction by adding 100 μl of stop solution to each well. The color will change to yellow.
8. Read the absorption at 450 nm in the ELISA plate reader.

3.4 Data Analysis and Sample Calculation

The concentration of the Abs is calculated based on a standard curve (from serial dilutions of 1:2,000–1:32, with blank subtraction) using the binding of known concentration of specific Ab to the protein of interest. The slope of the standard curve is determined from the straight line curve fit ($y = mx + c$; where y is optical density; *m* is the slope of equation; *x* is the concentration of standard protein; and *c* is the *y*-intercept) equation. Use this equation to determine the concentration of the Abs present in the sample from the optical density obtained at 450 nm in the ELISA plate reader. A sample is considered as positive for autoAbs if the values are over the average cutoff values obtained from normal ($n = 28$) human subjects (+/−: between 1 SD and 2 SD above mean; ++: >2 SD above mean).

4 Notes

1. Aliquot the serum samples on arrival. Avoid repeated freeze–thaw as this can destroy the Abs.
2. Store the antigen solutions at −20 to −80 °C in aliquots. Antigens like K- 1T and vimentin are prepared in our lab as recombinant proteins expressed in bacteria. The other antigens including various collagens are commercially purchased (mentioned above) and are aliquoted to 200 μl of 100 μg/ml and stored in −80 °C until used.
3. The optimal concentration for antigen solutions and standard Abs as well as the incubation times vary from lab to lab and the quality of the reagents. It is critical to determine the optimal concentrations of each of the reagents before conducting the actual experiments.
4. Prepare the serum dilutions starting from higher concentrations to lower concentrations in blocking buffer.
5. Each sample, including serum, standards, and blanks, should be tested in triplicate.
6. The outcome of the analysis will be affected if the wells dry out during the course of the experiment. Therefore, it is highly recommended to process one plate at a time to avoid drying of the wells.
7. The TMB substrate and the secondary Abs are light sensitive. Therefore, one should avoid bright light while preparing the secondary Ab, during incubation and during development of the enzyme–substrate reaction.

Acknowledgments

This work was supported by NIH HL056643, HL092514, and the Barnes-Jewish Children's Foundation to T.M. The authors would like to thank Billie Glasscock for her assistance in submitting this manuscript.

References

1. Engvall E, Perlmann P (1971) Enzyme-linked immunosorbent assay (ELISA). Quantitative assay of immunoglobulin G. Immunochemistry 8:871–874
2. Shulman HM, Sullivan KM (1988) Graft-versus-Host disease: allo- and autoimmunity after bone marrow transplantation. Concepts Immunopathol 6:141–165
3. Bharat A, Fields RC, Steward N, Trulock EP, Patterson GA et al (2006) CD4+25+ regulatory T cells limit Th1-autoimmunity by inducing IL-10 producing T cells following human lung transplantation. Am J Transplant 6:1799–1808
4. Milne DS, Gascoigne A, Wilkes J, Sviland L, Ashcroft T et al (1992) The immunohistopathology of obliterative bronchiolitis following lung transplantation. Transplantation 54:748–750
5. Goers TA, Ramachandran S, Aloush A, Trulock E, Patterson GA et al (2008) De novo production of K-alpha1 tubulin-specific antibodies: role in chronic lung allograft rejection. J Immunol 180:4487–4494
6. Saini D, Weber J, Ramachandran S, Phelan D, Tiriveedhi V et al (2011) Alloimmunity-induced autoimmunity as a potential mechanism in the pathogenesis of chronic rejection of human lung allografts. J Heart Lung Transplant 30:624–631
7. Burlingham WJ, Love RB, Jankowska-Gan E, Haynes LD, Xu Q et al (2007) IL-17-dependent cellular immunity to collagen type V predisposes to obliterative bronchiolitis in human lung transplants. J Clin Invest 117:3498–3506
8. Seetharam AB, Borg BB, Subramanian V, Chapman WC, Crippin JS et al (2011) Temporal association between increased virus-specific Th17 response and spontaneous recovery from recurrent hepatitis C in a liver transplant recipient. Transplantation 92:1364–1370
9. Borg BB, Seetharam A, Subramanian V, Basha HI, Lisker-Melman M et al (2011) Immune response to extracellular matrix collagen in chronic hepatitis C-induced liver fibrosis. Liver Transpl 17:814–823
10. Kaczmarek I, Deutsch MA, Kauke T, Beiras-Fernandez A, Schmoeckel M et al (2008) Donor-specific HLA alloantibodies: long-term impact on cardiac allograft vasculopathy and mortality after heart transplant. Exp Clin Transplant 6:229–235
11. Rose ML, Smith JD (2009) Clinical relevance of complement-fixing antibodies in cardiac transplantation. Hum Immunol 70:605–609
12. Leong HS, Mahesh BM, Day JR, Smith JD, McCormack AD et al (2008) Vimentin autoantibodies induce platelet activation and formation of platelet-leukocyte conjugates via platelet-activating factor. J Leukoc Biol 83:263–271
13. Nath DS, Ilias Basha H, Tiriveedhi V, Alur C, Phelan D et al (2010) Characterization of immune responses to cardiac self-antigens myosin and vimentin in human cardiac allograft recipients with antibody-mediated rejection and cardiac allograft vasculopathy. J Heart Lung Transplant 29:1277–1285
14. Nath DS, Tiriveedhi V, Basha HI, Phelan D, Moazami N et al (2011) A role for antibodies to human leukocyte antigens, collagen-V, and K-alpha1-Tubulin in antibody-mediated rejection and cardiac allograft vasculopathy. Transplantation 91:1036–1043

Chapter 21

Cylex ImmuKnow Cell Function Assay

Adriana Zeevi and John Lunz

Abstract

The use of immunosuppression in solid organ transplantation is associated with increased morbidity and mortality. Monitoring trough immunosuppression levels alone in transplant recipients is insufficient to gauge the suppression of immune responses. The ImmuKnow Immune Cell Function Assay (Cylex, Inc., Columbia, MD, USA) has been developed to measure the activity of CD4+ T cells as a marker of global immune-competence. The changes in T cell activation were correlated with the relative risk of rejection and infection. However, the most significant utility of the ImmuKnow test, in combination with other clinical parameters, is to identify immune-compromised patients and to help to tailor individualized immunosuppression regimens.

Key words Solid organ transplants, Infection, ATP synthesis, Immune response

1 Introduction

Successful management of solid organ transplant recipients depends on long term exposure to one or more immunosuppressive drugs. Monitoring the trough levels of primary immunosuppressive agents (i.e., Tacrolimus, Cyclosporine) provides important data on potential drug toxicity and can be useful in gauging compliance, but it fails to correlate with the net effect of all the immunosuppression agents taken by transplant recipients. The ImmuKnow Immune Cell Function Assay (Cylex, Inc., Columbia, MD, USA) is designed to measure the bioactivity of immunosuppressive drugs alone or in combination by measuring their net effect on immune cells [1]. The ImmuKnow assay is a US Food and Drug Administration approved test for detecting cell-mediated immunity in an immunosuppressed patient [2]. The ImmuKnow test measures the early response of CD4 T cell activation after phytohemagglutinin (PHA) stimulation by detecting intracellular ATP synthesis [2]. As a control, for basal background ATP, cells are also assayed in the absence of stimuli. Anti-CD4 monoclonal antibody coated magnetic beads are added to PHA-stimulated and non-stimulated whole blood to

Andrea A. Zachary and Mary S. Leffell (eds.), *Transplantation Immunology: Methods and Protocols, Second Edition*,
Methods in Molecular Biology, vol. 1034, DOI 10.1007/978-1-62703-493-7_21,

select CD4+ T cells. A lysis reagent releases the intracellular adenosine triphosphate (ATP), which is quantified using a luminescent reagent (luciferin/luciferase) and measured with a luminometer (emission maximum 562 nm). The concentration of ATP (ng/ml) is calculated for both stimulated and non-stimulated wells.

By comparing the responses of healthy individuals and transplant recipients, three immune response stratifications were identified: low response (ATP < 225 ng/ml); moderate response (226 > ATP < 524 ng/ml), and strong response (ATP > 525 ng/ml) [2]. Global use of the ImmuKnow assay has been adapted in diverse adult and pediatric solid organ transplant recipients as a potential marker of the patient immunosuppressive state. Infections in lung [3, 4], heart [5, 6], liver [7, 8], renal [9], and pancreas [10] transplant recipients correlated with significant drop of activated CD4 ATP values as compared to the values obtained during clinical stability. Furthermore, solid organ transplant recipients exhibiting prolonged low ImmuKnow responses had a high risk for short-term mortality with the major cause for death being infections and cancer [11].

The ImmuKnow procedure detailed below was adopted by UPMC per the manufacturer's instructions for the Cylex Immune Cell Function Assay.

2 Materials

2.1 Specimen

The ImmuKnow™ assay is performed using whole blood from a tube containing sodium heparin as the anticoagulant. The sample cannot be more than 30 h old. The specimen must be shipped or stored at room temperature (18–28 °C). Any sample received that is hemolyzed, clotted, or older than 30 h will not be accepted for testing because these parameters are outside the scope of the test.

2.2 Reagents

1. ImmuKnow Immune Cell Function Assay Kit (Cylex Inc. Cat. # 4400).
2. Buffer to rinse the manifold head: this can be water or PBS.

2.3 Equipment

1. Luminometer (Turner Biosystems).
2. Computer to support Luminometer function.
3. 27 °C/5 % CO_2 humidified incubator (CO_2 measured).
4. Cylex® Magnet Tray (Cylex Inc. Cat. # 1040).
5. Microtiter plate shaker.
6. Adjustable pipettes and tips capable of delivering 25–1,000 μl volumes.
7. 8-channel multichannel pipettes and tips capable of delivering 50–200 μl volumes.

8. Reagent reservoirs.
9. 12 × 75 mm tubes (Falcon 2025).
10. 12 × 75 tube caps (Sarstedt).
11. Kimwipes (Kimberly-Clark).
12. Appropriate protective barriers (lab coat, gloves, etc.).
13. Microtiter Plate Shaker/Rotator (DPC).
14. Time.
15. Vacuum source.
16. Vacuum apparatus with disposable tubing and receiving flask.

3 Methods

3.1 Assay Procedure Part 1: Cell Stimulation

1. Using the ImmuKnow™ Data Analysis Software, create a worksheet to correspond with the run.
2. Gently invert each control and patient whole blood specimen several times to ensure uniform distribution of blood cells.
3. Prepare a 1:4 dilution of each whole blood specimen using Sample Diluent (e.g., 250 μl whole blood + 750 μl Sample Diluent).
4. Assemble the Assay Plate according to the worksheet, using one 8-well strip for each specimen.
   (a) Dispense 25 μl of Sample Diluent into the first four wells of each Assay Plate strip, designated as non-stimulated wells according to the Worksheet.
   (b) Dispense 25 μl of Stimulant into the remaining four wells of each Assay Plate strip, designated as stimulated wells according to the Worksheet.
   (c) Dispense 100 μl of each of the diluted specimens into the appropriate wells.
5. Replace the plate cover and shake the plate on a plate shaker for 30 s.
6. Incubate the covered Assay Plate in a 37 °C–5 % CO_2 incubator for 15–18 h (*see* **Notes 1** and **2**).

3.2 Assay Part 2: CD4 Cell Selection and ATP Release

1. Remove the Assay Plate from the incubator and shake on a plate shaker for 3 min.
2. Gently swirl to resuspend the magnetic beads and dispense 50 μl into each well using a single or repeating pipettor.
3. Cover the plate, shake on the plate shaker for 15 s, and incubate for 15 min at room temperature (18–28 °C).
4. Shake the plate for 15 s and continue to incubate the plate at room temperature (18–28 °C) for another 15 min.

5. Shake the plate for a final 15–30 s.
6. Take the strips from the Assay Plate and place into the Magnet Tray. Wait 1–2 min for the magnetic beads to collect on the side of the wells (the CD4 positive cells are bound to the magnetic beads).
7. Aspirate the whole blood from each well using an 8-channel aspiration manifold attached to a vacuum system.
8. Perform three wash steps to remove residual unbound cells and interfering substances from the wells.
   (a) Wash #1:
      - Dispense 200 μl Wash Buffer into each well; Wait for 1 min and aspirate.
   (b) Wash #2:
      - Dispense 200 μl Wash Buffer into each well.
      - Inspect the wells and use a pipette tip to dislodge any residual blood spots from the sides of the wells. Wait for 1 min and aspirate.
   (c) Wash #3:
      - Dispense 200 μl Wash Buffer into each well.
      - Remove the Strip Holder from the Magnet Base.
      - Shake the strips for 1 min on the plate shaker.
      - Replace the Strip Holder onto the Magnet Base.
      - Wait for 1 min and aspirate.
9. Dispense 200 μl of Lysis Reagent into each well. This will separate the CD4 positive cells from the magnetic beads and lyse the cells to release ATP.
10. Remove the Strip Holder from the Magnetic Base and shake the strips on the plate shaker for 5 min.
11. Place the Strip Holder onto the Magnetic Base and wait for 1–2 min. The ATP will be free in the solution and the beads will adhere to the sides of the tray (*see* **Notes 3–9**).

3.3 Assay Part 3: ATP Measurement

1. Refer to the assay worksheet and assemble the Measurement Plate to mimic the assay plate adding two strips for the calibrators:
   (a) One strip for the Control.
   (b) One strip for each patient.
   (c) Two strips for the Calibrator Panel.
2. Using a multichannel pipette, transfer 50 μl from each well of the Magnet Tray to the appropriate wells of the Measurement Plate according to the Worksheet. Change pipette tips for each strip.

3. Dispense 50 μl of each level of the Calibrator Panel into duplicate wells of the Measurement Plate according to the worksheet.
4. Using a multichannel pipette, dispense 150 μl of Luminescence Reagent to each well of the Measurement Plate and shake plate for 30 s. (It is of no consequence to add reagent to blank wells.) Following the luminometer manufacturer's instructions, read the plate between 3 and 10 min after the addition of the Luminescence Reagent (*see* **Notes 10** and **11**).

3.4 Calibration

1. The amount of ATP present in the cell lysate is calculated from an ATP calibration curve generated in each assay run. Relative light units (RLU) for control and patient samples are obtained from the luminometer and converted to ATP ng/ml.
2. The RLU data from the luminometer is converted and analyzed using the ImmuKnow™ Data Analysis Software. Luminometer RLU values provided in Microsoft® Excel or tabular formats can be directly copied and exported into the Data Analysis Software spreadsheet. ATP Calibrator concentrations vs. RLU values are plotted on a log-log scale, and linear regression analysis generates a calibration curve. To assess linearity of the curve, each Calibrator is reanalyzed by plotting RLU values on the curve and calculating corresponding ATP values. In addition, the correlation coefficient (r^2) of the calibration curve is calculated.

3.5 Result Interpretation

1. The ATP result for the non-stimulated control sample must be ≤60 mg/ml.
2. The ATP result for the stimulated control sample must be ≥240 ng/ml.
3. The linearity of the calibration curve must be accepted under the following criteria:
   (a) The calculated value for the 1,000 ng/ml ATP Calibrator must be 900–1,100 ng/ml (refer to result in the "Average" column in Table IV of the Data Analysis Software Report).
   (b) The Calculated value for the 100 ng/ml ATP Calibrator must be 85–115 ng/ml (refer to result in the "Average": column in Table IV of the Data Analysis Software Report).
   (c) The correlation coefficient (r^2) of the ATP Calibration Curve must be ≥0.97.

3.6 Calculation of Results

1. Calculate the ATP concentrations of the patient specimens using the ImmuKnow™ Data Analysis Software. After RLU values and specimen identification are entered into the spreadsheet and the calibration curve is generated, the following data are calculated and displayed in a Report:
   (a) ATP result for each replicate.
   (b) Average ATP value of replicates.

   (c) Standard deviation of replicates.
   (d) Coefficient of variance of replicates.
2. For each control and patient specimen, review the coefficient of variance (CV) for stimulated wells. If the CV is >20 %, apply the following outlier evaluation or your laboratory's accepted analytical method to identify outlier values which can be omitted. Recalculate results.
   (a) If the % CV of the sample quadruplicates is >20 %, review the data for suspected outliers.
   (b) Remove the suspected outlier (the value furthest from the mean) and recalculate the mean and SD of the triplicate results.
   (c) If the suspected outlier falls outside the new mean ±3 SD calculated from the triplicates, then the replicate was an outlier and should be eliminated from the result calculation.
   (d) If no outlier is identified and the %CV for the quadruplicates is >20 %, the laboratory should use its established procedures for determining reportability of the results.

3.7 Reporting Results

1. Reported ATP values must be limited to the defined range of the Calibrator Panel. Samples with ATP values above the highest calibrator are reported as >1,000 ng/ml. Samples with ATP values below the lowest calibrator are reported as <1 ng/ml.
2. The specimen acceptance criteria are as follows:
   (a) The ATP level for the non-stimulated sample should be ≤60 ATP ng/ml.
   (b) The ATP level for the non-stimulated sample must be less than the ATP level for the stimulated sample.
3. If the specimen meets these criteria, proceed with interpretation of the stimulated sample. If the non-stimulated sample is >60 ng/ml, the specimen may have no specific production of ATP and a new specimen should be drawn.

3.8 Interpretation of PHA Stimulated Sample Results

The summary of the interpretation of results is depicted in Table 1. Three ranges of immune response: Low, Moderate, and Strong are identified based on the ATP level following PHA stimulation (*see* **Notes 12** and **13**).

3.9 Quality Control

1. With every assay run, a control specimen must be collected from a healthy individual and tested with patient sample.
2. Each new shipment three patients are to be run with the old and new shipment.
3. With each new lot, three patients are to be run with the old and new lot (*see* **Notes 14** and **15**).

Table 1
Interpretation of PHA stimulated sample results

ATP level (ng/ml)	Result	Interpretation
≤225	Low immune cell response	The patient's circulating immune cells are showing low response to PHA stimulation.
226–524	Moderate immune cell response	The patient's circulating immune cells are showing moderate response to PHA stimulation.
≥525	Strong immune cell response	The patient's circulating immune cells are showing strong response to PHA stimulation.

4 Notes

1. Before removing the tray from the incubator, remove the kit from the refrigerator/freezer to allow reagents to come to room temperature for later use
2. Reagents should be thoroughly mixed immediately before pipetting.
3. The magnetic beads contain sodium azide. Upon disposal of material, flush with a large volume of water to prevent sodium azide accumulation.
4. Keep the Magnet Tray away from computer disks or other magnet sensitive materials.
5. The microtiter plate shaker must provide a vigorous mix to fully resuspend settled blood cells following incubation without visible loss of material from the wells. Once an appropriate setting is determined, use this setting throughout the assay and keep extraneous materials away from the rocker tray to allow for free movement.
6. A vacuum pump of 150–200 mmHg strength is recommended. Aspiration manifold tips should be held at a 90° angle or at a slight angle away from the magnet to assure that the magnetic beads are not aspirated.
7. The magnetic beads must be thoroughly suspended to ensure consistent addition to each well. Magnetic beads settle quickly. Do not use a multichannel pipette for this step.
8. Avoid dislodging the magnetic beads by holding the aspirator in an upright position or tilted slightly away from the magnet.
9. Use a multichannel pipette held in a straight vertical position to dispense Wash Buffer.
10. If there will be more than a 4 h delay in proceeding to "Assay Part 3: ATP Measurement" the strips should be frozen at this time. Once frozen, the strips are stable for 30 days. Remove

the strips from the Strip Holder and place in the Assay Plate frame. Seal the strips with Parafilm, place the cover on the Assay Plate and freeze at −20 °C. To continue, remove the plate from the freezer, allow to come to room temperature (18–28 °C), and repeat step. Continue with "Assay Part 3: ATP Measurement".

11. The control and patient samples are run in quadruplicate and the calibrators are run in duplicate.
12. This is a qualitative assay. Therefore, the result does not directly quantify the level of immunosuppression, but rather identifies the immune status of a patient and should be used in conjunction with clinical presentation.
13. Reported ATP values must be limited to the defined range of the Calibrator Panel. Samples with ATP values above the highest calibrator are reported as <1,000 ng/ml. Samples with ATP values below the lowest calibrator are reported as >1 ng/ml.
14. *High non-stimulated control values ATP >60 ng/ml*: can be the result of improperly diluted sample or the presence of clots. Repeat the test with fresh sample
15. *Low stimulated control values ATP <240 ng/ml*: can be the result of old blood sample or it was subjected to temperature changes, or it was collected with an anticoagulant other than sodium heparin. Repeat the test with fresh sample.

References

1. Kowalski R, Post D, Schneider MC, Britz J, Thomas J, Deierhoi M (2003) Immune cell function testing: an adjunct to therapeutic drug monitoring in transplant patient management. Clin Transplant 17:77–88
2. Kowalski RJ, Post DR, Mannon RB, Sebastian A, Wright HI, Sigle G (2006) Assessing relative risks of infection and rejection: a meta-analysis using an immune function assay. Transplantation 82:663–668
3. Husain S, Raza K, Pilewski JM, Zaldonis D, Crespo M, Toyoda Y (2009) Experience with immune monitoring in lung transplant recipients: correlation of low immune function with infection. Transplantation 87:1852–1857. doi:00007890-200906270-00015 [pii]
4. Bhorade SM, Janata K, Vigneswaran WT, Alex CG, Garrity ER (2008) Cylex ImmuKnow assay levels are lower in lung transplant recipients with infection. J Heart Lung Transplant 27:990–994
5. Israeli M, Klein T, Brandhorst G, Oellerich M (2012) Confronting the challenge: individualized immune monitoring after organ transplantation using the cellular immune function assay. Clin Chim Acta 413:1374–1378
6. Kobashigawa JA, Kiyosaki KK, Patel JK, Kittleson MM, Kubak BM, Davis SN (2010) Benefit of immune monitoring in heart transplant patients using ATP production in activated lymphocytes. J Heart Lung Transplant 29:504–508
7. Mendler M, Kwok H, Franco E, Baron P, Weissman J, Ojogho O (2008) Monitoring peripheral blood CD4+ adenosine triphosphate activity in a liver transplant cohort: insight into the interplay between hepatitis C virus infection and cellular immunity. Liver Transpl 14:1313–1322
8. Te HS, Dasgupta KA, Cao D, Satoskar R, Mohanty SR, Reau N (2012) Use of immune function test in monitoring immunosuppression in liver transplant recipients. Clin Transplant 26:826–832
9. Batal I, Zeevi A, Heider A, Girnita A, Basu A, Tan H (2008) Measurements of global

cell-mediated immunity in renal transplant recipients with BK virus reactivation. Am J Clin Pathol 129:587–591
10. Thai NL, Blisard D, Tom K, Basu A, Smetanka C, Tan H (2006) Pancreas transplantation under alemtuzumab (Campath-1H) and tacrolimus: correlation between low T-cell responses and infection. Transplantation 82: 1649–1652
11. Berglund D, Bengtsson M, Biglarnia A, Berglund E, Yamamoto S, von Zur-Muhlen B (2011) Screening of mortality in transplant patients using an assay for immune function. Transpl Immunol 24:246–250

Chapter 22

Detection of Intracellular Cytokines

Nancy L. Reinsmoen and Chih-Hung Lai

Abstract

The intracellular cytokine method allows for a multiparametric readout by flow cytometry with precise phenotyping of the responding T cells. The intracellular cytokine staining of cells that have been fixed and permeabilized following a short-term activation and staining with antibodies to cell surface markers allows for identification of the cellular origin of the cytokine accumulated product.

Key words Flow cytometry, Intracellular, Cytokines, Cell surface markers, Protein transport inhibitor, Cell permeabilization

1 Introduction

The immune response is regulated by a network of small molecular weight proteins termed cytokines that have potent biological effects. The study of these cytokines and their corresponding receptors has revealed insight into normal homeostasis as well as various disease processes. Methods have focused on determining accurate measurement of the cytokine production and on identifying the cell types producing them. Initially, the quantification of cytokine levels relied on the use of cytokine sensitive cell lines as biosensors of cytokine production. Bulk culture release assays such as enzyme-linked immunoassays and radioimmunoassays were also used to determine the total amount of cytokine being produced. These assay systems were prone to interference by naturally occurring biological inhibitors and to difficulty in quantification. Intracellular cytokine detection by flow cytometry avoids interference by many of these inhibitors and allows for the use of monoclonal antibodies to cell surface markers to identify the cytokine producing cells.

The basic methodology involves a short pulse activation by protein, peptides, or mitogens, in the presence of a protein transport inhibitor such as Brefeldin A or Monensin [1]. These agents prevent the export of the newly synthesized proteins by interfering

Andrea A. Zachary and Mary S. Leffell (eds.), *Transplantation Immunology: Methods and Protocols, Second Edition*, Methods in Molecular Biology, vol. 1034, DOI 10.1007/978-1-62703-493-7_22, © Springer Science+Business Media, LLC 2013

with the transport between the endoplasmic reticulum and the Golgi apparatus [2]. The incubation time is short enough to capture a sufficient number of responding cells prior to cell division or apoptosis. EDTA can be used to arrest activation and to remove the adherent cells. Paraformaldehyde is usually used to fix the cells, thereby maintaining membrane stability and cell morphology. The most common agent used for cell permeabilization is saponin, a plant glycoside that replaces cholesterol in the membrane forming ring-shaped structure with central pores [3]. Intracellular cytokine staining has been refined to detect the presence of cytokines that have not been secreted [4]. Access to the intracellular compartment can be confirmed by using antibodies to cytoskeletal components such as vimentin [5]. The cells can then be stained with fluorescent-labeled antibodies provided the antibodies do recognize epitopes after the cells have been fixed and permeabilized. The data acquired by flow cytometry can be analyzed by gating on the cell population of interest (CD3+/CD8+; CD3+/CD4+; CD14; etc.). Antibodies to CD69, an early activation marker, can be used in combination to identify more readily the activated cytokine-producing cells (reviewed in [3]). This chapter focuses on the methods used to determine intracellular cytokines and the responding cells that produce them.

2 Materials

2.1 Activation Components

1. Heparinized whole blood or separated peripheral blood mononuclear cells (PBMC) (*see* **Notes 1** and **2**).
2. Culture reagents: RPMI-1640 medium with HEPES, 10 % fetal bovine serum and antibiotic/antifungal solution (Sigma-Aldrich Chemical Co, St. Louis, MO).
3. Activation antigens selected based on the requirements of the investigator: staphylococcal enterotoxin B (SEB) (Sigma-Aldrich), Cytomegalovirus (CMV) lysate or peptides (Advanced Biotechnologies, BD Biosciences), custom peptides (synthesized by various vendors), phorbol myristate acetate (PMA, Sigma-Aldrich), and calcium ionophore A23187 (Sigma-Aldrich).
4. Optional Co-stimulatory antibodies: CD28 and CD49d, 0.1 mg/ml of each in sterile phosphate-buffered saline (PBS).

2.2 Fluorescence-Labeled Antibodies

1. Directly conjugated monoclonal antibodies: e.g., CD8 (mouse IgG2a anti-human), IFN-γ (mouse IgG1anti-human), IL-4 (rat IgG1anti-human), IL-10 (rat IgG2a anti-human). The cytokine monoclonal antibodies are phycoerythrin (PE) labeled.
2. Isotype control antibodies: e.g., FITC-conjugated mouse IgG1 anti-human, PE conjugated mouse IgG1 anti-human, and PE conjugated rat IgG2a anti-human.

3. Staining buffer (fluorescence activated cell sorter (FACS) medium). Dulbecco's PBS without Mg^{2+} or Ca^{2+}, 1 % heat inactivated fetal calf serum, and 0.1 % sodium azide. pH 7.4–7.6, store at 4 °C.
4. Wash buffer: PBS, 0.5 % bovine serum albumin and 0.1 % sodium azide.

2.3 Reagents

1. Brefeldin A: Make up a stock solution of 5 mg/ml in dimethyl sulfoxide (DMSO).
2. 20 mM EDTA in PBS, pH 7.4.
3. Erythrocyte lysis and cell fixation buffer (e.g., BD FACS Lysing Solution).
4. Cell permeabilization reagent (e.g., BD FACS Permeabilizing Solution 2).
5. Fixation buffer (1 % paraformaldehyde in PBS): Dilute 10 % paraformaldehyde (EMD Chemicals, Gibbstown, NJ) 1:10 with PBS.
6. Pooled Normal Human Serum (PHS) can be purchased commercially (Gemini Bioproducts, Sacramento, CA).

2.4 Equipment

1. Flow cytometer: FACscan or FACS Canto II (BD Biosciences, San Jose, CA).
2. Humidified incubator, 37 °C and 5 % CO_2.

3 Methods

3.1 Sample Collection for Assays

1. Collect whole blood in sodium heparin and store at room temperature for less than 8 h (*see* **Note 3**).
2. Prepare impermeable PBMC from the whole blood by Ficoll gradient separation methods and resuspended at 2.5×10^6–1×10^7 PBMC/ml.
3. Cryopreserve PBMCs by thawing briefly in a 37 °C water bath and diluting slowly with culture medium. Spin the thawed cells for about 10 min at 250 × *g* and wash twice more with culture medium. Incubate thawed cryopreserved PBMCs overnight at 37 °C prior to stimulation (*see* **Note 4**).

3.2 Activation of Cells

1. Activation of cryopreserved PBMC with peptides: The peptides can be dissolved to 5 mg/ml in DMSO and stored at −80 °C. After thawing dilute 1:10 with PBS and 5 mg/ml of Brefeldin A stock. Pipet 20 μl of appropriate mix into each well containing 200 μl/well of cells in a round-bottom 96-well plate at concentrations described above. Incubate at 37 °C in humidified 5 % CO_2 incubator for 6 h.
2. Activation of PBMC by PMA: Plate PBMC or cells of interest at 50,000–350,000 cells per well in 96-well "V" bottom plate

at a final volume of 100 μl of 5 % PHS RPMI-1640. The stimulated cells are cultured with PMA (50 ng/ml) and unstimulated cells are cultured without PMA and calcium ionophore (1 μg/ml) and Brefeldin A (1.5 μg/ml). Incubate at 37 °C in a humidified 5 % CO_2 incubator for 4 h.

3. Activation of whole blood: Whole blood (1 ml) is stimulated with and without PMA (50 ng/ml) and calcium ionophore (1 μg/ml) and Brefeldin A (1.5 μg/ml). Unstimulated whole blood is incubated with RPMI-1640 and Brefeldin A. The whole blood cultures are incubated for 4 h at 37 °C in a humidified 5 % CO_2 incubator (*see* **Notes 5** and **6**).

3.3 Staining Procedures

3.3.1 PBMC Cultures

1. Centrifuge the plates for 5 min at 250×*g*, flick the plate to remove the supernatant and blot dry. Add 150 μl of FACS medium, recentrifuge, and repeat as above (*see* **Notes 7** and **8**).
2. Surface stain with the desired antibodies. For example, add 10 μl of anti-CD8 FITC antibody/well. Resuspend the cells by gently pipetting up and down about 8–10 times. Incubate at 4 °C for 20 min in the dark.
3. Wash wells with 200 μl of FACS medium, centrifuge for 4 min at 250×*g*, and flick off supernatant.
4. Fix cells with 150 μl of 4 % paraformaldehyde and incubate overnight in the refrigerator.
5. Centrifuge plates as described before. Add 150 μl of permeabilization buffer to each well.
6. Recentrifuge and wash as described before.
7. Stain with selected intracellular cytokine antibody (10 μl of a 1:10 dilution in permeabilization buffer). For unstained wells, add the permeabilization buffer alone.
8. Wrap plate in foil and place at 4 °C for 30 min.
9. Wash plate with 200 μl of FACS medium and centrifuge for 4 min at 250×*g*.
10. Flick off supernatant and add 200 μl of FACS medium and prepare for FACS analysis.

3.3.2 Whole Blood

1. Perform the surface marker staining using activated whole blood (Subheading 3.2) with FITC-labeled anti-CD8 antibody prior to the intracellular staining.
2. Fix and permeabilize the cells as above.
3. Briefly, incubate 100 μl of whole blood culture mixed with 100 μl of the fixation medium in a 5 ml Falcon tube for 15 min at room temperature.
4. Wash the cells with PBS.
5. Add 100 μl of permeabilizing solution to the cells.

6. Add the intracellular cytokine-specific antibody (10 μl) and incubate the mixture in the dark at room temperature for 15 min.
7. Wash the samples once in PBS and once in FACS medium.
8. Resuspend the sample in 200 μl of FACS medium and analyze them on the flow cytometer.

3.4 Data Analysis

1. The flow cytometer must be calibrated either manually or using beads and calibration software (*see* **Note 9**).
2. For manual calibration, a sample stained with an isotype control cocktail is used to set each photomultiplier tube (PMT) value. Samples stained individually with each fluorochrome are used to set the compensation values.
3. For bead-based calibration, follow the manufacturer's protocols. Using BD setting entitled "lyse with no wash" and BD CaliBRITE beads.
4. Set forward and side scatter gates for lymphocytes such that the dead cells, debris, and nonlymphoid cells are excluded. Be sure to size these regions to include cells that may have downmodulated cell surface markers as a result of activation.
5. The number of events acquired within the specific gates can vary according to the investigator's requirements, but typically range from 10,000 to 40,000 events. Analyzing small populations of antigen specific cells will require that the larger number of events is acquired.
6. Create two parameter histograms showing cytokine staining.
7. Generate the quadrant statistics based on the staining of the negative control isotypes.
8. Analyze cytokine production by detection of PE staining.
9. The number of cells staining for each cytokine is expressed as a percentage of the cells of a particular cell surface marker (e.g., CD8+ and CD8− cells) and the total number of cells is expressed per million PBMC.

4 Notes

1. Selection of appropriate reagents is critical. The appropriate immunoglobulin isotype control should be performed with each assay. Recombinant cytokines should be used for blocking studies to confirm antibody specificity. Blocking Fc receptors such as with human AB serum (HAB) may reduce nonspecific staining. Titers of the antibodies should be determined for each cell type and for each source of stimulation.

2. Sodium heparin should be used for blood collection to maintain a functional response. Other anticoagulants such as acid citrate dextrose additives (ACD) can be used provided the isolation is followed by appropriate washing steps and resuspended in calcium-containing medium.
3. If the PBMC or whole blood samples cannot be processed within 24 h after phlebotomy, The PBMCs can be cryopreserved by reliable techniques and stored in vapor phase liquid nitrogen refrigeration units.
4. It is recommended that the thawed cryopreserved cells be "rested" overnight by incubating overnight (12–18 h) prior to stimulation. Some investigators have also found that fresh PBMC may show an increase in cytokine fluorescence intensity after resting overnight [6].
5. The plates can be kept overnight at 4 °C after fixation. This step may also decrease nonspecific staining.
6. Stimulation for 6 h is adequate for induction of IFN-γ, TNF-α, IL-2, and IL-4 [7]. Although incubation for longer periods of time may increase the cytokine fluorescence intensity for a while, the longer time may cause toxicity at >12 h.
7. The 96-well plate configuration allows for a higher throughput analysis; however, care must be taken such that there is no well-to-well contamination, especially with regard to the placement of the positive control on the plate.
8. A commercial intracellular cytokine detection kit is available testing for CD8 positive or CD4 positive cells (BD Fast Immune, San Jose, CA).
9. A study involving testing by multiple laboratories has been published investigating the standardization of the intracellular cytokine flow cytometry assay [8].

References

1. Picker LJ, Singh MK, Zdraveski Z, Treer JR, Waldrop SL, Bergstresser PR et al (1995) Direct demonstration of cytokine synthesis heterogeneity among human memory/effector T cells by flow cytometry. Blood 86:1408–1419
2. Nylander S, Kalies I (1999) Brefeldin A, but not monensin, completely blocks CD69 expression on mouse lymphocytes: efficacy of inhibitors of protein secretion in protocols for intracellular cytokine staining by flow cytometry. J Immunol Methods 224:69–76
3. Maecker HT (2004) Cytokine flow cytometry, chapter 5. In: Hawley TS, Hawley RG (eds) Flow cytometry protocols. Humana, Totowa, NJ, p 95
4. Ghanekar SA, Maecker HT (2003) Cytokine flow cytometry: multiparametric approach to immune function analysis. Cytotherapy 5:1–6
5. O'Mahony L, O'Donoghue M (2001) Assaying interleukins intracellularly by FACS, chapter 4. In: O'Neill LAJ, Bowie A (eds) Interleukin protocols. Humana, Totowa, NJ, p 41
6. Suni MA, Dunn HS, Orr PL, de Laat R, Sinclair E, Ghanekar SA et al (2003) Performance of plate-based cytokine flow cytometry with automated data analysis. BMC Immunol 4:9
7. Nomura LE, Walker JM, Maecker HT (2000) Optimization of whole blood antigen-specific cytokine assays for CD4(+) T cells. Cytometry 40:60–68
8. Maecker HT, Rinfret A, D'Souza P, Darden J, Roig E, Landry C et al (2005) Standardization of cytokine flow cytometry assays. BMC Immunol 6:13

Chapter 23

Tolerogenic Dendritic Cells and Induction of T Suppressor Cells in Transplant Recipients

George Vlad and Nicole Suciu-Foca

Abstract

Tolerogenic antigen presenting cells (APC), primarily dendritic cells (DC), are essential to the induction and maintenance of immunologic tolerance in clinical transplantation. They induce the differentiation of CD8+ T suppressor (Ts) and CD4+ T regulatory (Treg) or anergic cells, which prevent transplant rejection maintaining a state of quiescence. Tolerogenic APC express high levels of inhibitory receptors such as Immunoglobulin-like transcript (ILT)3 and 4 which inhibit the effector function of T cells that recognize HLA-peptide complexes on APC. Here, we describe the methods for detection of tolerogenic APC induced by allospecific Ts/Treg cells.

Key words Tolerogenic dendritic cells, T suppressor cells, Inhibitory receptors, Transplant quiescence

1 Introduction

Dendritic cells (DC) are key regulators of adaptive immunity promoting or suppressing T cell responses depending on their functional state. They are highly specialized APC that integrate a wide array of incoming signals and convey them to lymphocytes directing the appropriate immune response [1]. For the initiation of CD4 T cell responses, DC in different stages of maturation are present in the circulation, as well as in lymphoid and non-lymphoid organs, where they exert a sentinel function. After antigen uptake, DCs migrate through the afferent lymph to T-dependent areas of secondary lymphoid organs where they can prime naïve T cells [2].

Bidirectional interaction between DC and antigen experienced T cells initiate either a tolerogenic or immunogenic pathway [3].

The differentiation of CD8+ cytotoxic T cells (CTL) is conditioned upon recognition of MHC class I/peptide complexes on APC that have been "licensed" by cognate CD4 T helper cells (Th) via the CD40-signaling pathway [4–7]. For effective CTL priming different peptides of the same protein must be recognized

Andrea A. Zachary and Mary S. Leffell (eds.), *Transplantation Immunology: Methods and Protocols, Second Edition*, Methods in Molecular Biology, vol. 1034, DOI 10.1007/978-1-62703-493-7_23, © Springer Science+Business Media, LLC 2013

on the same APC "bridge" by CD4+ and CD8+ T cells with cognate specificity. DC are able to process exogenous antigens not only into MHC class II but also into the class I pathway. This endows them with the capacity of cross-priming CD8+ CTL [8]. Pathogens which trigger toll-like receptors and inflammatory cytokines can also license DC to mature and stimulate the differentiation of effector and memory T cells [9].

Conversely, CD8+ T cells which have been exposed to chronic antigenic stimulation, induce the upregulation of the inhibitory receptors ILT3/ILT4, downregulation of costimulatory molecules, and suppression of NF-kB activation, in the DC with which they interact [10, 11]. Such "tolerogenic" DC further elicit the differentiation of CD8+ Ts and CD4+ Treg [11, 12].

Exposure of APC to IL-10, IFN-alpha or -beta also results in the upregulation of the inhibitory receptors ILT3 and ILT4, the characteristic markers of tolerogenic APC [3, 12].

Similarly, several immunosuppressive agents such as 1,25-dihydroxy vitamin D3 and its analogues induce high expression of ILT3/4 and secretion of IL-10, while downregulating the expression of costimulatory molecules and production of IL-12 [13, 14]. Knock-down of ILT3 from DC (by transfection with siRNA ILT3 vectors) increased their capacity to prime T cells, produce inflammatory cytokines and migration factors, upon TLR-ligation [9]. This further demonstrates the importance of ILT3 for inhibiting the differentiation of mature, immunogenic DC.

Recipients of heart, kidney or liver transplants who remain rejection-free for 1 year or more, requiring minimal immunosuppression, were shown to develop allospecific Ts. CD8 T cells from the circulation of such patients, but not from patients with episodes of acute cellular rejection, induced the downregulation of costimulatory molecules and upregulation of ILT3/4 on donor APC or endothelial cells (EC) matched to the donor for HLA class I antigen(s) [11, 15, 16]. This suggests that ILT3/4-inducing Ts/Treg inhibit the direct allo-recognition of donor HLA antigens expressed by graft EC [17]. Hence, inflammation and necrosis promoted by CD4 and CD8 effector cells may be prevented from occurring in the presence of such regulatory T cells. Furthermore, in the absence of inflammation and necrosis within the graft, indirect allo-recognition may also be inhibited since host APC are unlikely to become activated, process graft alloantigens, and present immunogenic allopeptides to T helper cells. Experimental evidence to this effect has been provided by studies which demonstrated that without direct recognition, indirect recognition is of no consequence, since tolerated heart allografts can be transplanted into syngeneic naïve recipients without triggering rejection [17].

Hence both direct and indirect allo recognition are subjected to the inhibitory feedback loop created by Ts–APC interaction [18, 19].

The identification of T cells capable to induce tolerogenic DC relies on both phenotypic and functional tests. The most reliable phenotypic markers for tolerogenic DC induced upon co-incubation with recipient CD8+ CD28− T cells are the high expression of ILT3 and ILT4 and low expression of CD80, CD86, and CD40 on APC from the donor or HLA-matched surrogate [11, 20]. Implicitly, the low allostimulatory capacity of such tolerogenic APC can be measured in an optimized CFSE-based T-cell suppression assay which permits the evaluation of Ts/Treg in transplant patients [21].

Several immunosuppressive agents have been shown to induce DCs with tolerogenic phenotype and function. Glucocorticoids, mycophenolate mofetil (MMF) and sirolimus impair DC maturation and inhibit upregulation of costimulatory molecules, secretion of proinflammatory cytokines, in particular IL-12, and allostimulatory capacity [22–29]. Similar effects are exerted on DC by anti-inflammatory agents, such as acetylsalicylic acid [30, 31], butyric acid [32] and *N*-acetyl-l-cysteine [33].

Tolerogenic DC induced by vitamin D receptor ligands, display increased expression of ILT3 and lead to enhancement of regulatory T cells. Analysis of DC subsets showed that plasmacytoid DC (pDC) display a higher expression of ILT3 compared to myeloid DC (mDC) [34, 35]. CD40 ligation increases the expression of costimulatory molecules on mDC, yet has no effect on pDC. Maintaining high expression of ILT3 on pDC matured via CD40 ligation is of interest, because this cell population induces CD8 regulatory T cells through an IL-10 dependent pathway [36]. Of significance is also the finding that pDC are potent producers of IFN-alpha, a cytokine which induces ILT3 upregulation on mDC [12]. This dual role of certain inflammatory cytokines, such as IFN-alpha and -beta, is consistent with the immunosuppressive effect of IFN-beta in Multiple Sclerosis [3].

The notion that certain cytokines induce upregulation of inhibitory receptors on naïve APC implied the possibility of unraveling their presence by testing transplant patients' sera for their capacity to induce the upregulation of ILT3 and ILT4. Previous studies in patients with HIV support this possibility, since the high content of IL-10 sera from patients with poor outcome was shown to upregulate the expression of these inhibitory receptors on APC from healthy individuals.

Monitoring of cells or soluble factors that induce tolerogenic APC is of importance for identifying patients whose immunosuppression can be safely decreased. In the following sections, we shall describe the methods used for identification of tolerogenic DC in transplant patients.

2 Materials

2.1 Flow Cytometry

1. Phosphate buffered saline (PBS): 10 nM phosphate buffer, pH 7.4, 2.7 mM KCl, 150 mM NaCl.
2. FACS staining buffer: PBS, 2 % FCS, 2 mM EDTA.
3. Flow Cytometry antibodies:

   Phycoerythrin (PE)-conjugated monoclonal antibodies (mAbs) to CD3, CD28, CD16, CD56, and CD86 from (BD Bioscience); and ILT4 (Santa Cruz).

   Fluorescein isothiocyanate (FITC)-conjugated mAbs to CD14, CD11c, CD4, and CD8 (BD Biosciences); Phycoerythrin cyanine (PC5) conjugated anti-human ILT3 (Beckman-Coulter Inc., Miami, FL) and anti-CD86 (BD Biosciences).

   Mixtures of mAbs to FITC-CD3, PE-CD4, PerCP-CD8, APC-CD19.
4. Viability staining materials: Anti-Annexin V antibody and propidium iodide (Beckton Dickinson).
5. Lymphocyte separation medium (Mediatech, Inc., Manassas, VA).

2.2 Cell Sorting Using Magnetic Beads

1. CD4 and CD8 Magnetic separation kits (Miltenyi Biotec) containing beads coated with antibodies against CD4 or CD8, and CD15, CD16, CD19, CD34, CD36, CD56, CD123, TCRγ/δ, and CD235a (Glycophorin A).
2. CD14 Magnetic separation beads or a monocyte negative selection kit (Miltenyi Biotec).
3. MACS buffer: PBS, 0.5 % BSA, 2 mM EDTA.
4. Magnets and columns (Miltenyi Biotec).

2.3 Cell Culture Assays

1. Culture medium: RPMI 1640 (Gibco), 10 % heat inactivated fetal calf serum (FCS) from Gemini, 2 mM l-Glutamine, 50 mcg/ml of gentamicin (Gibco-BRL, Grand Island, NY).
2. Enzymatic digestion medium: Collagenase type VIII (Sigma Chemical Co), Tris–NOtCl: add 90 ml of 0.16 M NH_4Cl to 10 ml of 0.17 M Tris pH 7.65, and adjust to pH 7.2 with HCl.
3. D1.1 CD40L expressing Jurkat cell line (ATCC).
4. Carboxyfluorescein diacetate succinimidyl ester (CFSE) staining kit, such as CellTrace™ CFSE Cell Proliferation Kit (Invitrogen).
5. 3H-thymidine (3H-TdR) (Perkin Elmer).
6. Cytokines and soluble factors: GMCSF, IL-4, IL-1b, TNF-a, IL-10, IFN-a, and IFN-b (R&D Systems), PGE2 (Sigma Aldrich).

3 Methods

3.1 Induction of Tolerogenic Phenotypes in APC by CD8+ CD28– T Cells from the Peripheral Blood of Transplant Recipients

Carry out all procedures under sterile conditions.

1. Isolate PBMC from 50 ml of anti-coagulated (e.g., heparin, ACD, EDTA) fresh peripheral blood by gradient centrifugation over lymphocyte separation medium (Invitrogen).
   (a) Dilute the blood with 2–4 times volumes of RPMI 1640 medium.
   (b) Layer the diluted blood over 15 ml of lymphocyte separation medium in 50 ml tubes.
   (c) Centrifuge for 30 min at room temperature at 400 × *g* in a swing-bucket rotor without brake.
   (d) Aspirate the upper layer, leaving the interface layer undisturbed.
   (e) Transfer the mononuclear cell layer to a new 50 ml tube.
   (f) Fill the tube with medium and wash by centrifuging at 300 × *g* for 10 min at room temperature. Remove supernatant completely.
   (g) For removal of platelets, resuspend the pellet in medium and centrifuge at 200 × *g* for 10 min at room temperature (Repeat if needed).
   (h) Count the cells using Turks solution and adjust their concentration in RPMI 1640 to 10^7/ml.
2. Isolate CD4+ CD25– and CD8+ CD28– T cells from the recipient's PBMC suspension (prepared as above).

   CD4+ CD25– T cells are obtained by first sorting the CD4+ population using a negative selection CD4+ T cell isolation kit (as described in Notes 4.1), and then depleting the CD4+ CD25+ subset by use of anti-CD25 mAb coupled to MACS beads.

   CD8+ CD28– T cells are obtained by first sorting the CD8+ population using a negative selection CD8+ T cell isolation kit (as described in Notes 4.1), and then depleting the CD8+ CD28+ subset by use of anti-CD28 mAb coupled to MACS beads.

   The purity of sorted CD4+ CD25– and CD8+ CD28– T cells is measured by staining the cells with fluoresceinated anti-CD4 or CD8 mAb and CD28 or CD25-PE (Becton Dickinson) for 15 min at 4 °C followed by washing and analysis on a flow cytometry instrument. The purity should be higher than 95 %.
3. Isolate donor APC by magnetic sorting of monocytes from fresh PBMC or from spleen using MACS anti-CD14 coated magnetic beads (as described in Notes 4.1). Alternatively, in vitro generated myeloid DC can be used (see below).

Magnetic sorting of donor monocytes:

If spleen is used as a source of monocytes, the following preliminary steps are recommended for mobilizing CD14+ cells:

(a) Cut the splenic tissue into pieces in a petri dish containing 5–10 ml medium.

(b) Load the contents into a 50 ml syringe with an 18 gauge needle and homogenize the sample with eight to ten strokes.

(c) Place the homogenate in a sterile petri dish containing enzymatic digestion medium (collagenase VIII at 260 U/ml). Incubate at 37 °C, 5 % CO_2 for 30 min with occasional agitation.

(d) Decant the suspension and stroma through a 30 μm nylon mesh (Becton Dickinson) into a 50 ml polypropylene tube.

(e) Wash the suspension twice by centrifugation for 10 min at $400 \times g$ in culture medium at 4 °C.

(f) Resuspend the cells in culture medium.

(g) Use fresh or cryopreserve for later use. For cryopreservation cells are suspended on ice in 10 % DMSO, 70 % FCS, 20 % RPMI 1640, at 20×10^6/ml and placed in 0.5 ml aliquots in freezing vials. The vials are stored overnight at −80 °C in a methanol containing box and then transferred to liquid nitrogen tanks for permanent storage.

In vitro differentiation of dendritic cells from monocytes:

(a) Magnetically isolated monocytes are cultured in 6-well plates at a concentration of 2×10^6 cells per well for 7 days.

(b) GM-CSF and IL-4 (each at 1,000 U/ml, R&D Systems, Minneapolis, MN) are added on days 0, 2, 4, and 6.

(c) Immature DCs are CD14− CD11c+ HLA-DR+, as shown by flow cytometry analysis.

4. Purified CD8+ CD28− T cells from the recipient's blood are incubated for 24 h with monocytes from the transplant donor or unrelated controls in 24-well plates at 1×10^6 cells/ml in a total volume of 2 ml of culture medium. Parallel cultures contain:

   (a) APC alone.

   (b) APC + D1.1.

   (c) APC + D1.1 + CD8+ CD28− Ts, at a 1:1:1 ratio.

   If immature DC are used as APC, the ratio should be 0.2:1:1.

5. Collect the cells from the cultures and wash two times in FACS buffer at $300 \times g$ for 5 min. Divide the washed cells into three aliquots and stain with CD14-FITC (Fl-1 channel) and CD40

or ILT4 PE-conjugated mAb (Fl-2 channel), and ILT3 or CD86 PC5-conjugated mAbs (Fl-3 channel).

Costimulatory molecules staining:	CD14-FITC	CD40-PE	CD86-PC5.
Inhibitory receptors staining:	CD14-FITC	ILT4-PE	ILT3-PC5.

If immature DC are used as APC, an anti-CD11c FITC mAb should be used in the Fl-1 channel.

6. Controls. Mouse IgG conjugated with the same fluorophores as those used for staining serve as isotype controls for nonspecific binding of test reagents, and as a marker for delineating the positive and negative populations. Viability of the APC under all three culture conditions is tested in a separate tube using CD14-FITC or CD11c-FITC mAb and PI staining (Becton Dickinson) to assess the fact that the CD8+ CD28− putative Ts were not cytotoxic.
7. Acquire the fluorescence data using a flow cytometry instrument and the appropriate acquisition software (i.e., FACScan and Cellquest, BD Biosciences).
8. Data analysis. To establish whether Ts inhibited costimulatory molecules and induced inhibitory receptors, the phenotype acquired by APC is analyzed by gating on the APC specific markers (i.e., CD14 for monocytes or CD11c for DC) for measuring the mean channel of fluorescence (MCF) in FL-2 and FL-3.

   Calculate the percent of change, using the mean channel of fluorescence (MCF), by the formula:

$$\%\text{Change} = ([\text{MCF}_{(\text{APC+D1.1+Ts})} / \text{MCF}_{(\text{APC+D1.1})}] - 1) \times 100$$

   An increase of MCF of ILT3 and ILT4 by more than 100 % accompanied by a decrease of MCF of CD40 and CD86 by more than 50 % is considered indicative of suppression.

3.2 Proliferation Assay

1. Obtain CD4+ CD25− responder T cells by first sorting the CD4+ population using a negative-selection CD4+ T cell isolation kit, and then depleting the CD4+ CD25+ subset by use of anti-CD25 mAb coupled to MACS beads (as indicated in Notes 4.1 and 4.2).
2. Label the CD4+ CD25− responder T cells by incubation with 3 mM CFSE ("CellTrace," Invitrogen) for 10 min in PBS/0.1 % BSA at room temperature. Stop the reaction by addition of ice-cold culture medium containing 10 % FCS for 5 min, followed by three repeat washes at 300 × *g* for 5 min in cold culture medium.

3. Incubate monocytes from the donor or HLA-mismatched control with recipient CD4 T cells alone or together with an equal number of CD8+ CD28− putative Ts sorted from the PBMC of the same recipient. The culture conditions are:
   (a) CD4+ CD25− Th responders, alone.
   (b) CD4+ CD25− Th + allogeneic Monocytes (from the donor or control).
   (c) CD4+ CD25− Th + Monocytes + putative CD8+ CD28− T suppressor cells (autologous to the responder).
4. After 5 days, collect the cultures and analyze on a flow cytometry instrument to determine the proliferation based on the number of cells showing CFSE dye-dilution.
5. Alternatively, to measure proliferation by scintillation counting, incubate triplicate cultures containing 1×10^5 responder CD4 T cells alone or with an equal number of putative CD8+ CD28− T suppressors and monocytes in 96-well U-bottom plates at 37 °C, in a humidified, 5 % CO_2 atmosphere. Label the cultures on day 5 with 1 μCi/ml 3H-thymidine (3H-TdR) for 18 h, harvest and count in a beta scintillation counter to measure 3H-TdR uptake.

3.3 Measurement of the ILT3/ILT4 Inducing Capacity of Recipient Sera

1. Test recipient sera for ILT3/ILT4 inducing factors by incubating 1×10^6 APC (monocytes or dendritic cells) from a healthy blood donor in culture medium (RPMI 1640, l-glutamine, gentamicin) containing 10 % serum from the transplant patient.
2. As a negative control, incubate APC with 10 % serum from the APC donor.
3. As a positive control, incubate APC in 10 % FCS culture medium supplemented with human recombinant IL-10 (hrIL-10) at 100 U/ml or IFN-beta at 20 ng/ml.
4. After 24 h of incubation at 37 °C, in a humidified 5 % CO_2 incubator, stain the cells with mAbs for ILT3 and ILT4. Analyze the ILT3 and ILT4 surface expression by flow cytometry.

As an alternative to flow cytometry testing, RT-PCR can be used to quantify the expression of ILT3 and ILT4.

1. Isolate total RNA from cultured APC using the RNEasy Kit (Qiagen). Detailed instructions are provided in Notes 4.3.
2. Synthesize cDNA using the 1st Strand cDNA Synthesis Kit for RT-PCR (Roche Diagnostics, Basel, Switzerland or equivalent). Detailed instructions are provided in Notes 4.4.
3. Perform quantitative real-time PCR using Taqman gene expression primer/probes (Applied Biosystems, Foster City, CA) specific for ILT3, ILT4, and GAPDH as a "housekeeping gene"

control. Forward and reverse primers contained in different exons should be used to prevent amplification of genomic DNA. Detailed instructions are provided in Notes 4.5.

4. Calculate the relative amount of gene expression according to the formula: $2^{-\Delta\Delta Ct}$, where $\Delta\Delta Ct = [Ct_{(gene)} - Ct_{(GAPDH)}]$ and Ct is the "crossing threshold" value returned by the PCR instrument for every gene amplification.
5. A doubling of the amount of ILT3/ILT4 in APC incubated in the presence of patient serum is considered indicative of the presence of soluble factors inducing tolerogenic APC.

4 Notes

4.1 Magnetic Sorting of CD4, CD8, CD14 Cells by Negative Selection

1. Prepare an MACS buffer consisting of 0.5 % BSA and 2 mM EDTA in PBS and cool it to 4 °C.
2. Resuspend cell pellet to a concentration of 10^7 cells per 40 μl separation buffer (e.g., for 3×10^7 cell, 120 μl of buffer are needed).
3. Add 10 μl of biotin-antibody cocktail per 10^7 cells. For CD8 T cell purification, the cocktail contains biotin conjugated antibodies against CD4, CD14, CD16, CD19, CD36, CD56, CD123, TCRγδ, and Glycophorin A. For CD4 T cell purification, the CD4 antibody in the cocktail is replaced by anti-CD8, and for monocyte purification the CD14 antibody is removed from the cocktail.
4. Mix well and incubate for 10 min at 2–8 °C.
5. Add 30 μl of MACS buffer per 10^7 cells.
6. Add 20 μl of anti-biotin microbeads per 10^7 cells.
7. Mix well and incubate for 15 min in the refrigerator (2–8 °C).
8. Wash cells with 2 ml of buffer per 10^7 cells and centrifuge at $300 \times g$ for 5 min.
9. Aspirate the supernatant completely and resuspend in 500 μl per 10^7 cells.
10. Apply the suspension to an MACS LS column which is prerinsed with 3 ml of MACS buffer and securely placed in a magnet.
11. Allow the suspension to drain through the column and collect unlabeled cells that pass through in a clean 15 ml tube labeled appropriately.
12. Wash column three times with 3 ml of buffer. Add new buffer when the reservoir is empty.
13. Remove column from the magnet and place it in an empty 15 ml tube labeled appropriately.

14. Pipette 5 ml of buffer in to the column and immediately use the plunger to flush out the magnetically labeled cells retained in the column.
15. Count the cells and resuspend them at a concentration of 1×10^6/ml in RPMI 1640 culture medium containing 10 % FCS and antibiotics.

4.2 Depletion of Cell Subsets from Magnetically Sorted T cells

1. To obtain CD8+ CD28− T cells magnetically sorted CD8 T cells are resuspended in MACS buffer at 10^7 per 80 μl.
2. Add 20 μl anti CD28 microbeads.
3. Incubate for 15 min at (2–8 °C).
4. Proceed with magnetic separation as described in Note 4.1 from **steps 8** to **15**.

4.3 RNA Extraction Using the RNEasy Kit (Qiagen)

1. Determine the number of cells. Pellet the number of cells by centrifugation oat 300 × *g*. Carefully remove the supernatant by aspiration.
2. Disrupt the cells using Buffer RLT. Use 350 μl buffer per less than 5×10^6 cells and 600 μl per $5–10 \times 10^6$ cells. Vortex or pipet to mix.
3. Homogenize the lysate using a QIAshredder column. Pipet the lysate directly into a QIAshredder spin column placed in a 2 ml collection tube, and centrifuge for 2 min at full speed.
4. Add 1 volume of 70 % ethanol to the homogenized lysate and mix well by pipetting. Do not centrifuge.
5. Transfer the lysate, to an RNeasy spin column placed in a 2 ml collection tube (supplied by the manufacturer). Close the lid gently and centrifuge for 15 s at 8,000 × *g* (10,000 rpm). Discard the flow-through. Retain the collection tube.
6. Add 700 μl Buffer RW1 to the RNeasy spin column. Close the lid gently and centrifuge for 15 s at 8,000 × *g* (10,000 rpm) to wash the spin column membrane. Discard the flow-through. Retain the collection tube.
7. Add 500 μl Buffer RPE to the RNEasy spin column. Centrifuge for 15 s at 8,000 × *g* (10,000 rpm) to wash the spin column membrane. Discard the flow-through. Retain the collection tube.
8. Add 500 μl Buffer RPE to the RNEasy spin column. Centrifuge for 2 min at 8,000 × *g* (10,000 rpm) to wash the spin column membrane. Discard the flow-through. Retain the collection tube.
9. Place the RNeasy spin column in a new 1.5 ml collection tube (supplied). Add 30–50 μl RNase-free water directly to the spin

column membrane. Close the lid gently and centrifuge for 1 min at 8,000 × *g* (10,000 rpm) to elute the RNA.

4.4 cDNA Preparation

1. Mix the following components in a sterile microcentrifuge tube for each sample to be processed:
   (a) 10× reaction buffer, 2 μl.
   (b) 25 mM $MgCl_2$, 4 μl.
   (c) Deoxynucleotide mix, 2 μl.
   (d) Oligo dT primer, 2 μl.
   (e) RNase inhibitor 1 μl.
   (f) AMV reverse transcriptase, 0.8 μl.
   (g) RNA sample, 1 μl.
   (h) Water, PCR grade, up to 20 μl total volume.
2. Vortex and centrifuge the mixture to collect the sample at the bottom of the tube.
3. Incubate the reaction at 25 °C for 10 min, then at 42 °C for 60 min.
4. Incubate the reaction at 99 °C for 5 min, then cool it to 4 °C for 5 min.

4.5 Real-Time PCR

1. Mix the following components in a 96-well plate compatible with the Applied Biosystems 7300 real-time PCR instrument:
   (a) 25 μl 2× Master Mix reaction buffer (Applied Biosystems).
   (b) 1 μl cDNA.
   (c) 2.5 μl gene specific primers (Taqman primer/probes, Applied Biosystems).
   (d) 21.5 μl Water, PCR grade, up to 50 μl total volume.
2. Spin the plate to ensure the collection of the components at the bottom.
3. Place the plate in the RT PCR instrument and turn it on.
4. Start the 7300 SDS 1.3.1 software (Applied Biosystems) and set up the following temperature cycling:
   (a) 50 °C, 2 min.
   (b) 95 °C, 10 min.
   (c) 95 °C, 15 s.
   (d) 60 °C, 1 min.

   Set **steps c** and **d** to repeat 40 times.
5. Initiate data acquisition.

References

1. Vlad G, Cortesini R, Suciu-Foca N (2005) License to heal: bidirectional interaction of antigen-specific regulatory T cells and tolerogenic APC. J Immunol 174:5907–5914
2. Penna G, Giarratana N, Amuchastegui S et al (2005) Manipulating dendritic cells to induce regulatory T cells. Microbes Infect 7:1033–1039
3. Vlad G, Chang CC, Colovai AI et al (2009) Immunoglobulin-like transcript 3: a crucial regulator of dendritic cell function. Hum Immunol 70:340–344
4. Lanzavecchia A (1998) Immunology. Licence to kill. Nature 393:413–414
5. Ridge JP, Di Rosa F, Matzinger P (1998) A conditioned dendritic cell can be a temporal bridge between a CD4+ T-helper and a T-killer cell. Nature 393:474–478
6. Bennett SR, Carbone FR, Karamalis F et al (1998) Help for cytotoxic-T-cell responses is mediated by CD40 signalling. Nature 393:478–480
7. Schoenberger SP, Toes RE, van der Voort EI et al (1998) T-cell help for cytotoxic T lymphocytes is mediated by CD40-CD40L interactions. Nature 393:480–483
8. Heath WR, Carbone FR (2001) Cross-presentation in viral immunity and self-tolerance. Nat Rev Immunol 1:126–134
9. Chang CC, Liu Z, Vlad G et al (2009) Ig-like transcript 3 regulates expression of proinflammatory cytokines and migration of activated T cells. J Immunol 182:5208–5216
10. Liu Z, Tugulea S, Cortesini R et al (1998) Specific suppression of T helper alloreactivity by allo-MHC class I-restricted CD8+CD28− T cells. Int Immunol 10:775–783
11. Chang CC, Ciubotariu R, Manavalan JS et al (2002) Tolerization of dendritic cells by T(S) cells: the crucial role of inhibitory receptors ILT3 and ILT4. Nat Immunol 3:237–243
12. Manavalan JS, Rossi PC, Vlad G et al (2003) High expression of ILT3 and ILT4 is a general feature of tolerogenic dendritic cells. Transpl Immunol 11:245–258
13. Adorini L, Giarratana N, Penna G (2004) Pharmacological induction of tolerogenic dendritic cells and regulatory T cells. Semin Immunol 16:127–134
14. Adorini L, Penna G (2009) Dendritic cell tolerogenicity: a key mechanism in immunomodulation by vitamin D receptor agonists. Hum Immunol 70:345–352
15. Ciubotariu R, Vasilescu R, Ho E et al (2001) Detection of T suppressor cells in patients with organ allografts. Hum Immunol 62:15–20
16. Manavalan JS, Kim-Schulze S, Scotto L et al (2004) Alloantigen specific CD8+CD28− FOXP3+ T suppressor cells induce ILT3+ ILT4+ tolerogenic endothelial cells, inhibiting alloreactivity. Int Immunol 16:1055–1068
17. Liu J, Liu Z, Witkowski P et al (2004) Rat CD8+ FOXP3+ T suppressor cells mediate tolerance to allogeneic heart transplants, inducing PIR-B in APC and rendering the graft invulnerable to rejection. Transpl Immunol 13:239–247
18. Liu Z, Colovai AI, Tugulea S et al (1996) Indirect recognition of donor HLA-DR peptides in organ allograft rejection. J Clin Invest 98:1150–1157
19. Ciubotariu R, Liu Z, Colovai AI et al (1998) Persistent allopeptide reactivity and epitope spreading in chronic rejection of organ allografts. J Clin Invest 101:398–405
20. Liu Z, Tugulea S, Cortesini R et al (1999) Inhibition of CD40 signaling pathway in antigen presenting cells by T suppressor cells. Hum Immunol 60:568–574
21. Boks MA, Zwaginga JJ, van Ham SM et al (2010) An optimized CFSE-based T-cell suppression assay to evaluate the suppressive capacity of regulatory T-cells induced by human tolerogenic dendritic cells. Scand J Immunol 72:158–168
22. Vieira PL, Kalinski P, Wierenga EA et al (1998) Glucocorticoids inhibit bioactive IL-12p70 production by in vitro-generated human dendritic cells without affecting their T cell stimulatory potential. J Immunol 161:5245–5251
23. Matasic R, Dietz AB, Vuk-Pavlovic S (1999) Dexamethasone inhibits dendritic cell maturation by redirecting differentiation of a subset of cells. J Leukoc Biol 66:909–914
24. Piemonti L, Monti P, Allavena P et al (1999) Glucocorticoids affect human dendritic cell differentiation and maturation. J Immunol 162:6473–6481
25. Woltman AM, de Fijter JW, Kamerling SW et al (2000) The effect of calcineurin inhibitors and corticosteroids on the differentiation of human dendritic cells. Eur J Immunol 30: 1807–1812
26. Mehling A, Grabbe S, Voskort M et al (2000) Mycophenolate mofetil impairs the maturation and function of murine dendritic cells. J Immunol 165:2374–2381
27. Colic M, Stojic-Vukanic Z, Pavlovic B et al (2003) Mycophenolate mofetil inhibits differentiation, maturation and allostimulatory function of human monocyte-derived dendritic cells. Clin Exp Immunol 134:63–69
28. Woltman AM, de Fijter JW, Kamerling SW et al (2001) Rapamycin induces apoptosis in monocyte- and CD34-derived dendritic cells

but not in monocytes and macrophages. Blood 98:174–180
29. Hackstein H, Taner T, Zahorchak AF et al (2003) Rapamycin inhibits IL-4–induced dendritic cell maturation in vitro and dendritic cell mobilization and function in vivo. Blood 101: 4457–4463
30. Matasic R, Dietz AB, Vuk-Pavlovic S (2000) Cyclooxygenase-independent inhibition of dendritic cell maturation by aspirin. Immunology 101:53–60
31. Hackstein H, Morelli AE, Larregina AT et al (2001) Aspirin inhibits in vitro maturation and in vivo immunostimulatory function of murine myeloid dendritic cells. J Immunol 166: 7053–7062
32. Millard AL, Mertes PM, Ittelet D et al (2002) Butyrate affects differentiation, maturation and function of human monocyte-derived dendritic cells and macrophages. Clin Exp Immunol 130:245–255
33. Verhasselt V, Vanden Berghe W, Vanderheyde N et al (1999) N-acetyl-L-cysteine inhibits primary human T cell responses at the dendritic cell level: association with NF-kappaB inhibition. J Immunol 162:2569–2574
34. Cella M, Jarrossay D, Facchetti F et al (1999) Plasmacytoid monocytes migrate to inflamed lymph nodes and produce large amounts of type I interferon. Nat Med 5:919–923
35. Penna G, Sozzani S, Adorini L (2001) Cutting edge: selective usage of chemokine receptors by plasmacytoid dendritic cells. J Immunol 167:1862–1866
36. Gilliet M, Liu YJ (2002) Generation of human CD8 T regulatory cells by CD40 ligand-activated plasmacytoid dendritic cells. J Exp Med 195:695–704

Chapter 24

Discovery and Customized Validation of Antibody Targets by Protein Arrays and Indirect ELISA

Tara K. Sigdel and Minnie M. Sarwal

Abstract

Because of our access to human genome data and ever improving genome sequencing and proteome analysis methods we are much better in terms of our understanding of biological processes. In addition to genomics, proteomics, and other "omics" methods, availability of more sophisticated molecular assaying methods have augmented our knowledge about immune processes towards autogeneic and allogeneic targets. High-density protein arrays are developed to analyze protein–small molecule interactions, enzyme–substrate profiling, protein–protein interaction, and immune monitoring by assessing antibodies in the serum.

Key words Antibodies, ELISA, Protoarray, Proteomics, Transplant, Urine, Biomarkers

1 Introduction

Organ transplantation is the optimal treatment for most end stage organ failure. However, due to lack of a specific and sensitive means to monitor graft injury long-term outcomes are not optimal [1]. Given the current status of organ shortage, advanced methods of organ monitoring and improving graft life expectancy is an unmet need in organ transplantation. Antibodies are known to be involved in acute and chronic rejection of transplanted organs, but their ability to predict graft injury events is poorly understood. Antibody's role in causing graft injury in different injury types has not been studied. Recently, microarray technology has evolved beyond nucleic acids hybridization to serve as a platform for detecting protein-specific antibodies [2]. Protein-array technology that can be used to analyze protein–small molecule interactions for identification of small molecules that have specific affinity to human antigens, enzyme–substrate profiling to identify novel substrates for enzymes, and protein–protein interaction, has also been used to assess antibody level in the blood collected from transplant

Andrea A. Zachary and Mary S. Leffell (eds.), *Transplantation Immunology: Methods and Protocols, Second Edition*, Methods in Molecular Biology, vol. 1034, DOI 10.1007/978-1-62703-493-7_24, © Springer Science+Business Media, LLC 2013

patients to identify reactive antigens activated in different graft injury phenotypes.

We have used the protein array platform to develop an immunogenic and anatomic roadmap of the most likely non-HLA antigens that result in serological responses in kidney transplantation [3]. We have also identified a number of antigens that are associated with kidney transplantation, end stage renal disease, and IgA nephropathy [4–7]. A successful study requires well designed experiments and optimized methods, sophisticated data analysis and subsequent validation of findings made by high-throughput "omic" platform. This chapter provides two independent platforms for identification and validation of antibody levels in human sera. First, we provide a detailed method of identification of increased antibody response against auto/allo antigens by assaying antibodies against ~9,500 human antigens using high-density protein arrays (ProtoArray®, Life technologies, Carlsbad, CA). Then we present protocols for antibody ELISA methods to validate the discovery made by protein arrays. Protein array and MSD ELISA protocol (Meso Scale Discovery, Gaithersburg, MD) include methods that are based on our protocol adopted from corresponding manufacturer's protocols.

2 Materials

2.1 Protein Arrays (ProtoArray®, Life Technologies, Carlsbad, CA)

1. Human serum or plasma sample (dilute the sample 1:150 in washing buffer, store on ice until use).
2. ProtoArray® Human Protein Microarray v5.0.
3. Alexa Fluor® 647 Goat Anti-Human IgG (Life Technologies, Cat. no. A21445).
4. Blocking buffer: either ProtoArray® Blocking Buffer Kit (Life Technologies, Cat. no. PA055) or 10× Synthetic Block (Life Technologies, Cat. no. PA017). *See* Table 1 for preparation using Synthetic Block.
5. Clean, 4-chamber incubation tray with cover (QuadriPERM® Culture Dish. 4-chamber polystyrene culture dish, VWR, San Francisco, CA), chilled on ice Forceps and deionized water Shaker (capable of circular shaking at 50 rpm, set the shaker at 4 °C).
6. Microarray slide holder and centrifuge equipped with a plate holder.
7. Fluorescence microarray scanner (e.g., GenePix 4000B Microarray Scanner or equivalent).
8. Microarray data acquisition software (e.g., GenePix® Pro from Molecular Devices).

Table 1
Recipe to prepare blocking buffer and wash buffer using 10× Synthetic Block

Blocking Buffer (50 mM HEPES, pH 7.5, 200 mM NaCl, 0.08 % Triton® X-100, 25 % Glycerol, 20 mM Reduced glutathione, 1× Synthetic Block, 1 mM DTT) *5 ml buffer required per microarray.*	*Washing Buffer* (1× PBS, 0.1 % Tween 20, 1× Synthetic Block) *60 ml buffer required per microarray.*
1. Prepare 50 ml Blocking Buffer fresh as follows: 1 M HEPES, pH 7.5, 2.5 ml 5 M NaCl, 2 ml 10 % Triton® X-100, 0.4 ml 50 % Glycerol, 25 ml Reduced glutathione, 305 mg 10× Synthetic Block 5 ml Deionized water to 50 ml 2. Adjust pH to 7.5 with NaOH. 3. Mix reagents, chill to 4 °C, and add 50 µl of 1 M DTT prior to use. 4. Use buffer immediately. Store any remaining buffer at 4 °C for <24 h.	1. Prepare 600 ml washing buffer fresh as follows: 10× PBS 60 ml 10 % Tween 20 6 ml 10× Synthetic Block 60 ml Deionized water to 600 ml 2. Mix reagents and cool to 4 °C. 3. Use buffer immediately. Store any remaining buffer at 4 °C for <24 h.

9. Data analysis software (ProtoArray® Prospector recommended, available from www.invitrogen.com/protoarray, Significant Analysis of Microarray (SAM) software [8], GraphPad Prism (GraphPad Software, La Jolla, CA), or equivalent software for basic statistics and visualization and presentation).

2.2 ELISA Assays

Conventional ELISA

1. Coating buffer: 15 mM Na_2CO_3, 30 mM $NaHCO_3$, 0.02 % NaN_3.
2. Nonfat dry milk powder (BioRad, Blotting Grade Blocker Non Fat Dry Milk Cat. no. 170-6404XTU).
3. PBST buffer (1× PBS, 0.05 % tween 20).
4. Primary antibody (positive control) and secondary antibody (anti human IgG AP).
5. AP-PNPP liquid substrate (Sigma, Cat. # 7998).
6. The standard for UV-visible microplate reader absorbance (absorbance detection in the UV-visible wavelength range 190–1,000 nm).

MSD Platform

1. The SECTOR Imager 2400 reader or 6000 reader (Meso Scale Discovery, Gaithersburg, MD).
2. Standard and/or High Bind Plates (Meso Scale Discovery, Gaithersburg, MD).

3. Blocker A (Meso Scale Discovery, Gaithersburg, MD).
4. Read Buffer T (Meso Scale Discovery, Gaithersburg, MD).
5. SULFO-TAG labeled antibody (Meso Scale Discovery, Gaithersburg, MD).

3 Methods

3.1 Serum and Plasma Processing and Sample Preparation

3.1.1 Serum Processing

1. Collect a blood sample in a red top tube with blood using standard venipuncture technique. Let the tube stand in upright position for 20–30 min until clot forms.
2. Centrifuge blood at 800 ×*g* for 10 min and aliquot serum and store at −80 °C until ready to use.

3.1.2 Plasma Processing

1. Collect blood sample into commercially available anticoagulant-treated tubes, e.g., EDTA-treated (lavender tops) or citrate-treated (light blue tops). Heparinized tubes (green tops) are indicated for some applications.
2. Centrifuge tubes for 10 min at 1,000–2,000 ×*g* using a refrigerated centrifuge and aliquot the upper plasma portion and store at −80 °C until ready to use.

3.1.3 Sample Preparation (Serum or Plasma)

1. Prior to use, process the sample to remove any aggregates by centrifugation (12,000 ×*g* for 30 s in a microcentrifuge).
2. Recommended dilution is 1:500 by the manufacturer but in our hands 1:150 dilution in washing buffer works the best. Users may have to optimize dilution based on their initial results.

3.2 ProtoArray

A summary of the probing method is presented in Fig. 1a.

3.2.1 Blocking and Detecting

1. Thaw the protein array slides by placing them at 4 °C for at least 15 min.
2. Place the protein array slides with barcoded side facing up into each well of a 4-chamber tray.
3. Pipet 5 ml blocking buffer (cooled to 4 °C) into each chamber, avoiding any direct pipetting onto the slides.
4. Incubate the slides for 1 h at 4 °C on a shaker set at 50 rpm (circular shaking preferred).
5. After the incubation step, aspirate blocking buffer using vacuum or a pipette.
6. Wash the slides with 5 ml washing buffer by incubating the tray for 5 min at 4 °C on a shaker set at 50 rpm (circular shaking).

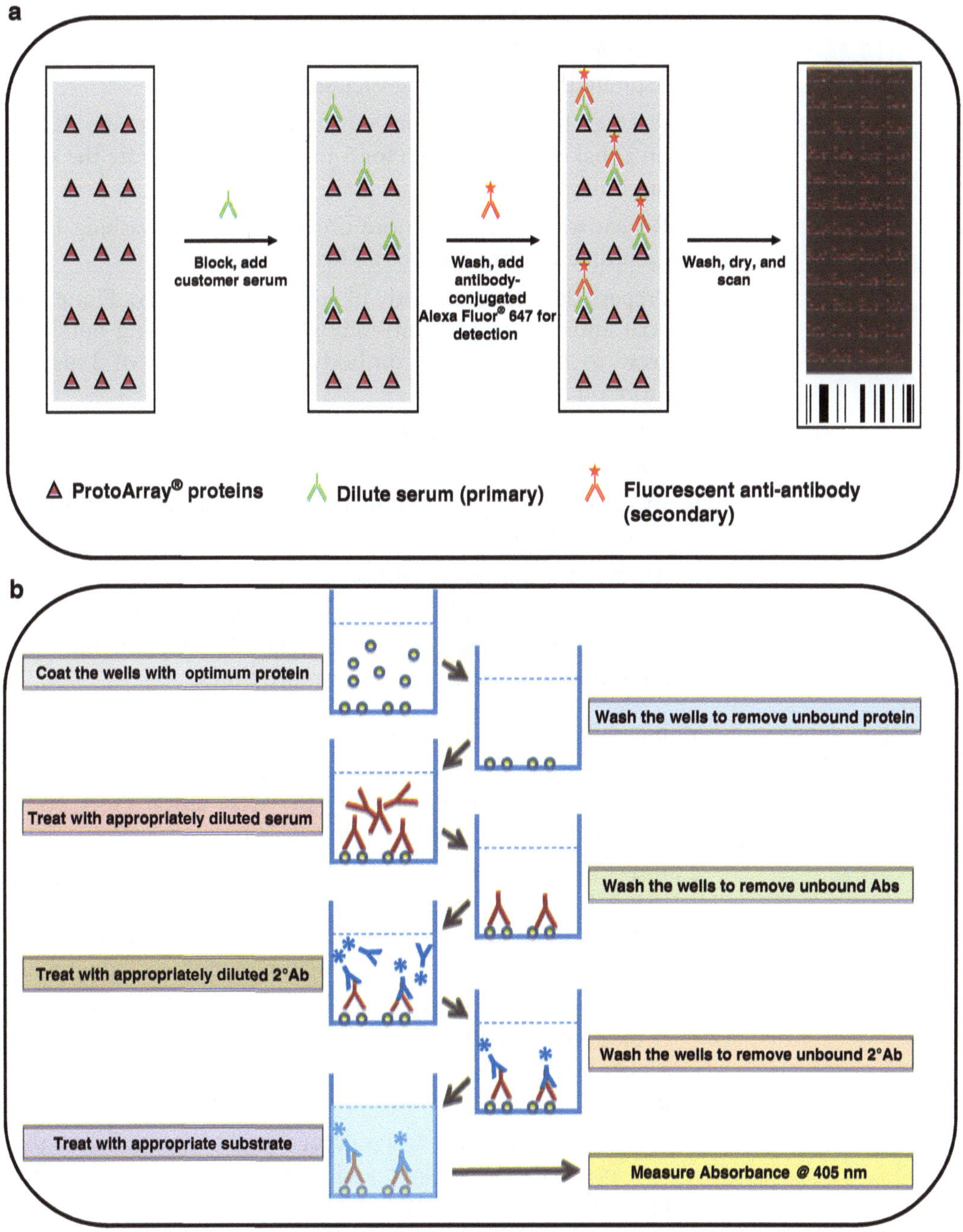

Fig. 1 Overview of ProtoArray methodology. A summary of the probing method is presented in (**a**). The indirect ELISA is shown in (**b**)

7. Aspirate the buffer using vacuum or pipette.
8. Add 5 ml serum or plasma sample diluted (1:150 or 1:500 or project specific optimized dilution) in washing buffer without touching the slide surface.

9. Incubate the tray for 90 min at 4 °C on a shaker set at 50 rpm (circular shaking).
10. Aspirate the sample using vacuum or pipette.
11. Wash each array with 5 ml washing buffer with gentle shaking on a shaker set at 50 rpm for 5 min at 4 °C. Aspirate the washing buffer.
12. Repeat wash step four more times using fresh washing buffer each time to obtain a total of five washes.
13. Prepare detection antibody by mixing 2.5 μl Alexa Fluor® 647 goat anti-human IgG antibody with 5 ml washing buffer per array to obtain a final antibody concentration of 1 μg/ml. Store on ice until use.
14. Add 5 ml Alexa Fluor® 647 antibody solution to the incubation tray.
15. Incubate the tray for 90 min at 4 °C on a shaker set at 50 rpm (circular shaking).
16. Aspirate the antibody solution.
17. Wash each array with 5 ml washing buffer with gentle shaking on a shaker set at 50 rpm for 5 min at 4 °C. Aspirate the washing buffer and repeat wash four more times.

3.2.2 Drying of Slides and Scanning

1. Remove slides from the 4-chamber incubation tray by inserting the tip of the forceps into the indentation at the numbered end of the slides and gently pry the array upward pick up the array by holding the array by its edges only.
2. Insert the array into a slide holder and quickly rinse by dipping the slides into a large beaker filled with deionized water five times. It is important to properly place the slides in the slide holder to prevent damage to the array during centrifugation.
3. Immediately centrifuge the array in the slide holder or 50 ml conical tube at 200 × *g* for 1 min in a centrifuge (equipped with a plate rotor, if you are using the slide holder) at room temperature. Ensure the array is completely dry.
4. After drying, store the arrays vertically or horizontally in a slide box protected from light and avoid prolonged exposure to light. To obtain the best results, scan the array within 24 h of probing.
5. To scan the array, start the appropriate array acquisition and analysis software on the computer connected to the fluorescence microarray scanner (GenePix 4000B Microarray Scanner or equivalent).
6. Follow the instrument manufacturer's protocol to scan the slides with the following setting: Wavelength: 635 nm, Pixel

Size: 10 μm, PMT Gain: 700, Lines to Average: 1.0 Laser Power: 100 %, Focus Position: 0 μm.

7. Save the image to a suitable location as "multi-image TIFF" file.

3.2.3 Data Generation

1. Use GenePix® Pro microarray data acquisition software or equivalent on the computer. Open the saved image (.tiff) and open the .GAL files downloaded from ProtoArray® Central (Life Technologies, Carlsbad, CA).
2. Adjust the subarray grid to ensure the grid is in proper location for each subarray. After the grid is properly adjusted and all features are aligned save .GPS file.
3. Once the gridding is completed acquire the pixel intensity data for each feature by clicking the Analyze button in GenePix® Pro, and save/export the results as a .GPR (GenePix® Results) file.

3.2.4 Data Analysis (Using Prospector Analyzer®, Life Technologies)

1. Install ProtoArray® Prospector (www.invitrogen.com/protoarray).
2. Start ProtoArray® Prospector from the desktop icon. Set the Application to Immune Response Profiling (for serum samples), or Immune Response Profiling with Plasma (for plasma samples).
3. Select the Load and Analyze button from the Tool Bar to normalize single protein arrays by selecting .GPR files with immune response profiling option selected from Application pull down menu.
4. Single array analysis generates a list of human proteins having significant IgG antibodies against them.
5. After single array analysis, group normalize group of array data by grouping the arrays from same sample type (i.e., disease group or control).
6. Once multiple arrays of the same phenotype/class are group normalized perform group comparison analysis. This allows identifying significantly increased antibodies in case of disease or injury.
7. Group normalization provides normalized data for further analysis.
8. Once the result is generated, users can see what antibodies are increased in how many samples per phenotype (% increase) and Chebyshev's Inequality (CI) *P* value.

3.2.5 Data Analysis Using Significant Analysis of Microarrays (SAM)

1. The SAM software is available at http://www-stat.stanford.edu/~tibs/SAM/
2. Normalized protein array data output from Prospector Analyzer (Life Technologies, Carlsbad, CA) can be used.

3. Data should be cube root transferred as the software does not handle a wide range of data such as that from ProtoArray very well.
4. SAM allows performance of a number of analyses such as two class unpaired (control and treatment groups with samples from different patients), two class paired (samples before and after treatment from the same patients), multiclass (more than two groups with each containing different experimental units), time course (each experimental units is measured at more than one time point; experimental units fall into a one or two class design), etc.

3.3 Conventional ELISA Method (A Summary of Indirect ELISA Is Presented in Fig. 1b)

1. Coat the plates by pipetting 50 μl protein/coating buffer mixture onto each well of Nunc-Immuno™ Plates (Thermo Scientific, Cat. no. 449824). Seal the plate with clear sealing film.
2. Store the plates at 4 °C at least overnight.
3. Dump the protein and the coating buffer out of the plates by dabbing it on a pad of absorbant paper stack. Briefly blot on paper to remove excess protein on the surface.
4. Wash the plates five times with PBST (1× PBS, 0.05 % tween 20).
5. To block nonspecific protein binding, coat wells with 100 μl per well 2 % milk in PBST. Allow the plate to incubate at room temperature for at least 1 h.
6. Add primary antibody as a positive control and standard or diluted serum in 2 % dry milk in PBST and incubate at 4 °C overnight or 1 h at room temperature.
7. Wash the plates five times with PBST with 200 μl buffer per well.
8. Without letting the plate go dry add the secondary antibody, Anti-IgG-alkaline phosphatase(AP) diluted 1:1,000 in 2 % milk in PBST.
9. Incubate for 1 h at room temperature and wash the plates five times with PBST.
10. Prepare developing reagent with PNPP tablets using manufacturer's protocol.
11. Add 75 μl of developing reagent per well and incubate the plates for 30 min.
12. Read the plate using a standard UV-visible microplate reader at 405 nm.

3.4 MSD ELISA

Protocol overview of MSD antibody ELISA.

1. Coat Hi Bind microwell plate with target protein diluted in PBS. If it is spot coat, pipet 5 μl of target protein and dry on plate. If it is solution, coat the wells by pipetting 30 μl of target protein per well.
2. Block with 150 μl per well of Blocking solution (either 5 %(w/v) Blocker A or 3 % nonfat dry milk in PBS) 1 h at RT with shaking (300–600 rpm).
3. Wash the plate once with PBS or PBST.
4. Perform a titration for serum dilution optimization by comparing different fold dilutions (1:10, 1:100, 1:500 fold dilution in sample dilution buffer) e.g., 1 % Blocker A in PBS-T, Low Cross Buffer (Candor BioScience).
5. Seal the plate and shake for 1–2 h at RT.
6. Wash the plate three times with PBST.
7. Add 25 μl per well detection antibody+**(diluted in 1 % Blocker A, seal, and shake for 1 h at RT.

   +Concentration of detection antibody, e.g., 0.25 or 1 μg/ml.

   **Source of detection antibody, e.g., using a biotinylated version of the antibody you are using for ELISA in conjunction with an equal concentration of SULFO-TAG streptavidin or use the catalog MSD SULFO-TAG goat anti-human IgG).
8. Wash the plates three times with PBST.
9. Add 150 μl Read BufferT per well and read plate immediately using The SECTOR Imager 2400 reader or 6000 reader (Meso Scale Discovery, Gaithersburg, MD) following manufacturer's manual.

4 Notes

4.1 Protein Arrays

1. If multiple experiments are to be run for a project, it is very critical that all experiment conditions are maintained as consistent as possible. Especially, the incubation time, number and wash techniques and times, shaker speed, sample and antibody dilutions must be maintained consistently.
2. Proper laboratory precautions are critical such as wearing a laboratory coat, disposable gloves, and eye protection.
3. Temperature of the arrays and reagents should be kept at 2–8 °C throughout the experiment.
4. Never touch the surface of the array as it will scratch and damage surface of the array which will contribute to smears and scratches.

5. It is critical to keep the arrays wet all the time during the experiment. Make sure the slides are submerged in the appropriate reagent.
6. A clean dust free experiment location helps to reduce high background signals.
7. Arrays must be dried prior scanning and scanning must be performed immediately after the experiment is completed.
8. Protect the arrays from direct light after probing with the fluorescent detection reagent and before scanning.
9. *Probing other immunoglobulins such as IgA, IgM*: The Protoarry® design favors measurement of IgGs as the platform contains internal control IgGs that can be used for linear normalization. However, measurement of other immunoglobins using this platform is possible. The measurement of other immunoglobin requires, labeling of detection antibodies such as anti-human IgA, anti-human IgM by an Alexa Fluor tag. These antibodies and Alexa Fluor labeling kits are commercially available. Once the detection antibodies are labeled, the experiment described in this protocol are equally applicable to measure other antibodies other than IgG.
10. *Strengths*: ProtoArray enables us to assay antibodies against almost 10,000 human antigens in one single experiment. The method is robust, reproducible and has a potential to provide us with information that otherwise would have taken years by conventional low throughput methods. This sophistication has provided researchers a quick screening of reactive antigens and move on to validation steps which consists fewer number of antigen–antibody pairs.
11. *Issues*: The arrays and reagents involved are expensive. There is no way to determine specificity of antibody–antigen. Even though it includes almost 10,000 antigens it still doesn't provide information on reactivity of other remaining thousands of antigens.

4.2 ELISA

4.2.1 Conventional ELISA Method

1. It is important to determine the appropriate dilution of protein in coating buffer to achieve desired protein concentration.
2. Coated plates can be kept for a prolonged period up to 12 months at 4 °C. However, it is recommended to assess quality of the plate using a positive control.
3. It is important that once plates are coated the plates are never allowed to sit dry for more than a minute or two as this could disrupt binding of protein with the surface at the bottom of the well. If there is a possibility of either of the blocking buffer or the primary antibody remaining on the plates for more than a week, use 0.1 % sodium azide.
4. *Strength*: It is simple to set up and does not require specific equipment. Reagents and scanner are readily available.

5. *Issues*: Since protein arrays use fluorescence detection system, discovery made by protein array is difficult to reproduce using conventional chromophores AP or HRP. Since the detection is not sensitive it requires relatively concentrated sample which contributes to high background.

4.2.2 MSD ELISA Method

1. MSD method is preferred for validation because of its sensitivity to low abundance analytes and its electrochemiluminescence detection system.
2. While coating standard plates, the coating buffer is PBS + 0.03 % Triton X-100. No Triton should be added to the PBS coating buffer for spot coating standard plates or for solution coating high bind or standard plates.
3. The amount of protein to be tested for optimal amount is 10, 40, 160 ng protein per well.
4. *Strength*: Because of its electrochemiluminescence detection system it is sensitive and is compatible with ProtoArray detection system. MSD provides multiplexed ELISA option that enables users to perform ELISA on as many as ten antibodies on a single plate thereby saving time and reagents to be used in the assays.
5. *Issues*: It requires specific reagents compatible with electrochemiluminescence detection system. The scanner for this detection system is expensive and may not be available to many researchers readily.

Acknowledgments

The authors would like to acknowledge NIH (R01 DK083447-01A2, U01 AI063594-06), and California Pacific Medical Center Research Institute San Francisco, CA for funding support.

References

1. Sigdel TK, Lee S, Sarwal MM (2011) Profiling the proteome in renal transplantation. Proteomics Clin Appl 5(5–6):269–280. doi:10.1002/prca.201000117
2. Mattoon D, Michaud G, Merkel J, Schweitzer B (2005) Biomarker discovery using protein microarray technology platforms: antibody-antigen complex profiling. Expert Rev Proteomics 2(6):879–889
3. Li L, Wadia P, Chen R, Kambham N, Naesens M, Sigdel TK et al (2009) Identifying compartment-specific non-HLA targets after renal transplantation by integrating transcriptome and "antibodyome" measures. Proc Natl Acad Sci USA 106(11):4148–4153
4. Li L, Chen A, Chaudhuri A, Kambham N, Sigdel T, Chen R et al (2010) Compartmental localization and clinical relevance of MICA antibodies after renal transplantation. Transplantation 89(3):312–319. doi:10.1097/TP.0b013e3181bbbe4c
5. Li L, Sigdel T, Vitalone M, Lee SH, Sarwal M (2010) Differential immunogenicity and clinical relevance of kidney compartment specific antigens after renal transplantation. J Proteome Res 9(12):6715–6721. doi:10.1021/pr1008674

6. Sigdel TK, Li L, Tran TQ, Khatri P, Naesens M, Sansanwal P et al (2012) Non-HLA antibodies to immunogenic epitopes predict the evolution of chronic renal allograft injury. J Am Soc Nephrol 23:750–763. doi:10.1681/ASN.2011060596
7. Sutherland SM, Li L, Sigdel TK, Wadia PP, Miklos DB, Butte AJ et al (2009) Protein microarrays identify antibodies to protein kinase Czeta that are associated with a greater risk of allograft loss in pediatric renal transplant recipients. Kidney Int 76(12):1277–1283. doi:ki2009384 [pii], 10.1038/ki.2009.384
8. Tusher VG, Tibshirani R, Chu G (2001) Significance analysis of microarrays applied to the ionizing radiation response. Proc Natl Acad Sci USA 98(9):5116–5121

Chapter 25

RNA Purification and Expression Analysis Using Microarrays and RNA Deep Sequencing

Steven R. Head, Tony Mondala, Terri Gelbart, Phillip Ordoukhanian, Rebecca Chappel, Gilberto Hernandez, and Daniel R. Salomon

Abstract

Transcriptome analysis or global gene expression profiling is a powerful tool for discovery as well as understanding biological mechanisms in health and disease. We present in this chapter a description of methods used to isolate mRNA from cells and tissues that has been optimized for preservation of RNA quality using clinical materials and implemented successfully in several large, multicenter studies by the authors. In addition, two methods, gene expression microarrays and RNAseq, are described for mRNA profiling of cells and tissues from clinical or laboratory sources.

Key words RNA Purification, mRNA, Global gene expression profiling, Microarrays, Next generation sequencing, Deep sequencing, RNAseq

1 Introduction

The application of transcriptome analysis, essentially global gene expression profiling, using microarrays as a method for identification of biomarkers as well as revealing insights into biological mechanisms has been well documented [1, 2]. Newer technologies for transcriptome analysis include the use of high throughput or "Next Generation" deep sequencing. A major question at this point is the value and optimal applications for these newer technologies [3]. In this chapter, we will describe protocols for gene expression profiling using microarrays and RNA deep sequencing. We cannot answer the question for the reader about what is the optimal technology for their purposes. The choice really depends on multiple factors at this point including both strategy and costs. However, while neither approach is dramatically superior to the other for straightforward gene expression profiling, we will comment on the relative merits of each.

Andrea A. Zachary and Mary S. Leffell (eds.), *Transplantation Immunology: Methods and Protocols, Second Edition*, Methods in Molecular Biology, vol. 1034, DOI 10.1007/978-1-62703-493-7_25, © Springer Science+Business Media, LLC 2013

Critical to generating useful and reproducible data is the extraction of high quality RNA so this subject is covered in the first section. We describe methods for preserving and extracting high quality RNA from various commonly used sources including tissue samples such as biopsies, cell pellets collected from cultured cells or peripheral blood mononuclear cell preparations. Whole blood RNA, commonly used for clinical studies and biomarker discovery projects, is prepared from blood drawn into specialized vacutainer tubes (PaxGene Blood RNA Tubes, Qiagen) designed specifically for preserving total RNA from all the cells comprising whole blood. The PaxGene Blood RNA preparation protocol described here utilizes the automated Qiacube robotic workstation to facilitate more efficient processing of multiple samples. As a general comment, when properly implemented, automated methods have the specific value of reducing the impacts of human errors and the inevitable variations in data, a common source of batch effects, when multiple technicians are doing individual parts of a complicated experiment.

In the second section of this chapter, we describe the gene expression profiling of high quality RNA preparations using high-throughput microarray technology—specifically the Affymetrix Gene 1.1 ST Array Plates processed on the GeneTitan system. The Affymetrix GeneTitan is a high throughput automated array system that is capable of processing two plates in a single run where each plate is comprised of 16, 48 or 96 arrays. However, the methods described here for RNA labeling are also applicable to the use of the older, single cartridge arrays.

Finally, we describe a protocol for gene expression profiling by deep RNA sequencing. This involves preparation of an RNAseq library from high quality total RNA samples using a specific NuGEN (San Carlos, CA) kit for analysis on the Illumina HiSeq2000 deep sequencing platform. One key advantage of RNAseq relative to microarray technology is that sequencing generates data free from any bias of what may or may not be represented with specific probes on any given commercial microarray. RNAseq can also provide the opportunity to run multiple samples in parallel in a single lane through the use of barcoded libraries—libraries with short sequence tags that identify their original sample source. Thus, we routinely run 6–12 samples per lane on an 8 lane HiSeq2000 flow-cell. At this depth of coverage, we have determined that the results from RNAseq are comparable to the gene expression profiling results obtained with the Affymetrix 1.1 ST Arrays. Nonetheless, these two technologies are in such constant evolution that it is not possible yet to conclude which of these two approaches to expression profiling is the best.

An important point is that we recognize that many readers are not going to be performing the entire workflow from RNA purification to the actual microarrays or RNA deep sequencing. In most instances, the latter stages of the pipeline will be done by trained technicians in specialized Core facilities. However, we strongly believe that investigators need to understand many of the details of the workflow in order to take responsibility for experimental design, effectively communicate with Core facility staff, and ultimately to understand the value and the limitations of the data obtained.

2 Materials

2.1 RNA Purification from Various Samples

2.1.1 RNA Extraction from Cells and Tissue

1. Trizol Reagent (Life Technologies).
2. Battery Operated Hand Homogenizer/Pellet Mixer (VWR).
3. 1.5 ml Pestle RNase and DNase free (Fisherbrand).
4. Chloroform (Sigma).
5. Ethanol 100 % (Sigma).
6. RNase Zap (Life Technologies).

2.1.2 RNA Extraction from Blood PaxGene Tubes

1. PAXgene Blood RNA Tubes (Qiagen).
2. PAXgene Blood miRNA Kit (Qiagen).
3. QIAcube Rotor Adaptors (Qiagen).
4. Isopropanol (Sigma).
5. Ethanol 100 % (Sigma).

2.2 Global Gene Expression Profiling Using Affymetrix DNA Microarrays: Gene 1.1 ST Array Plates

1. Ambion WT Expression Kit (Life Technologies).
2. Affymetrix WT Labeling and Controls Kit (Affymetrix).
3. Affymetrix HT HWS Kit for GeneTitan and WT Array Plates.
4. NuGEN Ovation Pico WTA System V2 (NuGEN).
5. NuGEN Encore Biotin Module (NuGEN).
6. Affymetrix GeneChip Expression Hybridization Controls (Affymetrix).
7. Affymetrix HT HWS Kit for GeneTitan and WT Array Plates.

2.3 Target Hybridization and Processing for Gene 1.1 ST Peg Arrays on the Affymetrix GeneTitan Instrument

1. Gene Titan Hybridization, Wash, and Stain Kit (Affymetrix).
2. Gene Titan 1.1 ST Peg arrays in 16, 24, or 96-array formats (Affymetrix).
3. 96-well PCR plate that can withstand heating to 95 °C (e.g., BioPioneer, GSO2918).
4. 8 or 12 strip caps for PCR plates (e.g., BioPioneer, PCR-SCF-SRCAP).
5. Centrifuge equipped with microtiter plate rotor (e.g., Eppendorf 5810R).

2.4 Global Gene Expression Profiling Using RNA Deep Sequencing (RNAseq) on an Illumina HiSEQ2000

1. Total RNA sample.
2. NuGen Encore® Complete RNA-Seq DR kit—provides all reagents, enzymes, buffers, barcoded adapters, and beads for library prep (NuGEN, Santa Carlos, CA, USA).
   (a) Multiplex barcode system 1–8 (PN 0333-32).
   (b) Multiplex barcode system 9–16 (PN0334-32).
3. Covaris S2 sonication system (Covaris, Woburn, MA, USA).
4. Covaris microTUBE (Covaris, Woburn, MA, USA).
5. 0.2 ml PCR tubes (Corning Thermowell®, Tewksbury, MA).
6. Ethanol for bead purifications (Pharmco-AAPER, Brookfield, CT).
7. Magnetic separation stand (Invitrogen™, Life Technologies, Carlsbad, CA).
8. Qubit® Fluorometer 2.0 (Invitrogen™, Life Technologies, Carlsbad, CA).
9. Agilent 2100 Bioanalyzer (Agilent Technologies, Santa Clara, CA, USA).
10. E-Gel® with SYBR Safe™ precast gel (Invitrogen™, Life Technologies, Carlsbad, CA, USA).
11. TrackIt™ 100 bp DNA Ladder (Invitrogen™, Life Technologies, Carlsbad, CA, USA).
12. Scalpel for gel excision.
13. Zymoclean™ Gel DNA Recovery Kit (Zymo Research, Irvine, CA, USA).
14. Illumina SR or PE Cluster Kit (Illumina, Inc., San Diego, CA, USA).
15. Illumina Cbot.
16. Illumina HiSeq 2000.

3 Methods

3.1 RNA Extraction from Cells and Tissues

RNA purified from cultured cells, cells isolated by flow cytometry, as well as peripheral blood mononuclear cells obtained from Becton Dickinson Vacutainer Cell Preparation Tubes (CPT) are performed using the Trizol hybrid protocol. This hybrid protocol allows the purification of total RNA, comprised of both mRNAs as well as small RNAs (e.g., microRNAs). The latter are important to researchers interested in the expression and functional roles of regulatory, noncoding small RNA. This protocol can also be used to isolate RNA from tissues preserved in the commercial preparation, RNAlater (available from both Qiagen and Ambion/ Life Technologies). The extraction of total RNA including small

RNA from whole blood stabilized in Qiagen RNA Blood PAXgene tubes is performed using the Qiagen miRNA Blood Extraction Kit. This is an automated protocol available on the QIAcube, a robotic workstation. We also recommend that users have access to an Agilent BioAnalyzer or equivalent instrument in order to determine RNA quality and estimate fragmentation after purification protocols.

3.1.1 Trizol Hybrid Protocol

1. Homogenize tissue samples (up to 100 mg) in 0.2 ml of Trizol reagent with battery operated hand homogenizer (VWR Pellet Mixer Cat # 47747-370 and Fisherbrand 1.5 ml Pestle RNase and DNase free Cat #V7339-901). Then bring to 1 ml with Trizol. Aspirate through 21g syringe several times. Incubate for 5 min at room temperature (*see* **Note 1**).
2. Add 200 μl of Chloroform. Shake vigorously for 15 s and incubate at room temperature for 3 min.
3. Centrifuge at 12,000 × *g* for 15 min at 4–8 °C.
4. Transfer the top aqueous phase to fresh tube and save remaining sample for DNA and/or protein extraction (*see* **Note 2**).
5. For small RNA inclusion slowly add 1.4 volumes of 100 % RNase-free EtOH instead of equal volume. Need at least 60 % EtOH, mixing as needed.
6. Load the sample (up to 700 μl) into an RNeasy column seated in a collection tube and spin for 30 s at 8,000 × *g*. Discard flow-through (*see* **Note 3**).
7. For small RNA inclusion add 700 μl of RPE Buffer onto the column and spin 30 s at 8,000 × *g*. DO NOT USE RW1 use only RPE. Make sure that ethanol has been added to the RPE buffer. Discard flow-through.
8. Transfer column into a new collection tube, add 500 μl buffer RPE and spin for 30 s at 8,000 × *g*. Discard flow-through. Make sure that ethanol has been added to the RPE buffer before use.
9. Add 500 μl buffer RPE and spin 2 min at 8,000 × *g*. Discard flow-through.
10. Spin the column for 1 min at 8,000 × *g* to get rid of remaining buffer in the column.
11. Transfer the column to a new 1.5 ml collection tube and pipet 30–50 μl of RNase-free water directly onto the column membrane. Allow the sample to sit at room temperature for 1–2 min and then spin 1 min at 8,000 × *g* to elute RNA. Quantitate on a NanoDrop spectrophotometer and check the quality on an Agilent Bioanalyzer.
12. Store RNA at −80 °C until use.

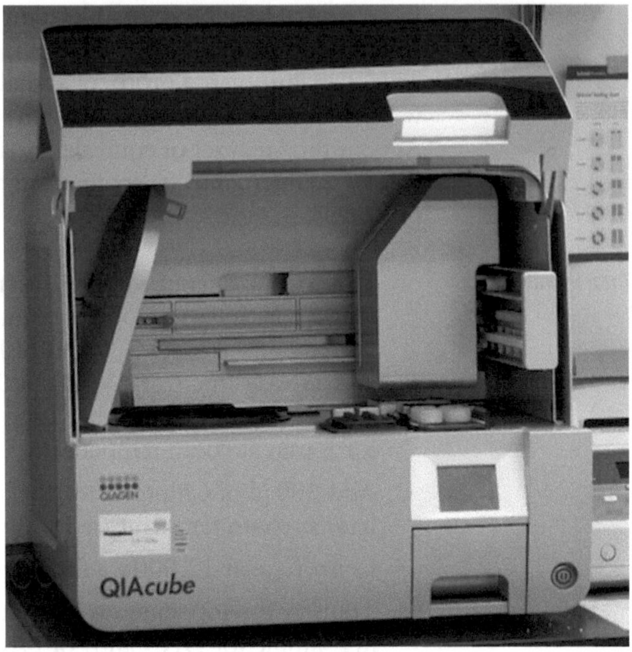

Fig. 1 The QIAcube, a robotic workstation from Qiagen

3.1.2 RNA Extraction from Blood PaxGene Tubes Using the QiaCube Robot (Fig. 1)

The PAXgene Blood RNA tubes collect 2.5 ml of whole blood into a sterile vacutainer tube containing a proprietary additive that near instantly stabilizes the in vivo gene transcription profile by blocking RNA degradation while preventing the cellular gene induction that otherwise occurs *ex vivo* following blood drawing. Blood samples collected in PAXgene tubes can be stored at room temperature for 72 h, at 2–8 °C for up to 5 days, or at −20 or −80 °C for at least 50 months without significant RNA degradation. After blood collection the PAXgene tube should be well mixed and incubated at room temperature for 2 h with occasional mixing to ensure that all the cells lyse.

Samples are processed using the Qiagen PAXgene miRNA kit that preserves both mRNA and miRNA after purification. Several manual steps are involved prior to placing the samples on the robot including centrifuging, washing and resuspending the nucleic acid pellet (**steps 1–6** below). Batches of 12 samples can be run in less than 3 h. Typical total RNA yield from healthy human whole blood is 3–7 μg (*see* **Note 4**).

1. Thaw the PAXgene tubes if frozen. The thawed tubes should then be mixed and stored at room temperature for 2 h with occasional mixing by gentle inversion or using a motorized rotator at the lowest speed.
2. Centrifuge the mixed PAXgene tubes for 10 min at 3,000–5,000 × *g* using a swinging bucket rotor.

3. Remove the supernatant by decanting. Add 4 ml RNase-free water to the pellet and close the tube with a clean cap.
4. Vortex until the pellet is dissolved and centrifuged for 15 min at 3,000–5,000 × *g*. Our centrifuge is limited to a maximum of 3,500 × *g*. Remove the supernatant completely and let the tube drain to remove all traces of liquid.
5. Add 350 μl of BM1 Buffer reagent. Vortex until the pellet is dissolved.
6. Pipet the sample into a 2 ml processing tube and load onto the QIAcube shaker.
7. The QIAcube is loaded with the remaining buffers, Proteinase K, DNase I, and Buffer BR5 for elution.
8. The QIA cube rotor adaptor is loaded with a PAXgene RNA spin column, PAXgene Shredder spin column, and a microfuge sample tube in the designated positions.
9. The PAXgene miRNA protocol A is begun. When Protocol A is complete the microfuge tube containing the eluted RNA is transferred to the heating block in the QIAcube and a short 10 min Protocol B is run to heat the sample for 5 min at 65 °C to denature the RNA for downstream reactions.
10. The RNA is then quantified on a NanoDrop spectrophotometer and the quality is assessed on an Agilent Bioanalyzer (Fig. 2).

Additional Considerations for RNA Purification

The current trend in profiling clinical samples for global gene expression analysis is to isolate total RNA including small or microRNAs. The co-isolation of protein as well as DNA and RNA from cells and tissues can also be done by including additional steps into the Trizol hybrid method [4]. These combination protocols were designed to take maximal advantage of precious clinical samples. They also represent the increasing and strategic use of multiple orthogonal technologies to advance a research objective (e.g., gene profiling and proteomics).

We exclusively use RNAlater for the preservation of RNA in tissue samples. One important consideration is that it takes some time for the RNAlater to permeate a tissue section or biopsy core to work optimally. Thus, it is important to consider the manufacturers guidelines for tissue size and volumes of RNAlater. Also, to insure the preservation of tissue RNA, we routinely leave a sample in RNAlater for at least 30 min at room temperature before freezing though it can sit overnight and be absolutely fine. In situations where we are sorting cells by flow cytometry or separating by magnetic beads and when using non-adherent cell lines, we go directly into Trizol instead. The disadvantage of Trizol is mainly the fact that it is a hazardous material and, while not an issue in a single laboratory setting, it can be a serious challenge in a multicenter clinical study where shipping samples for archiving and analysis is necessary.

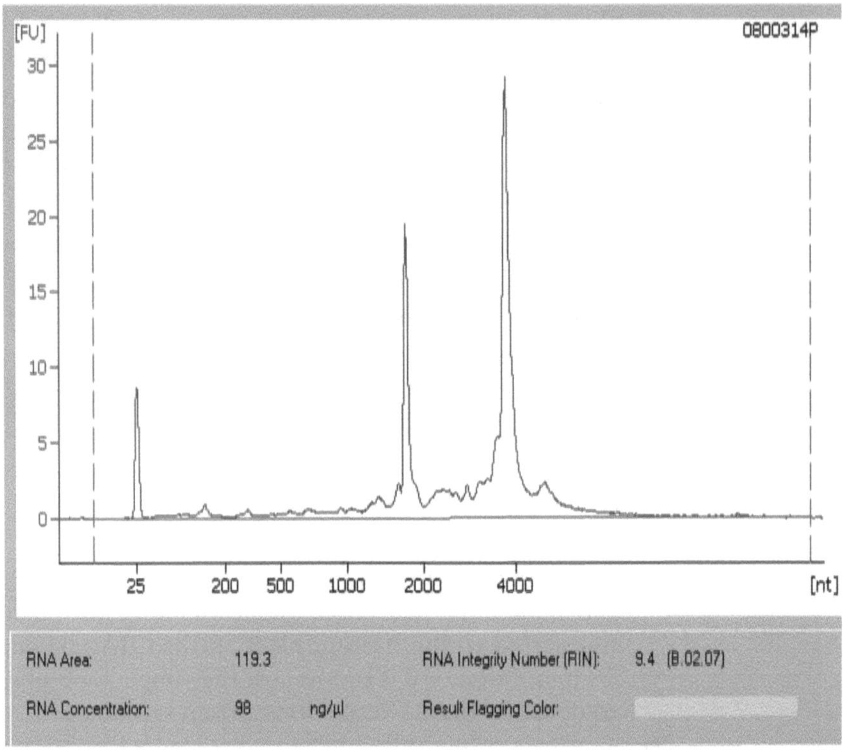

Fig. 2 BioAnalyzer (Agilent) trace of high quality RNA sample. *X*-axis shows size in bases (*nt* nucleotides), *Y*-axis shows relative fluorescent units. The peak at approximately 25 nt is a size marker. The larger peaks near 1,700 and 4,000 nt show the two major ribosomal RNA transcripts

Whole blood samples present a unique challenge to mRNA expression due to the huge number of red blood cells containing hemoglobin-related transcripts in proportion to the relatively small number of other circulating, nucleated cells. The concern has been that these globin transcripts reduce the sensitivity and signals of the other RNA transcripts that are the target for most gene expression profiling experiments. The good news is that we have demonstrated in our laboratory that globin reduction does not give additional benefits in terms of signal intensities or the sensitivity of differential gene expression when using the Affymetrix 1.1 ST peg arrays in combination with the current generation of labeling kits (unpublished data: http://www.genetics.ucla.edu/transplant-genomics/protocols/). Considering the added cost, time, effort and additional loss of RNA during the globin reduction steps, we don't recommend this procedure.

The next question is whether globin reduction is currently required for gene expression profiling by RNAseq experiments. One recent paper suggested there was a value in globin reduction resulting in increased sensitivity [5]. We are currently in the process of testing this in our laboratory and the results will be posted at our Web site when available (see URL above).

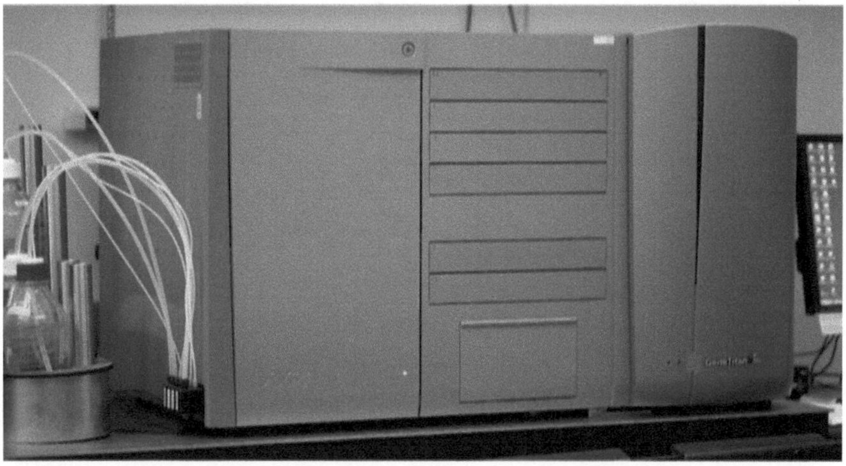

Fig. 3 The GeneTitan system (Affymetrix) used to hybridize, wash, stain and scan labeled samples to Affymetrix 1.1 ST array plates in 16, 24, and 96 Peg array formats

3.2 Global Gene Expression Profiling Using Affymetrix DNA Microarrays: Gene 1.1 ST Array Plates

Gene expression profiling on the Affymetrix GeneTitan system requires that high quality total RNA samples be prepared for hybridization to the expression arrays (Fig. 3). This involves following either one of the target preparation protocols described below (the Ambion WT Expression kit with the Affymetrix GeneChip WT Terminal Labeling Kit or the NuGEN Ovation Pico WTA V2 System with Biotin Module). We generally use the Ambion WT Expression kit when we have adequate amounts of total RNA. As little as 50 ng of starting material can be used. When only limited amounts of total RNA are available, we use the NuGEN Ovation Pico WTA V2 system with Biotin Module. We have used this protocol successfully with as little as 0.5 ng total RNA.

Finally, once the target RNA has been prepared and labeled, it is ready to hybridize to Affymetrix 1.1 ST array plates available in 16, 24, and 96 peg formats.

3.2.1 Ambion WT Expression Kit

The WT Expression Kit is designed to generate amplified sense-strand cDNA ready for fragmentation and labeling using the Affymetrix GeneChip WT Terminal Labeling Kit. The labeled product is generated in about 3 days at which point it is for ready for hybridization to the Affymetrix GeneChip ST (Sense Target) Arrays. The starting requirement is 50–500 ng of total RNA. For example, some sources suggest a yield of 10 pg total RNA/cell; thus, approximately 5,000–50,000 cells would be required using this protocol for global expression profiling. In our experience a more reasonable expectation for yield is 1–5 pg per cell. The key is to determine this yield experimentally for your chosen cell and protocol.

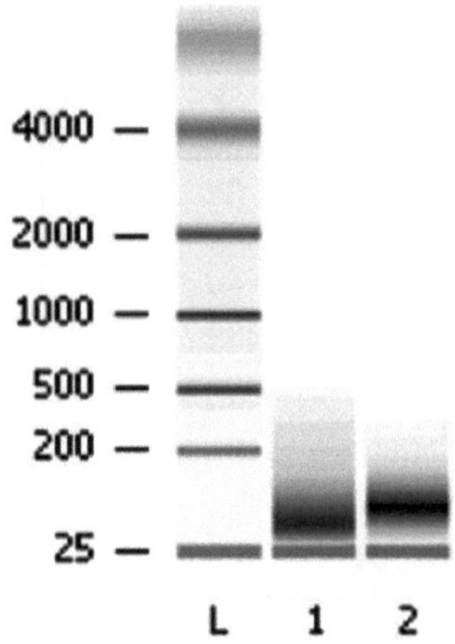

Fig. 4 BioAnalyzer trace showing the fragmented samples, before (*lane 1*) and after labeling (*lane 2*). A sizing ladder is also shown (*lane L*). The fragmentation results in a band with the size of 40–70 nucleotides (i.e., bases; nt) and the subsequent fragmented and labeled cDNA shows a slight shift to a larger size due to attachment of the labels

The WT Expression Kit uses a reverse transcription priming method that specifically primes non-ribosomal RNA from your sample. This is important because otherwise ribosomal RNA is so abundant in all cells that it would interfere with detection of mRNAs in the sample. The cDNA is then in vitro transcribed (IVT) to amplify the target and finally the RNA generated in the IVT reaction is copied back into cDNA with dUTP incorporated for the downstream fragmentation step described below (*see* **Note 5**).

3.2.2 Fragmentation and Labeling of the cDNA generated from the WT Expression Kit

In the next step of the process, the Affymetrix WT Labeling and Controls Kit (Affymetrix) is used to fragment and label the cDNA generated from the Ambion WT Expression Kit. Fragmentation is accomplished through treatment of the cDNA with *uracil-DNA Glycosylase* (UDG) and apurinic/apyrimidinic endonuclease (APE), which effectively cleave the cDNA wherever a uracil was incorporated during cDNA synthesis. After fragmentation, the cDNA fragments are labeled using terminal deoxynucleotidyl transferase (TdT) to incorporate a biotin label onto the 3′ ends. At each step 1 μl of the sample should be saved so that the fragmentation and labeling steps can be checked on the Bioanalyzer (*see* Fig. 4). The fragmented sample, before and after labeling, should be run side by side for comparison. The fragmentation should result in a band with the size of 40–70 nucleotides and the subsequent fragmented and labeled cDNA should show a slight shift to a larger size due to attachment of the labels. The amount of fragmented and labeled cDNA needed for each Affymetrix ST Peg array is 2.8 μg (*see* **Note 6**).

3.2.3 NuGEN Ovation Pico WTA System V2

As an alternative to the protocol described above for preparation of total RNA samples for hybridization to Affymetrix gene expression arrays, the NuGEN Ovation Pico WTA V2 System can be used to prepare labeled cDNA from a range of 0.5–50 ng of total RNA input. The NuGEN Encore Biotin Module is used to fragment and label the target in a manner analogous to the Affymetrix WT Labeling protocol described above in Subheading 3.2.2. The labeled product is ready for hybridization to microarrays in about 2 days.

The primer mix contains a unique mixture of random and oligo dT primers such that priming occurs across the whole transcript. The NuGEN kits use a linear amplification Ribo-SPIA technology based on SPIA (Single Primer Isothermal Amplification) for amplification. This method uses DNA/RNA chimeric primers (SPIA primers), DNA polymerase and RNase H in an isothermal assay. Since many NuGEN protocols for RNA amplification use their universal SPIA primers it is important to note that there is a potential for the generation of nonspecific amplification products from carry-over (contamination) of previously amplified SPIA cDNA. Thus, care must be taken to avoid this pitfall if the laboratory chooses to adopt this approach. Precautions similar to those used to prevent PCR contamination are absolutely required (see **Note 7**).

3.2.4 Target Hybridization and Processing for Gene 1.1 ST Peg Arrays on the Affymetrix GeneTitan Instrument

Preparation of Hybridization Cocktail (*see* **Note 8**).

1. Prepare master mix consisting of the components of the GeneTitan Hybridization kit following kit instructions for the number of samples being hybridized.
2. Add 39.2 μl master mix to the wells of a 96-well plate followed by addition of 2.8 μg of the fragmented and labeled cDNA in 32.8 μl volume from each sample. Bring volume in each well to 120 μl by addition of 48 μl of the *2.5X WT Hyb Add 6* reagent that comes in the GeneTitan Hybridization kit.
3. Seal 96-well plate with strip caps and vortex briefly to mix. Briefly centrifuge plate to bring liquid to bottom of wells.
4. Heat the sealed 96-well plate to 95 °C for 5 min and then 45 °C for 5 min and centrifuge at high speed for 1 min.
5. Transfer 90 μl of each sample into each well of the hybridization plate included in the Hybridization kit.

3.2.5 Preparation of GeneTitan Instrument

The GeneTitan integrates hybridization, washing, and imaging in a single instrument. It supports many types of Peg arrays including 3′ expression arrays, whole transcript arrays, SNP genetics arrays and genome-wide screening arrays. In addition, there are three formats of Peg plates comprised of 16, 24 or 96-arrays per plate. We will limit our current discussion to global gene expression profiling using the Whole Transcript 1.1 ST Peg arrays.

The instrument is initialized, which turns on the hybridization oven, prepares the fluidics for staining and washing and subsequently prepares the laser for scanning. Plate and sample identification files are uploaded to the instrument's computer system. Trays and lids are treated with an anti-static gun. Three stain trays are prepared with 105 µl of stain in each well and a scan tray is filled with 150 µl per well of an array holding buffer. The three stain plates, scan plate, hybridization plate, and the peg array plate are loaded into the GeneTitan instrument as prompted by the running computer program. The sample will now automatically be incubated at 48 °C for 17 h, then stained and washed and scanned. The initial hybridization cocktail preparation and loading of the plates into the Titan takes about an hour and then the entire time for hybridization, staining, and scanning is 20 h for a 16 or 24 Peg array plate and 24 h for a 96 Peg array plate. A second Peg array plate can be loaded once the first Peg array has begun the process. A delay in starting the process for the second Peg plate is necessary since each array should be scanned immediately after the stain and wash step is completed and there is only one scanning station. The delay is 5 h if the first plate is a 96 Peg array and the delay is 2½ h if the run is started with 16 or 24 Peg arrays.

Additional Considerations for Global Gene Expression Profiling Using Affymetrix DNA Microarrays

While a comprehensive discussion of experimental design for microarray (and RNAseq) experiments is beyond the scope of this book chapter, a few important principles should be noted. The principles of a good experimental design will apply to any microarray experiment whether using the Affymetrix arrays described here or alternative array technologies from companies such as Illumina and Agilent.

Good experimental design dictates the use of adequate sample sizes for statistical analysis and statistical power. We have found in practice with real clinical samples that a minimum of 20 samples per group in a study is necessary for statistical power. That does not mean that a trial or discovery run cannot be done with as few as five samples per group but care should be taken in not over-interpreting the significance of any specific result obtained unless these are validated using another technology (e.g., quantitative PCR or proteomics) or multiple replications of the same experiment are done with many more samples.

Another important consideration is proper organization of samples and controls for processing to mitigate batch effects while effectively addressing the biological questions of interest. The entire process from RNA isolation to labeling to hybridization to the actual printing of the plate by the manufacturer can contribute different kinds of technical noise. This noise creates bias in the data that is not reflecting the biology that is being studied. This kind of data bias or batch effects can result from many different choices made in the process. For examples, when all the controls are done on one plate and all the experimental samples on another. Even if all samples are done on a single plate but they are prepared and labeled for hybridization on different days or by different technicians or even different kit lots, batch effects will result. It is critical for the investigator to plan out the entire organization of processing all the experimental samples before starting. However, a key point is that even given all this care, the nature of these highly complex technologies is that they generate some batch effects and these must be effectively compensated for during the statistical analysis of the data later.

A number of new protocols are being developed to allow successful profiling of samples obtained from biopsies that have already been fixed and embedded. These allow access to large archives of samples that are clinically invaluable such as tumor biopsies and autopsy specimens and this is especially important for profiling rare samples. However, the analysis of formalin fixed paraffin embedded (FFPE) samples or other samples with degraded RNA presents unique challenges and requires alternative approaches to preparing the RNA for hybridization to microarrays and will not be discussed here.

Finally, the analysis of microarray data is complex and the reader is advised to involve an experienced statistician/bioinformatics expert for this task. Standardized analysis methods are frequently used for identification of differentially expressed genes, determination of *p*-values and false discovery rates as well as clustering, generation of heat maps and running class prediction algorithms.

3.3 Global Gene Expression Profiling Using RNA Deep Sequencing (RNAseq) on an Illumina HISEQ2000

The rapid evolution of high-throughput deep sequencing technology has created new opportunities to do global gene expression profiling using RNAseq. A number of issues must be considered by investigators before deciding on whether to do any given experimental study using this new approach. The isolation and required amounts of total RNA is roughly the same for both microarrays and deep sequencing. However, as can be clearly seen when the previous section is reviewed, the workflows are very different. Microarrays take total RNA, label the mRNA transcripts, hybridize them to arrays of printed probes and then detect the amount of fluorescent signal excited by a laser scan to reveal the level of gene expression in the pool of RNA. Deep RNA sequencing starts with creating a tagged library of all the mRNA transcripts in the RNA pool.

The preparation of the sequencing library adds two key elements. The first is a set of adaptors on each end of the double stranded cDNA created that is required for binding to complementary oligonucleotides attached to the surface of the sequencing flow cell. Binding to these oligonucleotides positions each transcript in the library in the correct orientation for sequencing.

The second element added is the unique barcodes. These are short DNA sequences that uniquely identify the sample and are subsequently decoded in the statistical analysis of the sequencing data. The use of barcodes enables the sequencing of multiple samples in a single lane on the flow cell and that ability to multiplex has made RNAseq a cost-effective alternative to microarrays. Nonetheless, the workflow for RNAseq is more complicated, operating the technology platforms is considerably more demanding and the initial stages of data analysis are more computationally intensive. Another key point is that gene expression data obtained by deep RNA sequencing compared to the latest generation of microarrays reveals that both are highly correlated and valuable. Thus, there is no reason for an a priori decision to choose RNAseq over microarrays.

Though beyond the scope of the present chapter, RNAseq can go far beyond just gene expression profiling. Using long paired-end reads a novel transcriptome can be studied and this is now driving new research into viral, bacterial and fungal microbiomes. Paired-end reads can also be used to align intron-exon boundaries to reveal alternative splicing, a major source of transcriptional and proteomic diversity in eukaryotic biological systems. Because RNAseq provides the actual sequences of the mRNA transcripts, there is a potential to discover genetic mutations (e.g., single nucleotide polymorphisms) in transcribed regions. Finally, we believe that the quality of the data and the economics of doing miRNA profiling by miRNAseq using high levels of barcode multiplexing is now the best approach.

The RNAseq library is generated using the NuGen Encore Complete DR kit following their recommended protocol (URL: www.nugeninc.com/nugen/).

1. After initial QC of RNA by Bioanalyzer tracing, 100–150 ng of total RNA is taken into the Encore Complete prep.
2. First strand cDNA is generated from the total RNA using the provided first strand primer, buffer, and enzyme mix in the Encore Complete kit. The first strand primer is annealed at 65 °C for 5 min. The enzyme and buffers are added to the sample and incubated at 40 °C for 30 min.
3. Immediately following, second strand cDNA is generated using the provided second strand buffer and enzyme mix. The reaction is held at 16 °C for 60 min. A stop solution from the kit is added to stop the enzymatic reaction.
4. The now double stranded cDNA is fragmented using an S2 Covaris to a median size of 200 bp.
5. The fragmented cDNA is purified using 1.8 volumes of Agencourt RNAClean XP beads and a 70 % ethanol bead wash solution.

6. End repair buffer and enzyme mix from the kit are added to the sample and incubated at 25 °C for 30 min and then 70 °C for 10 min. This step creates blunt ends of the cDNA allowing for efficient ligation of adapters.
7. Barcoded adapters are ligated to the cDNA using 1 of the 16 barcoded adapters provided in the kit along with the ligation buffer and enzyme mix. The reaction is held at 25 °C for 30 min.
8. After ligation, two strand selection steps are completed to end up with only one cDNA strand with adapters. The first step is completed with strand selection I enzyme mix and buffer provided in the kit. The reaction is held at 72 °C for 10 min.
9. The sample is then purified using 1.8 volumes of Agencourt RNAClean XP beads and a 70 % ethanol bead wash solution.
10. The second strand selection step is completed with strand selection II enzyme mix and buffer provided in the kit. The reaction is held at 37 °C for 30 min and then 95 °C for 30 s.
11. The library is amplified using the DR primer mix, DMSO, buffer and enzyme mix provided in the kit. 20 total cycles; 5 with an annealing temperature of 55 °C and 15 with an annealing temperature of 63 °C are completed.
12. A final bead purification of the amplified library is completed using 1.2 volumes of Agencourt RNAClean XP beads and a 70 % ethanol bead wash solution.
13. The library is run on an Agilent 2100 Bioanalyzer DNA 1000 chip (Fig. 5). The final product has a size range of 200–400 bp with characteristic peaks around 285 bp. The spectra are used to validate the library as well as determine the presence or absence of adapter dimer. The dimer has a size of around 130 bp.
14. Qubit fluorometer is used to measure the concentration of the final library.
15. For multiplex sequencing, Qubit concentrations are used to equally pool the libraries. Each pool is gel purified and size selection is used to obtain the desired insert size for sequencing. Paired-end 2 × 100 sequencing, for example, would require an insert size of >200 bp. Material would be cut from the gel between 330 and 430 bp to obtain insert sizes of 200–300 bp including 130 bp of adapter.
16. Using 2 % Invitrogen precast gels, the samples are loaded into 2–3 lanes alongside a 100 bp DNA Track-It ladder.
17. The gel is ran for 20 min and viewed under a transilluminator. Using a scalpel, the section of gel is selected between 330 and 430 bp for a 200 bp insert (Fig. 6).

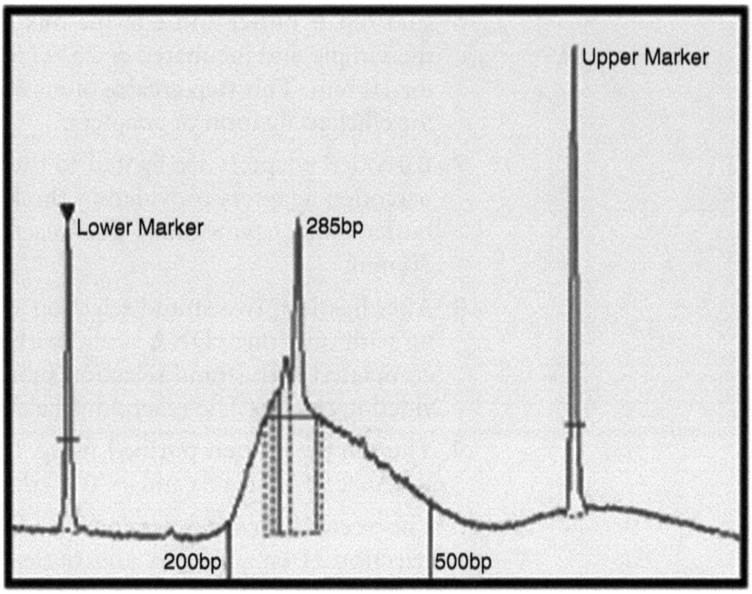

Fig. 5 Bioanalyzer trace of a successfully completed Nugen Encore Complete DR RNAseq library

18. The gel slice after excision is dissolved using Zymo ADB buffer and purified using a Zymo (25 μg) column and eluted in water.
19. A final QC of the library is done using the Bioanalyzer and quantified using the Qubit fluorometer.
20. The libraries for each lane are placed into the cBot (Fig. 7a) that loads the flow cell and begins the process of clustering required to initiate the sequencing protocol.
21. The clustered flow cell is then loaded onto the Illumina HiSeq 2000 for sequencing (Fig. 7b).

3.3.1 Additional Considerations for Global Gene Expression Profiling Using RNA Deep Sequencing (RNAseq)

One important question for any new technology is what metrics can be used to judge the quality of an RNA deep sequencing run. The Illumina HiSeq system provides real-time information on read quality as it is being generated and these will be monitored by the technical staff in the Core facility. When the data is delivered to investigators the important metrics to review include pass filter rate (ideally above 85 %), total number of reads per lane (ideally 150–200 million per lane) and alignment to the genome (can vary with preparation but should be 70–80 % using the protocol described here). However, it is worth noting that if a project involves less standard protocols or sample sources then the expectations for results must be adjusted. For example, we do a challenging protocol called RIPseq that first involves the immunoprecipitation of RNA-binding proteins bound to mRNA transcripts and then deep RNA sequencing of the target mRNAs and the extremely low yields of mRNA presents challenges at multiple points in the workflow.

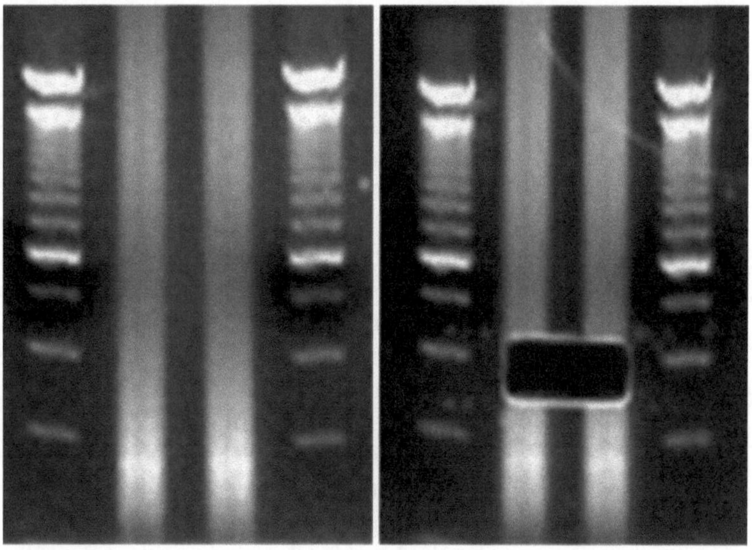

Fig. 6 Gel purification of a library for paired-end 2 × 100 sequencing run on a 2 % agarose gel

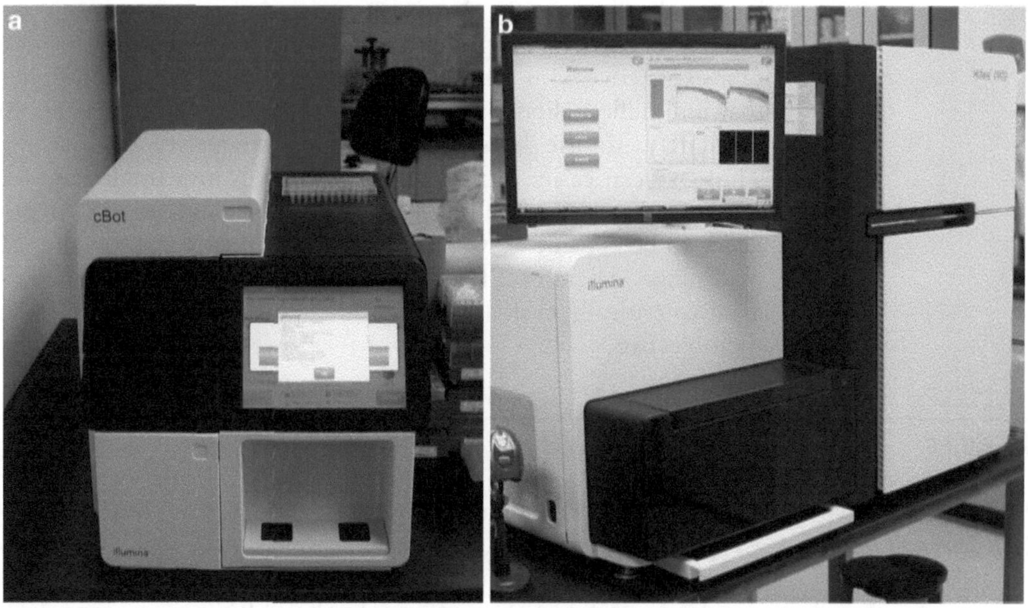

Fig. 7 (**a**) The Illumina cBot used to cluster libraries onto flow-cells for sequencing and (**b**) the Illumina HiSeq 2000 sequencing system used to generate deep sequencing data

A decision that must be made at the start of every sequencing project is the read length. For simple RNA expression profiling, the objective is to detect an mRNA and determine relative abundances. This can be done with single reads of 50–100 bp in length. However, in other situations, we choose to do paired-end read sequencing, usually at 100 bp each (e.g., 2 × 100). For example, we routinely do paired-end reads for alternative splicing analysis because it is very useful in identifying intron/exon splice junctions during analysis. We also use paired-end sequencing for RNA expression profiling of nonhuman primates because the analysis pipeline requires alignment to much less complete maps of the nonhuman primate genomes. A key step in the process is matching sequence reads to annotated genes based on homology to their human counterparts and longer, paired-end reads improve the alignment quality.

The last major issue to note is that of "read depth." This term is calculated by the total number of reads multiplied by the fraction (%) of reads that align to the genome. The key point is that deep sequencing generates a huge amount of data but the important data is only that which contributes to your experimental objective. For example, we can generate a billion reads with one RNAseq sample in a single run. The opportunity to do multiple samples in a single lane using barcodes allows considerable cost savings and increased efficiency. So the real question is how many reads are actually needed to determine the global gene expression profile? Our experience with activation of purified human T cells indicates that ten million aligned reads gives results that are comparable to profiling with the latest generation of Affymetrix microarrays. Thus, we can easily run 12 different samples in a single lane for RNAseq. For the profiling of alternative splicing the read depth needs to be considerably greater, at least in the 30 million aligned read range. Therefore, for each project, investigators are encouraged to critically evaluate the required read depth to accomplish the objective.

4 Notes

4.1 RNA Extraction from Cells and Tissues

1. Bring Trizol reagent to room temperature. RPE Buffer is supplied as a concentrate in the RNeasy kit. Add appropriate volume of 100 % ethanol before using for the first time. Work in the fume hood. Do not worry about RNases in **steps 1–3**. Your sample is full of them anyway. They are inhibited as long as they are in the Trizol.
2. From **step 4** you should be careful to not contaminate the samples with RNases. Keep cleaning your gloves with RNase Zap through the whole process. The main source of contamination

comes from your fingers by accidentally touching the inner part of the tube caps.

3. While discarding flow-through in **steps 6–9**, avoid touching the mouth of the collection tubes with anything.
4. Please refer to the Qiagen PAXgene Blood miRNA Kit Handbook for the latest information available. This is available at the Qiagen Web site: http://www.qiagen.com/. If a QiaCube Robot is not available, simply follow the workflow described for the manual version of the protocol at the same site. In this case, it is recommended that all samples in one phase of a study be done by the same person and in a random order to minimize technical batch effects.

4.2 Global Gene Expression Profiling Using Affymetrix DNA Microarrays

5. Please refer to the manufacturer's literature: "The Ambion® WT Expression Kit: For Affymetrix® GeneChip® Whole Transcript (WT) Expression Arrays" available on the Life Technologies Web site for current protocol details and instructions (URL: www.lifetechnologies.com/).
6. Please refer to the manufacturer's literature: "GeneChip® WT Terminal Labeling and Controls Kit" available on the Affymetrix Web site for the most current protocol instructions (URL: www.affymetrix.com/).
7. Please refer to the NuGEN Ovation Pico WTA System V2 User Guide available on the NuGEN Web site for the most current protocol instructions (URL: www.nugeninc.com/nugen/).
8. Please refer to the Affymetrix "Target Hybridization for Gene 1.1 ST Array Plates Processed on the GeneTitan Instrument" user guide from the Affymetrix Web site for the most current protocol instructions.

References

1. Verweij CL (2009) Transcript profiling towards personalized medicine in rheumatoid arthritis. Neth J Med 67(11):364–371
2. Cooper-Knock J, Kirby J, Ferraiuolo L, Heath PR, Rattray M, Shaw PJ (2012) Gene expression profiling in human neurodegenerative disease. Nat Rev Neurol. doi:10.1038/nrneurol.2012.156
3. Malone H, Oliver B (2011) Microarrays, deep sequencing and the true measure of the transcriptome. BMC Biol 9:34
4. Bai B, Laiho M (2012) Efficient sequential recovery of nucleolar macromolecular components. Proteomics. doi:10.1002/pmic.201200071
5. Mastrokolias A, den Dunnin JT, van Ommen GB, 't Hoen PA, van Roon-Mom WMC (2012) Increased sensitivity of next generation sequencing-based expression profiling after globin reduction in human blood RNA. BMC Genomics 13:28

INDEX

Andrea A. Zachary and Mary S. Leffell (eds.), *Transplantation Immunology: Methods and Protocols, Second Edition*, Methods in Molecular Biology, vol. 1034, DOI 10.1007/978-1-62703-493-7, © Springer Science+Business Media, LLC 2013

U

V

W

MIX
Papier aus verantwortungsvollen Quellen
Paper from responsible sources
FSC® C105338

If you have any concerns about our products,
you can contact us on
ProductSafety@springernature.com

In case Publisher is established outside the EU,
the EU authorized representative is:
Springer Nature Customer Service Center GmbH
Europaplatz 3, 69115 Heidelberg, Germany

Printed by Libri Plureos GmbH
in Hamburg, Germany